Food Counter's Pocket Companion

FIFTH EDITION

**Calories · Carbohydrates · Protein · Fats
Fiber · Sugar · Sodium · Iron · Calcium
Potassium · Vitamin D**

JANE STEPHENSON
REBECCA LINDBERG, MPH, RDN

THE EXPERIMENT
NEW YORK

THE FOOD COUNTER'S POCKET COMPANION, FIFTH EDITION: *Calories, Carbohydrates, Protein, Fats, Fiber, Sugar, Sodium, Iron, Calcium, Potassium, and Vitamin D*
Copyright © 1999 by Jane Stephenson and Bridgett Wagener, RD
Copyright © 2001, 2003, 2004, 2008, 2010, 2012, 2014, 2016, 2018, 2019 by Jane Stephenson and Diane Bader
Copyright © 2022 by Jane Stephenson and Rebecca Lindberg, MPH, RDN

Originally published as *HealthCheques™: Carbohydrate, Fat & Calorie Guide* by Appletree Press, Inc., in 1999. First published in revised form by The Experiment, LLC, in 2022.

The authors and publisher have made every effort to provide accurate data based on values that are current as of 2021. Nutrient values and product availability are subject to change; in cases where the Nutrition Facts differ from the data provided, defer to the label. This book is sold with the understanding that the authors and publisher are not engaged in rendering medical, health, or any other kind of personal or professional services in the book. The author and publisher specifically disclaim all responsibility for any liability, loss, or risk—personal or otherwise—that is incurred as a consequence, directly or indirectly, of the use and application of any of the contents of this book.

All rights reserved. Except for brief passages quoted in newspaper, magazine, radio, television, or online reviews, no portion of this book may be reproduced, distributed, or transmitted in any form or by any means, electronic or mechanical, including photocopying, recording, or information storage or retrieval system, without the prior written permission of the publisher.

The Experiment, LLC | 220 East 23rd Street, Suite 600 | New York, NY 10010-4658 | theexperimentpublishing.com

THE EXPERIMENT and its colophon are registered trademarks of The Experiment, LLC. Many of the designations used by manufacturers and sellers to distinguish their products are claimed as trademarks. Where those designations appear in this book and The Experiment was aware of a trademark claim, the designations have been capitalized.

The Experiment's books are available at special discounts when purchased in bulk for premiums and sales promotions as well as for fundraising or educational use. For details, contact us at info@theexperimentpublishing.com.

Library of Congress Cataloging-in-Publication Data

Names: Stephenson, Jane, author. | Lindberg, Rebecca, author.
Title: The food counter's pocket companion : calories, carbohydrates, protein, fats, fiber, sugar, sodium, iron, calcium, potassium, and vitamin D / Jane
    Stephenson, Rebecca Lindberg, MPH, RDN.
Other titles: Carbohydrate, fat & calorie guide
Description: Fifth edition. | New York, NY : The Experiment, 2022. |
    Revision of: Carbohydrate, fat & calorie guide / Jane Stephenson, Diane
    Bader.
Identifiers: LCCN 2021055556 (print) | LCCN 2021055557 (ebook) | ISBN
    9781615198122 (paperback) | ISBN 9781615198139 (ebook)
Subjects: LCSH: Food--Composition--Tables. | Nutrition--Tables. |
    Food--Caloric content--Tables. | Food--Carbohydrate content--Tables. |
    Food--Fat content--Tables. | Food--Cholesterol content--Tables. |
    Food--Cholesterol content--Tables.
Classification: LCC RA784 .S73 2022 (print) | LCC RA784 (ebook) | DDC
    613.202/1--dc23/eng/20211220
LC record available at https://lccn.loc.gov/2021055556
LC ebook record available at https://lccn.loc.gov/2021055557

ISBN 978-1-61519-812-2
Ebook ISBN 978-1-61519-813-9

Cover and text design by Jack Dunnington
Cover photo from Shutterstock/monticello

Manufactured in the United States of America

First printing March 2022
10 9 8 7 6 5 4

Contents

About This Book 5

Personalize Your Nutrition Goals 6

MyPlate 9

Abbreviations 10

Alcohol 12

Beverages 14

Breads & Bread Products 15

Candy 18

Cereal Bars & Cereals 21
Cereal Bars 21
Hot Cereal 22
Ready-to-Eat Cereal 22

Cheese 25

Combination Foods,
Frozen Entrées & Meals 26

Condiments, Sauces
& Baking Ingredients 31

Crackers, Dips & Snacks 35

Desserts, Sweets & Toppings 41
Bars 41
Cakes, Pastries & Sweet Breads . . . 41
Cookies 43

Frozen Yogurt 44
Ice Cream 44
Other Sweets 46
Pies 46
Syrups & Toppings 47

Eggs, Egg Dishes & Egg Substitutes . . . 47

Fats, Oils, Cream & Gravy 48

Fish & Seafood 51

Fruit & Vegetable Juices 54

Fruits 55

Meats 58
Beef & Veal 58
Game 59
Lamb 59
Pork 59
Processed & Luncheon Meats 59
Specialty & Organ Meats 60

Milk & Yogurt 61

Nuts, Seeds & Nut/Seed Butters 63

Pasta, Rice & Other Grains 64

Poultry 65
Chicken 65
Game 66
Turkey 66

Restaurant Favorites 67

  Appetizers. 67

  Desserts 67

  Entrées 68

    American. 68

    Asian. 68

    Italian/Mediterranean. 68

    Mexican & Tex-Mex. 69

  Salads 69

  Side Dishes 69

  Soups 70

Restaurant & Fast Food Chains 70

  A&W 70

  Arby's 72

  Boston Market 75

  Burger King. 76

  Chick-fil-A 79

  Chili's. 80

  Chipotle 84

  Country Style. 86

  Dairy Queen 90

  Denny's 93

  Domino's 97

  Dunkin'. 99

  Hardee's. 104

  IHOP 107

  KFC 110

  Little Caesars 112

  McDonald's. 114

  Olive Garden. 117

  P.F. Chang's 119

  Panda Express. 122

  Panera Bread 124

  Pizza Hut. 127

  Popeyes 128

  Sonic 129

  Starbucks 131

  Subway 136

  Taco Bell. 138

  Tim Hortons 140

  Uno Pizzeria & Grill 144

  Wendy's 147

Salads 149

Salad Dressings 150

Soups 151

Vegetables 154

Vegetarian Foods & Legumes 157

Nutrients 161

  Choline. 161

  Fiber 162

  Iron 163

  Magnesium. 164

  Omega-3 Fatty Acids. 165

  Omega-6 Fatty Acids. 166

  Potassium 167

  Sodium. 168

  Vitamin A 169

  Vitamin B12 170

  Vitamin C. 171

  Vitamin D 172

  Vitamin E. 173

  Water. 174

References 175

About the Authors 176

About This Book

The Food Counter's Pocket Companion, Fifth Edition, is a resource to help you make healthy food choices at home or on the go. The more you are aware of what is in the foods and beverages you choose, the better choices you can make for your overall well-being—no matter what type of eating pattern you follow.

This book lists the calories, fat, saturated fat, sodium, carbohydrate, fiber, sugar, protein, vitamin D, calcium, iron, and potassium content of over 4,500 common foods. Additionally, it highlights 13 important nutrients, each of which includes practical tips to help you make healthier choices every day based on your individual needs. You can also learn how to customize your personal daily nutrient goals in three easy steps on page 6.

Keep this pocket companion in your purse, pocket, desk drawer, or glove compartment and pull it out whenever and wherever you need it. It's not a guide to restricting food or strictly counting calories—it's a tool for learning how to incorporate healthier food choices into whatever eating plan you follow, enjoy what you eat, nourish your body, and feel great.

Personalize Your Nutrition Goals

1. Estimate your calorie needs. Your calorie needs vary based on age, sex, body size, genetics, and activity level. This type of estimation is not a perfect science, but it will give you a good starting point for making informed decisions. You can use online calculators such as the Mifflin-St. Jeor (calculator.net/bmr-calculator .html) or National Institutes of Health Body Weight Planner (niddk.nih.gov/bwp) to calculate your personal needs.

Below are estimates of calorie needs based on the Dietary Guidelines for Americans, 2020–2025. Keep in mind that individual needs fluctuate. The best way to know how many calories your body needs is to monitor how you feel along with your food intake, activity, and weight.

Activity Level	Men (calories)	Women (calories)
Sedentary	2,000–2,600	1,600–2,000
Moderately Active	2,200–2,800	1,800–2,200
Active	2,400–3,200	2,000–2,400

2. Determine your nutrient needs. Your personal needs depend on the type of eating pattern you follow as well as your health history, goals, and activity level. Working with a registered dietitian is the most precise way to determine your needs. However, you can start by estimating using the table below.

Calorie goal	Fat (g) 20–35% daily calories	Saturated fat (g) 7–10% daily calories	Sodium (mg)	Carbohydrates (g) 45–65% daily calories	Fiber (g) 14 g per 1,000 calories	Sugar (g/tsp) <10% daily calories	Protein (g) 10–35% daily calories
1,600	36–62	12–18	2,300	180–260	22	40/10	40–140
1,800	40–70	14–20	2,300	203–293	25	45/11	45–158
2,000	44–78	16–22	2,300	225–325	28	50/13	50–175
2,400	53–93	19–27	2,300	270–390	34	60/15	60–210
2,800	62–109	22–31	2,300	315–455	39	70/18	70–245
3,200	71–124	25–36	2,300	360–520	45	80/20	80–280

3. Eat and drink to improve health and prevent disease.

Aim to increase fiber. Most people don't get enough fiber in their diets. For tips on boosting your intake, see page 162.

Cut down on sugar. Many experts recommend eating less sugar because a high sugar intake has been linked to obesity, high blood sugar, high blood pressure, inflammation, and fat buildup on artery walls. The American Heart Association suggests no more than 6 tsp for women and 9 tsp for men per day.

Choose good fats. You need fat to absorb vitamins, feel full after eating, and reduce disease risk. The key is eating good fats (like avocados, nuts, seeds, and olives, including oils from these foods) and staying clear of the bad fats (like trans fat). The American Heart Association recommends you get only 5 to 6 percent of calories from saturated fat. There's no need to monitor your cholesterol intake from food, as it has little to no effect on your blood cholesterol levels.

Reduce sodium. Most Americans eat too much sodium. Use herbs and spices in place of salt and limit processed and ultra-processed foods high in sodium. See page 168 for more tips.

Eat fruits and vegetables. You can reduce your risk of heart disease, stroke, and some types of cancers by eating at least 5 servings of fruits and vegetables every day.

Pick healthy drinks. Make water your beverage of choice—you can learn more about its importance on page 174. Limit alcohol intake to no more than 1 drink a day for women and 2 drinks a day for men.

Counting carbohydrates: Carbohydrate counting may be recommended for certain health conditions like diabetes. While some people stick to counting total grams of carbohydrate, there are others who count carbohydrate choices: One choice contains about 15 grams of carbohydrate.

Total carbohydrate in grams / 15 = Number of carb choices

MyPlate

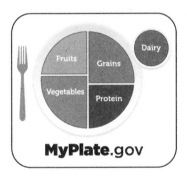

MyPlate is a visual way to design your breakfast, lunch, and dinner plates for better health. It recommends filling half your plate with fruits and vegetables, choosing whole grains over refined grains, and prioritizing high-quality, protein-rich foods. You can find resources for setting food goals, identifying tools to personalize your plate, and discovering new recipes at myplate.gov.

Abbreviations

Nutrient values have been rounded to the nearest calorie, gram, milligram, or microgram (with the exception of saturated fat values, which have been rounded to the nearest 0.5 gram). Apparent inconsistencies may result from rounding off numbers. Values may have been obtained from more than one source, recipe, or sample of the same food, and they may vary due to seasonal and manufacturer differences.

Nutrient values change as products and recipes are reformulated and reanalyzed. Menu items listed may not be available at all restaurants, and nutrient values for fast-food restaurants are meant for general information purposes only. Nutrient values are subject to change; values are current as of 2021. If the information you find on a label differs significantly from the data in this book, please use the label as your guide.

This book includes many trademarked company and product names. Where the authors and publisher were aware of a trademark, all such names have been capitalized.

Imperial	Metric
1 oz	28 g
1 fl oz	30 ml
1 in	2.5 cm

Abbreviation	Stands for . . .
fl oz	fluid ounce
g	gram
in	inch
mcg	microgram
mg	milligram
n/a	not available
oz	ounce
pc	piece
pkg	package
pkt	packet
tsp	teaspoon
T	tablespoon
w/	with
w/o	without
/	or

RDA: The Recommended Dietary Allowance is the average daily level of intake sufficient to meet nutrient requirements for nearly all healthy people.

AI: Adequate Intakes are established when evidence is insufficient to develop an RDA; they are set at a level that ensures nutritional adequacy.

ALCOHOL	Amount	Calories	Fat (g)	Saturated Fat (g)	Sodium (mg)	Carbohydrate (g)	Fiber (g)	Sugar (g)	Protein (g)	Vitamin D (mcg)	Calcium (mg)	Iron (mg)	Potassium (mg)
Alabama Slammer	5 fl oz	318	0	0.0	5	32	0	30	0	0	7	0	111
B-52	1.5 fl oz	154	2	1.0	14	17	0	15	0	0	0	0	5
Bahama Mama	5 fl oz	243	0	0.0	6	21	0	20	0	0	6	0	56
Beer	12 fl oz	146	0	0.0	11	11	0	0	1	0	14	0	118
light	12 fl oz	99	0	0.0	11	5	0	0	1	0	11	0	92
nonalcoholic	12 fl oz	133	0	0.0	47	29	0	29	1	0	25	0	29
Black Russian	4 fl oz	335	0	0.0	5	25	0	21	0	0	0	0	18
Bloody Mary	8 fl oz	165	1	0.0	497	8	1	5	2	0	24	1	439
Bourbon & club soda	6 fl oz	139	0	0.0	1	0	0	0	0	0	0	0	1
Brandy	1 fl oz	70	0	0.0	0	0	0	0	0	0	0	0	1
Brandy Alexander	3 fl oz	272	11	7.0	11	15	0	12	1	0	20	0	38
Champagne	4 fl oz	98	0	0.0	6	3	0	1	0	0	11	0	85
Cordials/liqueurs, 53-proof	1 fl oz	117	0	0.0	3	16	0	13	0	0	0	0	10
Cosmopolitan	6 fl oz	281	0	0.0	7	16	0	14	0	0	0	0	46
Daiquiri	6 fl oz	228	0	0.0	73	27	0	27	0	0	5	0	50
Fuzzy Navel	6 fl oz	380	0	0.0	6	48	0	45	1	0	10	0	166
Gimlet	2.5 fl oz	141	0	0.0	1	4	0	3	0	0	2	0	22
Gin & tonic	8 fl oz	187	0	0.0	20	15	0	15	0	0	2	0	1
Gin fizz	8 fl oz	158	0	0.0	38	5	0	5	0	0	10	0	22
Gin/rum/vodka/whiskey													
80-proof	1 fl oz	64	0	0.0	0	0	0	0	0	0	0	0	1
86-proof	1 fl oz	70	0	0.0	0	0	0	0	0	0	0	0	1
90-proof	1 fl oz	73	0	0.0	0	0	0	0	0	0	0	0	1
100-proof	1 fl oz	82	0	0.0	0	0	0	0	0	0	0	0	1
Grasshopper	4 fl oz	340	4	2.5	28	39	0	35	1	0	40	0	61
Harvey Wallbanger	6 fl oz	167	0	0.0	4	16	0	11	1	1	76	0	241
Highball	4 fl oz	71	0	0.0	19	0	0	0	0	0	5	0	2
Hot buttered rum	4 fl oz	191	5	3.5	5	6	0	6	0	0	10	0	13
Hot toddy	8 fl oz	158	0	0.0	10	18	0	17	0	0	6	0	22
Hurricane	8 fl oz	196	0	0.0	5	23	0	0	0	0	0	0	0
Irish coffee													
w/ whipped cream	8 fl oz	193	4	2.0	4	14	0	14	0	0	4	0	95
w/o whipped cream	8 fl oz	143	0	0.0	4	12	0	12	0	0	4	0	95
Irish cream	1 fl oz	97	4	2.5	24	7	0	6	1	0	5	0	10
Jack & Coke	6 fl oz	185	0	0.0	16	13	0	13	0	0	0	0	1
Kahlua	1 fl oz	101	0	0.0	2	14	0	11	0	0	0	0	9
Kamikaze	4 fl oz	241	0	0.0	6	10	0	8	0	0	4	0	24
Long Island Iced Tea	6 fl oz	193	0	0.0	29	16	0	15	0	0	2	0	13
Mai Tai	4 fl oz	187	0	0.0	6	21	0	17	0	0	8	0	81
Manhattan	2.5 fl oz	167	0	0.0	2	1	0	1	0	0	1	0	11

ALCOHOL

	Amount	Calories	Fat (g)	Saturated Fat (g)	Sodium (mg)	Carbohydrate (g)	Fiber (g)	Sugar (g)	Protein (g)	Vitamin D (mcg)	Calcium (mg)	Iron (mg)	Potassium (mg)
Margarita													
w/ salt	6 fl oz	220	0	0.0	369	29	0	29	0	0	4	0	40
w/o salt	6 fl oz	220	0	0.0	10	29	0	29	0	0	4	0	40
Martini													
Appletini	2.5 fl oz	142	0	0.0	1	5	0	4	0	0	2	0	20
Chocolate	2.5 fl oz	142	0	0.0	1	5	0	4	0	0	2	0	20
traditional	2.5 fl oz	151	0	0.0	2	0	0	0	0	0	1	0	10
Melon Ball	4 fl oz	205	0	0.0	16	20	0	15	1	0	8	0	177
Mimosa	8 fl oz	156	0	0.0	7	17	0	11	1	0	78	0	302
Mint julep	4 fl oz	223	0	0.0	5	7	0	7	0	0	0	0	1
Mojito	6 fl oz	205	0	0.0	26	28	1	26	0	0	20	0	45
Mudslide	4 fl oz	411	20	12.5	38	22	0	18	2	1	30	0	52
Old Fashioned	4 fl oz	194	0	0.0	5	7	0	7	0	0	12	0	42
Piña Colada	6 fl oz	272	4	3.5	11	35	0	32	1	0	14	0	162
Rob Roy	2.5 fl oz	165	0	0.0	3	3	0	2	0	0	2	0	22
Rum & cola	8 fl oz	214	0	0.0	7	19	0	18	0	0	2	0	10
Rusty Nail	4 fl oz	322	0	0.0	2	13	0	13	0	0	0	0	1
Screwdriver	8 fl oz	223	0	0.0	5	21	0	15	1	1	101	0	322
Sex on the Beach	6 fl oz	242	0	0.0	4	28	0	25	0	0	9	0	124
Singapore Sling	6 fl oz	176	0	0.0	27	14	0	12	0	0	9	0	56
Sloe Gin Fizz	8 fl oz	158	0	0.0	38	5	0	5	0	0	10	0	22
Sloe Screw	8 fl oz	223	0	0.0	5	21	0	15	1	1	101	0	322
Tequila Maria	8 fl oz	158	0	0.0	500	6	1	4	1	0	24	1	20
Tequila Sunrise	6 fl oz	202	0	0.0	7	24	0	17	1	0	68	0	220
Toasted Almond	4 fl oz	420	11	7.0	14	41	0	37	1	0	20	0	42
Tom Collins	8 fl oz	175	0	0.0	29	12	0	12	0	0	7	0	4
Vodka Red Bull	8 fl oz	203	0	0.0	67	17	0	17	1	0	10	0	6
Whiskey sour	4 fl oz	181	0	0.0	24	16	0	9	0	0	0	0	6
White Russian	4 fl oz	211	9	5.5	52	14	0	11	3	0	88	0	115
Wine													
cooking													
Marsala	2 T	45	0	0.0	190	4	0	4	0	0	2	0	28
red/white	2 T	20	0	0.0	190	1	0	0	0	0	3	0	26
sherry	2 T	45	0	0.0	190	2	0	2	0	0	2	0	26
table													
dessert, dry	4 fl oz	179	0	0.0	11	14	0	1	0	0	9	0	109
dessert, sweet	4 fl oz	189	0	0.0	11	16	0	9	0	0	9	0	109
red/rosé	4 fl oz	100	0	0.0	5	3	0	1	0	0	9	1	149
sangria	8 fl oz	230	0	0.0	24	20	0	17	0	0	14	1	163
sherry, dry	4 fl oz	102	0	0.0	5	3	0	1	0	0	10	1	152
white, dry/medium	4 fl oz	96	0	0.0	6	3	0	1	0	0	11	0	83
Wine cooler	12 fl oz	245	0	0.0	18	36	0	35	0	0	14	0	97
Wine spritzer	8 fl oz	118	0	0.0	26	4	0	1	0	0	17	1	144

BEVERAGES

	Amount	Calories	Fat (g)	Saturated Fat (g)	Sodium (mg)	Carbohydrate (g)	Fiber (g)	Sugar (g)	Protein (g)	Vitamin D (mcg)	Calcium (mg)	Iron (mg)	Potassium (mg)
Café latte													
w/ skim milk	8 fl oz	68	0	0.0	76	10	0	9	6	2	190	0	373
w/ whole milk	8 fl oz	120	6	3.5	77	9	0	9	7	2	200	0	334
Café mocha w/ whipped cream													
w/ skim milk	8 fl oz	180	6	4.0	70	23	2	18	7	2	200	2	346
w/ whole milk	8 fl oz	207	11	6.0	73	23	2	19	7	2	200	2	317
Cappuccino													
w/ skim milk	8 fl oz	47	0	0.0	67	7	0	7	5	1	153	0	250
w/ water, flavored mix	8 fl oz	70	4	3.5	170	9	0	5	0	0	5	0	104
w/ whole milk	8 fl oz	72	4	2.5	58	6	0	6	4	1	136	0	240
Capri Sun													
orange	6 fl oz	50	0	0.0	15	14	0	13	0	0	0	0	0
Roarin' Waters	6 fl oz	30	0	0.0	15	8	0	8	0	0	0	0	0
Club soda/seltzer	8 fl oz	0	0	0.0	115	0	0	0	0	0	12	0	5
Coconut water	8 fl oz	45	0	0.0	25	11	0	11	0	0	40	0	470
Coffee													
brewed/instant	6 fl oz	2	0	0.0	5	0	0	0	0	0	4	0	118
flavored mixes	6 fl oz	60	2	0.5	40	10	0	0	0	0	5	0	111
Crystal Light	8 fl oz	5	0	0.0	75	3	0	0	0	0	0	0	175
Espresso	3 fl oz	2	0	0.0	10	0	0	0	0	0	5	0	111
Frappuccino	9.5 fl oz	200	3	2.0	100	37	0	0	6	0	0	0	0
Fruit20 flavored water	8 fl oz	0	0	0.0	38	0	0	0	0	0	0	0	0
Fruit punch	8 fl oz	90	0	0.0	15	25	0	24	0	0	20	1	164
Gatorade													
Bolt24	16.9 fl oz	45	0	0.0	230	11	0	9	0	0	0	0	60
G Series	12 fl oz	80	0	0.0	160	21	0	21	0	0	0	0	45
G2 Series	12 fl oz	30	0	0.0	160	8	0	7	0	0	0	0	45
Zero w/ protein	16.9 fl oz	50	0	0.0	230	1	0	0	10	0	0	0	70
Hawaiian Punch	8 fl oz	60	0	0.0	105	15	0	15	0	0	0	0	0
light	8 fl oz	10	0	0.0	105	2	0	2	0	0	0	0	0
Hi-C	8 fl oz	53	0	0.0	20	15	0	13	0	0	0	0	0
Hot cocoa													
sugar-free, mix	8 fl oz	80	1	0.5	190	14	0	11	6	0	420	2	500
w/ water, mix	8 fl oz	80	2	1.5	190	15	1	12	0	0	10	1	140
w/ 1% milk, homemade	8 fl oz	220	3	2.0	260	38	1	32	9	2	312	0	558
w/ whole milk, homemade	8 fl oz	226	4	3.0	164	40	1	38	7	2	243	0	340
Kool-Aid	8 fl oz	60	0	0.0	0	16	0	16	0	0	0	0	0
sugar-free	8 fl oz	0	0	0.0	5	0	0	0	0	0	0	0	0
Lemonade	8 fl oz	110	0	0.0	15	29	0	28	0	0	5	0	25
sugar-free	8 fl oz	0	0	0.0	20	1	0	0	0	0	26	0	12
Quinine/tonic water	8 fl oz	90	0	0.0	0	23	0	23	0	0	2	0	0
Red Bull energy drink	8.4 fl oz	111	0	0.0	101	26	0	26	1	0	16	0	8
sugar-free	8.4 fl oz	13	0	0.0	208	2	0	0	1	0	33	0	8

BEVERAGES

	Amount	Calories	Fat (g)	Saturated Fat (g)	Sodium (mg)	Carbohydrate (g)	Fiber (g)	Sugar (g)	Protein (g)	Vitamin D (mcg)	Calcium (mg)	Iron (mg)	Potassium (mg)
Rockstar energy drink	8 fl oz	135	0	0.0	35	32	0	32	0	0	0	0	0
sugar-free	8 fl oz	13	0	0.0	120	1	0	0	0	0	0	0	0
Soda													
7 Up	12 fl oz	140	0	0.0	45	39	0	38	0	0	0	0	0
Coca-Cola/Coke	12 fl oz	140	0	0.0	45	39	0	39	0	0	0	0	0
cherry	12 fl oz	150	0	0.0	35	42	0	42	0	0	0	0	0
vanilla	12 fl oz	150	0	0.0	35	42	0	42	0	0	0	0	0
cream	12 fl oz	170	0	0.0	45	43	0	43	0	0	19	0	5
diet, most varieties	12 fl oz	0	0	0.0	35	0	0	0	0	0	0	0	0
Dr Pepper	12 fl oz	150	0	0.0	55	40	0	39	0	0	0	0	0
ginger ale	12 fl oz	140	0	0.0	50	36	0	36	0	0	11	1	4
grape	12 fl oz	150	0	0.0	51	38	0	38	0	0	0	0	0
Mello Yellow	12 fl oz	170	0	0.0	30	32	0	32	0	0	0	0	0
Mountain Dew	12 fl oz	170	0	0.0	65	46	0	46	0	0	0	0	0
Code Red	12 fl oz	168	0	0.0	108	46	0	46	0	0	0	0	0
Orange Crush	12 fl oz	160	0	0.0	70	43	0	43	0	0	0	0	0
Pepsi	12 fl oz	150	0	0.0	30	41	0	41	0	0	0	0	0
wild cherry	12 fl oz	160	0	0.0	30	42	0	42	0	0	0	0	0
root beer	12 fl oz	170	0	0.0	80	47	0	46	0	0	19	0	4
Sierra Mist	12 fl oz	140	0	0.0	35	37	0	37	0	0	6	0	4
Sprite	12 fl oz	140	0	0.0	70	38	0	38	0	0	0	0	0
Squirt	12 fl oz	140	0	0.0	55	39	0	38	0	0	0	0	0
Tang	8 fl oz	90	0	0.0	40	22	0	22	0	0	43	0	20
Tea													
brewed/instant	6 fl oz	0	0	0.0	0	0	0	0	0	0	0	0	0
iced, diet, w/ lemon	8 fl oz	0	0	0.0	0	0	0	0	0	0	0	0	0
iced, sweetened	8 fl oz	70	0	0.0	5	18	0	18	0	0	0	0	20
Vitaminwater	8 fl oz	40	0	0.0	0	11	0	11	0	0	110	0	220
Water, bottled	8 fl oz	0	0	0.0	0	0	0	0	0	0	0	0	0
Yoo-hoo, chocolate	8 fl oz	116	1	0.0	167	26	0	24	2	2	95	0	204

BREADS & BREAD PRODUCTS

Breads & Muffins

	Amount	Calories	Fat (g)	Saturated Fat (g)	Sodium (mg)	Carbohydrate (g)	Fiber (g)	Sugar (g)	Protein (g)	Vitamin D (mcg)	Calcium (mg)	Iron (mg)	Potassium (mg)
Bagels													
blueberry													
medium	1 (3 oz)	280	2	1.0	390	55	2	8	9	0	15	2	80
large	1 (5 oz)	382	3	0.0	616	78	5	17	14	0	47	4	173
cinnamon raisin													
medium	1 (3 oz)	280	2	0.0	390	56	2	11	9	0	20	3	120
large	1 (5 oz)	381	3	0.0	596	79	5	17	14	0	48	4	194
egg													
medium	1 (2 oz)	158	1	0.0	286	30	1	6	6	0	14	4	71

BREADS & BREAD PRODUCTS

Breads & Muffins	Amount	Calories	Fat (g)	Saturated Fat (g)	Sodium (mg)	Carbohydrate (g)	Fiber (g)	Sugar (g)	Protein (g)	Vitamin D (mcg)	Calcium (mg)	Iron (mg)	Potassium
large	1 (5 oz)	315	2	0.5	573	60	3	11	12	0	17	5	89
plain													
mini	1 (1.5 oz)	125	1	0.0	220	25	1	3	4	0	80	3	80
medium	1 (3 oz)	270	2	0.0	450	53	2	6	9	0	10	3	80
large	1 (5 oz)	330	3	0.5	600	66	2	8	10	0	24	5	132
Bialys	1 (2.5 oz)	190	2	0.5	590	36	2	0	6	0	40	1	114
Biscuits													
baking powder, can	1 (2 oz)	180	6	2.5	450	26	0	5	4	0	0	2	260
baking powder, homemade	1 (2 oz)	184	6	3.0	568	28	2	5	4	0	15	1	86
buttermilk, can	1 (2 oz)	170	8	3.5	550	23	0	2	4	0	30	2	78
buttermilk, homemade	1 (2 oz)	201	9	2.5	328	25	1	1	4	0	132	2	66
Breads													
Boston brown, can	1 slice (1 oz)	55	0	0.0	179	12	1	1	1	0	20	1	90
challah/egg	1 slice (1 oz)	81	2	0.5	108	14	1	1	3	0	25	1	33
chapati	1 slice (1 oz)	84	2	0.5	116	13	1	1	3	0	26	1	75
cracked wheat	1 slice (1 oz)	74	1	0.5	153	14	2	0	2	0	12	1	50
French/Vienna	1 slice (1 oz)	77	1	0.0	170	15	1	1	3	0	15	1	33
Ezekiel/sprouted	1 slice (1.2 oz)	80	1	0.0	75	15	3	0	5	0	9	1	81
fruit	1 slice (1 oz)	103	5	0.5	87	13	0	7	2	0	41	1	47
garlic	1 slice (1 oz)	170	6	3.5	260	23	1	0	4	0	6	1	14
Irish soda	1 slice (1 oz)	84	3	1.5	139	14	1	5	2	0	29	1	73
Italian	1 slice (1 oz)	77	1	0.0	156	14	1	1	2	0	22	1	31
multigrain	1 slice (1 oz)	60	1	0.0	110	11	2	0	4	0	50	1	82
low-carb	1 slice (1 oz)	70	4	0.5	130	7	4	0	5	0	30	0	40
oatmeal	1 slice (1 oz)	74	1	0.0	96	11	1	2	3	0	23	1	40
pita, white	1 (6 inch)	165	1	0.0	322	33	1	0	5	0	52	1	72
pita, whole wheat	1 (6 inch)	168	1	0.0	337	36	4	2	6	0	10	2	109
pumpernickel	1 slice (1 oz)	71	1	0.0	169	13	2	0	2	0	19	1	59
raisin	1 slice (1 oz)	78	1	0.0	98	15	1	2	2	0	19	1	64
rye	1 slice (1 oz)	73	1	0.0	171	14	2	1	2	0	21	1	47
sourdough	1 slice (1 oz)	77	1	0.0	17	15	1	1	3	0	15	1	33
wheatberry	1 slice (1 oz)	76	1	0.0	144	14	1	2	3	0	38	1	50
white	1 slice (1 oz)	79	1	0.0	153	15	1	2	2	0	41	1	36
light	1 slice (0.8 oz)	40	0	0.0	111	9	2	1	3	0	58	0	18
whole wheat	1 slice (1 oz)	73	1	0.0	105	14	2	3	3	0	18	1	82
light	1 slice (0.8 oz)	40	0	0.0	90	9	3	1	3	0	26	0	37
Breadsticks, soft	1 (2 oz)	150	5	1.0	270	23	1	2	4	0	10	2	59
Cornbread	1 (2 oz)	217	10	0.5	206	32	1	18	2	0	19	0	20
Croissants	1 (2 oz)	230	12	6.5	265	26	1	6	5	0	21	1	67
English muffins													
plain	1 medium	132	1	0.0	197	26	2	1	5	0	102	1	60
raisin	1 medium	140	1	0.0	170	29	1	8	4	0	40	1	90
whole wheat	1 medium	120	1	0.0	220	23	3	2	5	0	60	1	90
Melba toast	4	78	1	0.0	120	15	1	0	2	0	18	1	40

BREADS & BREAD PRODUCTS

Breads & Muffins

	Amount	Calories	Fat (g)	Saturated Fat (g)	Sodium (mg)	Carbohydrate (g)	Fiber (g)	Sugar (g)	Protein (g)	Vitamin D (mcg)	Calcium (mg)	Iron (mg)	Potassium (mg)
Muffins													
banana nut	1 (2 oz)	247	10	3.0	255	39	1	10	3	0	25	1	132
blueberry	1 (2 oz)	230	8	1.5	195	38	1	22	3	0	11	1	46
bran, w/ raisins	1 (2 oz)	153	4	0.5	223	27	3	5	4	0	36	2	287
chocolate chip	1 (2 oz)	275	10	3.0	200	43	1	25	4	0	15	2	87
corn	1 (2 oz)	230	8	1.5	335	36	1	15	4	0	9	1	43
cranberry nut	1 (2 oz)	212	9	1.5	191	30	1	18	3	0	25	1	69
lemon poppy seed	1 (2 oz)	229	12	2.5	178	27	1	16	3	0	23	1	18
pumpkin	1 (2 oz)	275	12	5.0	200	39	1	19	3	0	15	2	69
Popovers	1 (2 oz)	150	5	2.5	169	20	1	2	6	1	67	1	113
Rolls													
brown & serve	1 medium	78	2	0.5	134	13	1	2	3	0	45	1	35
crescent	1 medium	110	6	1.5	220	11	0	3	2	0	11	1	34
French	1 medium	105	2	0.5	231	19	1	0	3	0	41	1	51
hamburger/hot dog	1 medium	120	2	0.5	206	21	1	4	4	0	75	2	63
hard	1 medium	167	2	0.5	310	30	1	1	6	0	53	2	61
kaiser	1 medium	167	2	0.5	310	30	1	1	6	0	54	2	62
rye	1 medium	81	1	0.0	253	15	1	1	3	0	26	1	60
sesame seed	1 medium	140	3	1.5	240	23	0	0	5	0	36	1	59
sourdough	1 medium	100	1	0.0	240	19	1	2	4	0	16	1	36
submarine	1 (8 inch)	220	2	0.0	460	44	2	8	7	0	153	4	129
whole wheat	1 medium	75	1	0.0	136	14	2	1	2	0	76	2	49
yeast	1 medium	106	3	0.5	126	18	0	5	3	0	70	1	54
Scones	1 large	304	13	4.0	345	39	1	9	8	0	147	2	74

Bread Products

	Amount	Calories	Fat (g)	Saturated Fat (g)	Sodium (mg)	Carbohydrate (g)	Fiber (g)	Sugar (g)	Protein (g)	Vitamin D (mcg)	Calcium (mg)	Iron (mg)	Potassium (mg)
Corn fritters	1 (2 oz)	209	12	3.0	268	22	1	2	4	0	70	1	89
Crepes	1 (8 in)	144	7	2.0	187	14	0	3	6	1	60	1	101
Croutons	¼ cup	37	1	0.0	70	7	1	0	1	0	2	0	0
seasoned	¼ cup	37	1	0.0	131	7	1	0	1	0	3	0	2
French toast													
frozen	1 slice	126	4	1.0	292	19	1	0	4	0	63	1	79
homemade	1 slice	159	6	2.0	261	2	1	5	6	1	48	2	89
Lefse	1 (1.5 oz)	100	1	0.0	270	22	2	2	2	0	75	1	140
Pancakes													
blueberry, mix	2 (6 in)	342	14	3.0	634	45	2	10	9	0	317	3	213
buttermilk, mix	2 (6 in)	256	8	1.5	507	42	1	9	6	0	86	6	99
plain, frozen	2 (6 in)	340	10	1.5	673	55	1	12	8	0	114	8	131
plain, homemade	2 (6 in)	350	15	3.5	676	44	2	10	10	0	337	3	203
plain, low-fat, homemade	2 (6 in)	296	2	0.0	472	63	1	9	6	0	63	2	107
whole wheat, mix	2 (6 in)	252	11	2.0	673	32	4	7	8	1	216	2	240
Pizza crust, Boboli	½ (8 in)	190	4	1.5	380	34	1	1	6	0	90	2	8
Pretzels, soft													
shopping mall, salted	1 large	340	5	3.0	990	65	2	10	8	0	20	1	90
SuperPretzel, frozen	1 medium	160	0	0.0	890	34	1	1	4	0	7	3	50

BREADS & BREAD PRODUCTS

Bread Products

	Amount	Calories	Fat (g)	Saturated Fat (g)	Sodium (mg)	Carbohydrate (g)	Fiber (g)	Sugar (g)	Protein (g)	Vitamin D (mcg)	Calcium (mg)	Iron (mg)	Potassium
Stuffing, prepared													
bread, homemade	½ cup	177	9	1.5	472	22	1	2	3	0	30	1	72
cornbread, box	½ cup	179	9	2.0	526	22	3	0	3	0	26	1	62
Stove Top, box	½ cup	150	6	1.5	460	21	0	2	3	0	0	1	90
reduced sodium	½ cup	150	6	1.5	290	21	0	2	3	0	0	1	0
Taco shells, corn	3 (5 in)	150	8	3.0	130	19	2	0	2	0	30	1	65
Tortillas													
corn	2 (6 in)	100	2	0.0	10	20	3	2	2	0	60	1	80
flour	1 (8 in)	142	33	0.5	200	23	1	1	4	0	59	1	51
Waffles													
Belgian, mix	1 (8 in)	381	12	2.5	886	60	3	6	9	0	373	8	173
Eggo, Blueberry, frozen	1 (1.2 oz)	90	3	1.0	185	15	0	6	2	0	130	2	40
Eggo, Homestyle, frozen	1 (1.2 oz)	95	4	1.0	180	14	0	1	2	0	130	2	28
Eggo, Nutrigrain, frozen	1 (1.2 oz)	70	1	0.5	190	14	2	3	2	0	130	2	45
plain, homemade	1 (7 in)	218	11	2.0	383	25	1	2	6	0	191	2	119
plain, low-fat, frozen	1 (1.2 oz)	80	1	0.5	137	16	0	2	2	0	132	2	31

CANDY

	Amount	Calories	Fat (g)	Saturated Fat (g)	Sodium (mg)	Carbohydrate (g)	Fiber (g)	Sugar (g)	Protein (g)	Vitamin D (mcg)	Calcium (mg)	Iron (mg)	Potassium
Almonds													
candy coated	10	165	6	0.5	5	24	1	25	4	0	25	0	89
chocolate covered	10	145	11	3.5	4	14	2	9	3	0	36	1	136
Bit-o-Honey	6 small	150	3	2.0	120	32	0	19	1	0	20	0	50
Bridge mix	¼ cup	200	12	8.0	16	24	2	20	2	0	40	1	133
Boston Baked Beans	½ cup	160	2	0.0	420	31	5	13	7	0	60	2	390
Cadbury Eggs, creme	1 (1.4 oz)	150	6	4.0	15	24	0	20	2	0	37	0	41
Candy bars (average size)													
3 Musketeers	1 (1.4 oz)	240	7	5.0	90	42	1	36	1	0	20	0	80
5th Avenue	1 (1.4 oz)	260	12	4.5	115	38	2	29	4	0	31	1	170
100 Grand	1 (2.13 oz)	190	8	5.0	90	30	0	22	1	0	20	0	70
Almond Joy	1 (2 oz)	220	12	8.0	50	26	2	21	2	0	20	1	110
Baby Ruth	1 (1.5 oz)	280	14	8.0	140	39	1	33	4	0	40	1	149
Butterfinger	1 (2.1 oz)	250	10	5.0	100	39	1	24	3	0	0	1	143
Caramello	1 (1.7 oz)	180	8	5.0	35	24	0	21	2	0	70	0	14
Charleston Chew	1 (1.4 oz)	80	2	2.0	5	15	0	11	0	0	25	1	35
Chunky	1 (2.1 oz)	190	11	6.0	15	25	1	21	2	0	40	0	187
Heath Bar	1 (1.4 oz)	210	13	7.0	140	25	1	24	1	0	24	0	54
Hershey's													
Milk Chocolate	1 (1.4 oz)	220	13	8.0	35	26	1	25	3	1	60	1	160
Special Dark	1 (1.45 oz)	190	12	8.0	0	26	3	22	2	0	0	4	180
w/ almonds	1 (1.75 oz)	210	14	7.0	25	22	2	19	4	1	85	1	170
Kit Kat	1 (1.45 oz)	210	11	7.0	30	27	1	22	3	0	60	1	120
Milky Way	1 (1.5 oz)	240	9	7.0	75	37	1	31	2	0	40	0	72
Midnight	1 (1.76 oz)	220	8	5.0	65	36	1	29	1	0	20	0	98

CANDY

	Amount	Calories	Fat (g)	Saturated Fat (g)	Sodium (mg)	Carbohydrate (g)	Fiber (g)	Sugar (g)	Protein (g)	Vitamin D (mcg)	Calcium (mg)	Iron (mg)	Potassium (mg)
Mounds	1 (2.05 oz)	230	13	10.0	55	29	3	21	2	0	10	2	120
Mr. Goodbar	1 (1.76 oz)	260	17	8.0	50	27	2	23	5	0	50	1	240
Nestle Crunch	1 (1.75 oz)	240	13	13.0	65	32	1	21	3	0	40	0	134
Oh Henry!	1 (1.75 oz)	120	6	2.0	60	17	1	13	2	0	21	0	67
Pay Day	1 (1.55 oz)	240	13	2.5	120	27	2	21	7	0	51	1	200
Pearson's Nut Roll	1 (1.8 oz)	240	11	2.0	170	27	2	20	8	0	18	0	217
Skor	1 (1.85 oz)	210	12	7.0	135	25	0	24	1	0	26	1	94
Symphony	1 (1.35 oz)	200	12	7.0	40	22	1	21	3	0	91	0	163
Snickers	1 (1.8 oz)	250	12	4.5	120	33	1	27	4	0	50	0	150
Twix	1 (1.4 oz)	250	12	7.0	105	34	1	25	2	0	52	1	100
Whatchamacallit	1 (2.07 oz)	230	12	10.0	100	28	1	21	3	0	40	1	100
Candy corn	15	110	0	0.0	60	28	0	22	0	0	1	0	1
Caramels	4	130	3	1.5	80	24	0	21	1	0	44	0	88
Cherries, chocolate covered	2	110	5	2.5	10	19	0	15	1	0	21	0	31
Circus peanuts	6	160	0	0.0	0	39	0	34	1	0	0	0	0
Cotton candy	1 oz	110	0	0.0	0	28	0	28	0	0	0	0	0
Divinity, homemade	2 (0.4 oz)	83	0	0.0	8	20	0	10	0	0	2	0	10
Dots	12	150	0	0.0	15	36	0	23	0	0	1	0	2
Ferrero Rocher	3	230	16	5.0	25	18	1	15	3	0	31	1	132
Fondant	2 (0.5 oz)	106	0	0.0	5	26	0	12	0	0	0	0	1
Fudge, homemade													
chocolate													
w/ nuts	1 oz	131	5	1.5	12	19	1	14	1	0	13	0	40
w/o nuts	1 oz	117	3	1.5	13	22	0	16	1	0	11	0	30
vanilla													
w/ nuts	1 oz	123	4	1.0	13	21	0	16	1	0	10	0	23
w/o nuts	1 oz	109	2	1.0	14	23	0	18	0	0	8	0	11
Ghirardelli Chocolate Squares													
dark	4 squares	213	16	9.0	0	23	4	16	3	0	27	1	227
milk	4 squares	220	13	8.0	30	26	0	24	3	0	80	0	180
w/ caramel	3 squares	225	12	7.5	68	27	0	24	3	0	75	0	135
Goobers	¼ cup	220	13	5.0	10	22	2	18	5	0	40	0	187
Good & Plenty	33	131	0	0.0	18	33	0	25	0	0	5	0	5
Gum, regular/sugar-free	1 stick	5	0	0.0	0	2	0	0	0	0	0	0	0
Gumdrops	10	140	0	0.0	16	36	0	21	0	0	1	0	2
Gummy bears	15	115	0	0.0	6	27	0	16	2	0	1	0	2
Hard candies	3 small	35	0	0.0	3	9	0	6	0	0	0	1	15
sugar-free	3 small	34	0	0.0	0	8	0	0	0	0	0	0	0
Hershey's													
Hugs	7	160	9	6.0	30	19	0	16	2	0	60	0	105
Kisses	7	160	9	6.0	25	19	1	18	2	1	40	1	120
w/ almonds	7	160	10	5.0	20	16	3	15	3	0	40	1	130

CANDY

CANDY	Amount	Calories	Fat (g)	Saturated Fat (g)	Sodium (mg)	Carbohydrate (g)	Fiber (g)	Sugar (g)	Protein (g)	Vitamin D (mcg)	Calcium (mg)	Iron (mg)	Potassium (mg)
Hot Tamales	16	110	0	0.0	0	27	0	18	0	0	0	0	0
Jelly beans	35 small	140	0	0.0	15	37	0	28	0	0	1	0	14
Jolly Ranchers	3	70	0	0.0	0	17	0	11	0	0	1	0	0
Junior Mints	12	130	3	1.5	0	26	0	25	0	0	6	1	62
Licorice, black/red	3 (8 in)	120	1	0.0	70	27	0	16	1	0	0	0	15
Lifesavers	4	60	0	0.0	0	15	0	12	0	0	0	0	0
Lollipops													
Blow Pop	1	70	0	0.0	0	17	0	13	0	0	123	0	0
Dum • Dum	2	50	0	0.0	0	13	0	10	0	0	0	0	0
Saf-T-Pop	1	43	0	0.0	0	11	0	9	0	0	0	0	0
Tootsie Pop	1	60	0	0.0	0	15	0	11	0	0	0	0	1
M&M's	1 pkg	230	9	6.0	35	35	1	31	2	0	40	1	94
crispy	1 pkg	200	7	4.5	60	31	1	25	2	0	40	1	0
peanut	1 pkg	250	13	5.0	25	30	2	23	5	0	40	6	0
Malted milk balls	18	190	7	7.0	95	31	0	24	1	0	63	1	140
Marshmallows	4 large	100	0	0.0	25	24	0	17	1	0	1	0	1
Mike and Ike	16	110	0	0.0	10	27	0	18	0	0	0	0	0
Milk Duds	10	130	5	2.5	75	22	0	16	1	0	0	0	94
Mints													
Altoids	3	10	0	0.0	0	2	0	2	0	0	0	0	0
Breath Savers	1	5	0	0.0	0	2	0	0	0	0	0	0	0
butter	6	51	0	0.0	21	12	0	12	0	0	0	0	0
Nips, caramel	2	60	2	1.0	10	12	0	7	0	0	10	0	0
Nonpareils	15	200	10	6.0	15	28	0	27	1	0	54	1	133
Orange slices	2	130	0	0.0	10	32	0	23	0	0	0	0	0
Peanut brittle	1.5 oz	210	15	6.0	260	19	0	14	4	0	20	0	71
Peanuts, chocolate covered	¼ cup	210	14	7.0	15	20	2	16	4	0	40	1	187
Peeps	4	110	0	0.0	0	28	0	25	0	0	0	0	1
Pez	1 roll (12)	35	0	0.0	0	9	0	9	0	0	0	0	0
Praline, homemade	1 (1.4 oz)	173	10	3.0	40	22	1	30	1	0	42	0	77
Raisinets	10	40	2	0.5	4	7	1	0	1	0	0	0	51
Raisins, yogurt covered	¼ cup	120	4	4.0	15	21	1	18	1	0	20	0	160
Reese's													
Peanut Butter Cups	2 (0.8 oz)	210	12	4.5	150	24	2	22	5	0	39	1	150
Pieces	38	150	7	6.0	35	19	1	16	3	0	10	1	90
Rolos	5	140	6	4.5	50	20	0	19	1	0	40	0	70
Skittles	27	110	1	1.0	5	26	0	21	0	0	0	0	3
Sour Patch Kids	12	110	0	0.0	25	27	0	24	0	0	10	0	2
Starburst	6	120	3	2.5	0	24	0	16	0	0	0	0	0
Sugar Babies	21	120	1	0.5	25	28	0	22	0	0	0	0	0
Sugar Daddy	1 (1.7 oz)	200	3	1.5	70	44	0	29	1	0	20	0	31

CANDY

	Amount	Calories	Fat (g)	Saturated Fat (mg)	Sodium (mg)	Carbohydrate (g)	Fiber (g)	Sugar (g)	Protein (g)	Vitamin D (mcg)	Calcium (mg)	Iron (mg)	Potassium (mg)
Swedish Fish													
small	12 (1 in)	110	0	0.0	25	27	0	23	0	0	0	0	0
medium	19 (2 in)	140	0	0.0	30	36	0	29	0	0	0	0	0
Sweet Tarts	13	60	0	0.0	0	14	0	13	0	0	0	0	0
Taffy													
Airheads	2 (4 in)	130	1	0.0	5	30	0	21	0	0	0	0	0
saltwater	7 small	160	2	1.5	60	38	0	23	0	0	2	0	1
Tic Tacs	2	4	0	0.0	0	0	0	0	0	0	0	0	0
Toblerone	4 pcs	190	10	6.0	20	22	1	21	2	0	60	1	100
Tootsie Rolls	6 small	140	3	0.5	15	28	0	20	1	0	20	1	46
Truffles	3 (1.3 oz)	220	17	12.0	25	16	1	15	2	0	60	1	126
Turtles	2 (0.6 oz)	170	10	4.0	40	19	1	16	2	0	40	0	125
Whoppers	18	190	7	7.0	95	31	0	24	1	0	63	1	140
York Peppermint Pattie	1 (1.4 oz)	150	3	1.5	10	32	1	26	1	0	0	1	48

CEREAL BARS & CEREALS

Cereal Bars

	Amount	Calories	Fat (g)	Saturated Fat (mg)	Sodium (mg)	Carbohydrate (g)	Fiber (g)	Sugar (g)	Protein (g)	Vitamin D (mcg)	Calcium (mg)	Iron (mg)	Potassium (mg)
Fiber One Oats & Chocolate	1 bar	140	4	1.5	95	29	9	9	2	0	140	1	0
Kashi Chewy Granola													
chocolate almond sea salt	1 bar	130	5	1.0	125	23	4	7	3	0	20	1	120
chocolate peanut butter	1 bar	140	6	1.5	140	21	5	6	3	0	10	1	130
trail mix	1 bar	130	5	0.0	105	24	3	7	3	0	20	1	110
Milk 'n Cereal													
Cinnamon Toast Crunch	1 bar	180	4	2.0	150	33	1	14	3	0	290	2	110
Honey Nut Cheerios	1 bar	160	4	2.0	90	13	1	13	3	1	280	1	120
Nature Valley													
Crunchy Granola													
cinnamon	1 bar	90	4	0.0	75	15	1	6	2	0	0	1	0
maple brown sugar	1 bar	100	4	0.0	75	15	1	6	2	0	0	1	0
oats 'n honey	1 bar	100	4	0.0	70	15	1	6	2	0	0	1	0
peanut butter	1 bar	100	4	0.0	80	14	1	5	2	0	0	1	0
Sweet & Salty Nut Granola													
almond	1 bar	160	7	2.0	140	22	2	8	3	0	30	1	100
dark chocolate peanut & almond	1 bar	170	8	3.0	125	22	2	9	3	0	0	1	0
peanut	1 bar	170	8	2.5	140	20	1	7	4	0	0	0	0
Nutri-Grain Soft Baked													
apple cinnamon	1 bar	130	4	0.5	125	25	1	13	2	0	130	2	80
blueberry	1 bar	130	4	0.5	130	25	1	13	2	0	130	2	80
strawberry	1 bar	130	4	0.5	140	25	1	13	2	0	130	2	80
Power Bar Protein Plus													
chocolate peanut butter	1 bar	210	6	3.0	200	25	4	12	20	0	96	1	100
vanilla	1 bar	210	5	3.0	130	23	4	14	20	0	96	1	120

CEREAL BARS & CEREALS

Cereal Bars	Amount	Calories	Fat (g)	Saturated Fat (g)	Sodium (mg)	Carbohydrate (g)	Fiber (g)	Sugar (g)	Protein (g)	Vitamin D (mcg)	Calcium (mg)	Iron (mg)	Potassium (mg)
Quaker Chewy Granola													
chocolate chip	1 bar	100	4	1.5	70	17	1	7	1	0	80	1	60
cookies & cream, 25% less sugar	1 bar	90	3	0.5	85	18	3	5	1	0	110	1	50
oatmeal raisin	1 bar	90	2	0.0	80	19	1	7	1	0	90	1	60
peanut butter/chocolate chip	1 bar	100	3	1.0	95	17	1	7	2	0	100	1	60
Rice Krispies Treats	1 bar	90	2	0.5	105	17	0	8	0	0	0	1	0
Special K													
cranberry almond nut	1 bar	140	6	1.5	55	20	2	12	3	0	20	1	120
chocolate almond nut	1 bar	170	10	3.0	45	16	2	9	4	0	20	1	130
stawberry pastry crisps	1 bar	100	2	1.0	80	20	0	7	0	0	10	1	20
Hot Cereal (prepared)													
Cream of Rice	1 cup	150	0	0.0	0	35	0	0	2	5	340	13	30
Cream of Wheat	1¼ cups	120	0	0.0	100	25	1	0	3	4	260	9	30
Grits, corn													
instant	1 pkt	100	1	0.0	310	22	1	0	2	0	130	8	40
old fashioned	1 cup	140	1	0.0	0	32	2	0	3	0	0	2	60
quick	1 cup	130	1	0.0	0	29	2	0	3	0	0	2	50
Maltex	1 cup	180	1	0.0	0	38	5	2	5	0	0	9	200
Malt-O-Meal	1 cup	130	0	0.0	0	27	0	0	4	0	100	11	30
Maypo	1 cup	180	3	0.5	105	34	4	4	5	0	180	14	150
Oat bran	1 cup	140	3	0.5	0	26	5	1	6	0	30	3	240
Oatmeal													
apples & cinnamon, instant	1 pkt	160	2	0.5	160	33	4	11	4	0	20	1	150
cinnamon & spice, instant	1 pkt	160	3	0.5	200	32	3	10	4	0	20	1	130
maple & brown sugar, instant	1 pkt	160	2	0.5	260	33	3	12	4	0	20	1	110
regular, instant	1 pkt	100	2	0.5	75	18	3	0	4	0	120	8	100
regular, old fashioned/quick	1 cup	150	3	0.5	0	27	4	1	5	0	20	2	150
steel cut	1 cup	150	3	0.5	0	27	4	1	5	0	20	2	150
Wheatena	1 cup	143	1	0.0	5	30	5	1	5	0	22	1	200
Ready-to-Eat Cereal (w/o milk)													
All-Bran	½ cup	110	2	0.0	300	36	17	12	5	2	30	5	430
buds	½ cup	110	2	0.0	300	36	17	12	5	2	30	5	430
Amaranth flakes	1 cup	132	3	0.0	6	22	4	0	5	0	24	1	120
Apple Jacks	1 cup	120	1	0.0	146	29	3	15	2	2	0	5	50
Basic 4	1 cup	200	2	1.0	280	43	5	12	4	1	300	5	170
Bran flakes	1 cup	110	1	0.0	190	29	7	7	4	2	10	9	210
Cap'n Crunch	1 cup	150	2	0.5	290	33	0	17	2	0	0	8	50
Crunch Berries	1 cup	150	2	0.5	270	32	0	16	2	0	0	8	50
peanut butter crunch	1 cup	170	4	1.0	300	32	0	13	3	0	0	7	70

CEREAL BARS & CEREALS

Ready-to-Eat Cereal	Amount	Calories	Fat (g)	Saturated Fat (g)	Sodium (mg)	Carbohydrate (g)	Fiber (g)	Sugar (g)	Protein (g)	Vitamin D (mcg)	Calcium (mg)	Iron (mg)	Potassium (mg)
Cheerios	1½ cups	140	3	0.5	190	29	4	2	5	2	130	13	250
apple cinnamon	1 cup	150	3	0.0	150	30	3	12	3	2	130	4	99
banana nut	¾ cup	110	2	0.0	120	22	2	8	2	1	120	5	80
frosted	1 cup	140	2	0.0	200	29	3	12	3	2	130	4	94
honey nut	1 cup	140	2	0.0	210	30	3	12	3	2	130	4	152
multigrain	1⅓ cups	150	2	0.0	150	32	3	8	3	2	130	18	170
Chex													
cinnamon	1 cup	170	4	0.0	250	33	2	8	2	2	130	11	49
corn	1¼ cups	150	1	0.0	280	33	2	4	3	2	130	11	61
honey nut	1 cup	170	1	0.0	270	38	2	12	3	2	130	4	88
rice	1⅓ cups	160	1	0.0	330	35	2	3	3	2	130	13	51
wheat	1 cup	210	1	0.0	340	51	8	6	6	2	130	18	190
Cinnamon Toast Crunch	1 cup	170	4	0.0	230	33	2	12	2	2	130	4	80
Cocoa Pebbles	1 cup	140	2	0.0	220	31	0	12	2	2	9	3	60
Cocoa Puffs	¾ cup	100	2	0.0	100	23	1	9	1	1	120	5	85
Cocoa Rice Krispies	1 cup	160	1	0.0	140	37	0	13	3	2	190	5	70
Cookie Crisp	1 cup	140	2	0.0	150	31	2	2	2	1	120	4	81
Corn flakes	1½ cups	150	0	0.0	300	36	1	4	3	3	1	12	60
Corn Pops	1⅓ cups	150	0	0.0	160	36	0	15	2	2	2	5	30
Cracklin' Oat Bran	¾ cup	230	8	3.5	65	41	7	16	4	3	20	5	210
Crispix	1⅓ cups	150	0	0.0	260	34	0	5	3	3	3	11	20
Crunchy Oatmeal Squares	1 cup	210	3	0.5	190	44	5	9	6	0	30	17	200
Fiber One	⅔ cup	90	1	0.0	140	34	18	0	3	0	130	4	148
honey clusters	1 cup	170	2	0.0	200	45	10	10	4	0	130	16	193
Froot Loops	1⅓ cups	150	2	0.5	210	34	2	12	2	2	3	5	60
Frosted Flakes	1 cup	130	0	0.0	190	33	1	12	2	2	1	7	30
Fruity Pebbles	1 cup	140	2	0.0	190	31	0	12	1	2	8	1	20
Golden Crisp	1 cup	150	1	0.0	85	34	0	21	2	0	4	1	70
Golden Grahams	¾ cup	110	1	0.0	230	25	1	9	2	1	120	5	70
Granola, Bear Naked													
fruit & nut	½ cup	270	12	3.0	0	39	5	13	6	0	30	2	190
peanut butter	⅔ cup	290	13	2.0	55	42	5	13	6	0	20	2	210
protein original cinnamon	½ cup	260	12	1.0	100	31	5	12	11	0	40	2	240
Granola, Simply	⅔ cup	260	7	1.0	30	48	7	13	7	0	60	2	190
w/ raisins	⅔ cup	270	7	0.5	30	51	7	17	7	0	60	2	230
Grape-Nuts	½ cup	200	1	0.0	280	47	7	5	6	0	20	17	260
flakes	1 cup	150	2	0.0	200	34	5	7	4	2	10	13	160
Great Grains													
banana nut crunch	1 cup	230	5	0.5	240	45	5	10	6	2	20	17	295
blueberry morning	1 cup	220	3	0.0	200	48	4	16	4	2	20	3	150
cranberry almond crunch	1 cup	210	3	0.0	200	44	5	12	5	2	20	5	180
crunchy pecans	¾ cup	210	5	0.5	160	39	5	8	5	2	20	16	190
raisins, dates & pecans	¾ cup	200	4	0.0	140	40	5	13	4	2	20	11	210

Ready-to-Eat Cereal	Amount	Calories	Fat (g)	Saturated Fat (g)	Sodium (mg)	Carbohydrate (g)	Fiber (g)	Sugar (g)	Protein (g)	Vitamin D (mcg)	Calcium (mg)	Iron (mg)	Potassium
Honey Bunches of Oats													
honey roasted	1 cup	160	2	0.0	190	34	2	9	3	2	10	16	60
w/ almonds	1 cup	170	3	0.0	180	34	2	9	3	2	10	16	80
Honeycomb	1¾ cups	110	1	0.0	70	25	0	12	1	0	110	0	20
Kashi	1¼ cups	180	2	0.0	115	40	13	8	12	0	40	2	390
GO													
cinnamon crisp	1 cup	210	5	0.5	200	37	11	11	13	0	60	3	350
Organic													
blueberry clusters	1 cup	210	3	0.0	130	44	3	11	5	0	10	1	120
honey toasted oat	1 cup	150	2	0.0	65	35	6	7	4	0	10	12	100
Strawberry Fields	1 cup	200	0	0.0	180	46	3	11	5	0	0	1	110
Whole Wheat Biscuits													
cinnamon harvest	31 biscuits	200	1	0.0	0	48	7	9	7	0	10	2	190
simply raisin	30 biscuits	190	1	0.0	0	47	7	7	7	0	20	2	280
Kix	1½ cups	160	1	0.0	220	34	3	4	3	2	130	11	54
honey	1½ cups	160	2	0.0	190	34	2	3	2	2	130	11	100
Life	1 cup	160	2	0.0	210	33	3	8	4	0	150	13	110
Lucky Charms	1 cup	140	1	0.0	160	31	1	12	1	2	130	4	80
Mini-Wheats													
blueberry	25 biscuits	210	1	0.0	10	50	6	12	5	0	10	18	210
frosted bite-size	25 biscuits	210	2	0.0	10	51	6	12	5	0	0	18	160
Mueslix	1 cup	250	4	0.0	150	50	5	17	6	0	30	2	200
Nature's Patch Flax Plus													
maple pecan crunch	1 cup	230	7	1.0	210	39	6	10	6	0	30	3	250
multibran	1 cup	150	2	0.0	180	31	7	5	5	0	22	2	190
Oat bran flakes	1 cup	120	2	0.0	75	25	4	4	5	0	20	2	180
Oatmeal Squares w/ brown sugar	1 cup	210	3	0.5	190	44	5	9	6	0	30	17	200
Puffed rice	1 cup	60	0	0.0	0	14	1	0	1	0	0	0	50
Puffed wheat	1 cup	50	0	0.0	0	13	2	0	2	0	10	1	60
Raisin Bran	1 cup	190	1	0.0	200	47	7	17	5	0	20	2	280
Crunch	1 cup	190	1	0.0	200	46	4	19	4	0	20	1	280
Reese's Puffs	¾ cup	120	3	0.5	160	22	1	9	2	1	120	5	70
Rice Krispies	1½ cups	150	0	0.0	200	36	0	4	3	3	0	11	30
Shredded Wheat													
big biscuit	2 biscuits	170	1	0.0	0	41	7	0	6	0	20	2	230
regular, Spoon Size	1⅓ cups	210	2	0.0	0	49	8	0	7	0	20	2	250
Wheat 'N Bran, Spoon Size	1⅓ cups	210	2	0.0	0	49	8	0	7	0	20	2	240
Smart Start, Original Antioxidants	1¼ cups	240	1	0.0	260	56	3	18	5	2	10	8	130
Special K	1 cup	150	1	0.0	270	29	0	5	7	2	0	11	10
fruit & yogurt	1 cup	150	1	0.5	190	36	3	13	3	2	10	11	90
red berries	1 cup	140	1	0.0	250	34	3	11	3	2	10	11	80
Total whole grain	1 cup	140	1	0.0	190	33	4	6	3	2	40	18	140
Trix	1 cup	123	1	0.0	160	28	1	10	2	1	5	100	52

CEREAL BARS & CEREALS

Ready-to-Eat Cereal	Amount	Calories	Fat (g)	Saturated Fat (g)	Sodium (mg)	Carbohydrate (g)	Fiber (g)	Sugar (g)	Protein (g)	Vitamin D (mcg)	Calcium (mg)	Iron (mg)	Potassium (mg)
Weetabix	3 biscuits	180	1	0.0	190	43	6	2	5	0	20	7	230
Wheat bran flakes	1 cup	110	1	0.0	190	29	7	7	4	2	10	9	210
Wheat germ	3 T	60	1	0.0	0	8	2	1	4	0	10	1	141
Wheaties	1 cup	130	1	0.0	240	30	4	5	3	1	0	13	130

CHEESE

	Amount	Calories	Fat (g)	Saturated Fat (g)	Sodium (mg)	Carbohydrate (g)	Fiber (g)	Sugar (g)	Protein (g)	Vitamin D (mcg)	Calcium (mg)	Iron (mg)	Potassium (mg)
American	1 oz	106	9	5.0	474	1	0	1	6	1	300	0	37
fat-free	1 oz	36	0	0.0	373	3	0	1	6	1	220	0	110
low-fat	1 oz	68	4	2.5	340	3	0	2	5	2	150	0	94
singles	1 slice	95	6	4.0	297	3	0	1	5	1	270	0	59
fat-free	1 slice	37	0	0.0	373	3	0	2	6	0	224	0	83
reduced fat	1 slice	67	4	2.0	343	3	0	3	6	2	298	0	69
Blue	1 oz	100	8	5.0	325	1	0	0	6	0	150	0	73
Brick	1 oz	105	8	5.0	159	1	0	0	7	0	191	0	38
Brie	1 oz	95	8	5.0	178	0	0	0	6	0	52	0	43
Camembert	1 oz	85	7	4.0	239	0	0	0	6	0	110	0	53
Caraway	1 oz	107	8	5.0	196	1	0	0	7	0	191	0	26
Cheddar	1 oz	115	9	5.0	185	1	0	0	7	0	201	0	22
fat-free	1 oz	45	0	0.0	283	2	0	0	9	0	253	0	19
low-fat	1 oz	50	2	1.0	247	1	0	0	7	0	118	0	19
shredded	¼ cup	114	9	5.0	184	1	0	0	6	0	201	0	21
spread	2 T	80	7	5.0	150	1	0	1	2	0	40	0	69
Cheez Whiz	2 T	91	7	4.0	541	3	0	2	4	0	118	0	79
Colby	1 oz	112	9	6.0	171	1	0	0	7	0	194	0	36
Colby & Monterey Jack	1 oz	111	9	5.0	172	1	0	0	7	0	152	0	30
Cottage													
1% fat	½ cup	81	1	0.5	459	3	0	3	14	0	67	0	97
2% fat	½ cup	92	3	1.5	348	5	0	5	12	0	125	0	141
fat-free	½ cup	80	0	0.0	390	8	0	6	13	1	100	0	159
Cream cheese	2 T	102	10	6.0	91	2	0	1	2	0	28	0	38
fat-free	2 T	38	0	0.0	253	3	0	2	6	0	126	0	100
flavored													
onion & chive	2 T	80	7	5.0	150	2	0	1	2	0	40	0	68
strawberry	2 T	80	6	4.0	105	5	0	4	1	0	40	0	39
light	2 T	60	5	2.5	108	2	0	2	2	0	44	0	74
onion & chive	2 T	60	5	3.0	108	2	0	2	2	0	44	0	74
Easy Cheese, cheddar	2 T	87	6	4.0	488	3	0	2	5	0	169	0	72
Edam	1 oz	101	8	5.0	230	0	0	0	7	0	207	0	53
Feta	1 oz	75	6	4.0	260	1	0	1	4	0	140	0	18
Fondue	¼ cup	148	11	6.5	163	1	0	0	10	0	343	0	46
Fontina	1 oz	110	9	5.5	227	0	0	0	7	0	156	0	18
Goat, soft	1 oz	75	6	4.0	130	0	0	0	5	0	40	1	7
Gorgonzola	1 oz	100	8	5.5	325	1	0	0	6	0	150	0	73

CHEESE

	Amount	Calories	Fat (g)	Saturated Fat (g)	Sodium (mg)	Carbohydrate (g)	Fiber (g)	Sugar (g)	Protein (g)	Vitamin D (mcg)	Calcium (mg)	Iron (mg)	Potassium (mg)
Gouda	1 oz	101	8	5.0	232	1	0	1	7	0	198	0	34
Gruyère	1 oz	117	9	5.5	202	0	0	0	8	0	287	0	23
Havarti	1 oz	105	8	5.0	159	1	0	0	7	0	191	0	39
Jarlsberg	1 oz	111	9	5.0	53	0	0	0	8	0	252	0	20
Limburger	1 oz	93	8	5.0	227	0	0	0	6	0	141	0	36
Mascarpone	1 oz	120	12	7.0	10	0	0	0	2	0	40	0	70
Monterey Jack	1 oz	101	9	5.0	192	0	0	0	6	0	203	0	23
Mozzarella													
part-skim	1 oz	84	6	3.0	189	2	0	0	7	0	198	0	53
whole milk	1 oz	90	7	4.5	201	1	0	0	6	0	163	0	21
Muenster	1 oz	104	9	5.5	178	0	0	0	7	0	203	0	38
Neufchatel	1 oz	72	6	3.5	95	1	0	1	3	0	33	0	43
Parmesan, grated	1 T	30	2	1.5	113	0	0	0	3	0	90	0	9
reduced fat	1 T	19	1	1.0	107	0	0	0	1	0	78	0	9
Pepper Jack	1 oz	111	9	5.0	192	0	0	0	7	0	203	0	23
Port wine, cold pack	2 T	80	6	3.0	160	3	0	3	4	0	100	0	73
Provolone	1 oz	100	8	5.0	248	1	0	0	7	0	214	0	39
Ricotta													
fat-free	½ cup	100	0	0.0	130	10	0	4	10	0	200	0	316
low-fat	½ cup	120	6	4.0	140	6	0	4	14	0	200	0	280
part-skim	½ cup	140	9	6.0	170	6	0	6	12	0	200	0	155
whole milk	½ cup	180	12	8.0	150	6	0	6	14	0	300	0	219
Romano, grated	1 T	30	2	1.5	113	0	0	0	3	0	90	0	11
Roquefort	1 oz	105	9	5.5	513	1	0	0	6	0	188	0	26
Soy cheese	1 oz	43	2	0.5	6	2	0	0	4	0	53	2	56
String	1 oz	83	6	3.0	189	2	0	1	7	0	198	0	53
Swiss													
natural	1 oz	111	9	5.0	53	1	0	0	8	0	252	0	20
processed	1 oz	92	7	4.5	440	1	0	0	6	0	205	0	81
Velveeta	1 oz	81	5	3.5	415	2	0	2	5	0	203	0	94
Yogurt cheese	1 oz	26	2	1.0	22	2	0	2	1	0	50	0	61

COMBINATION FOODS, FROZEN ENTRÉES & MEALS

	Amount	Calories	Fat (g)	Saturated Fat (g)	Sodium (mg)	Carbohydrate (g)	Fiber (g)	Sugar (g)	Protein (g)	Vitamin D (mcg)	Calcium (mg)	Iron (mg)	Potassium (mg)
Bagel Bites, frozen													
cheese & pepperoni	4 pcs	190	6	3.5	380	29	2	2	8	0	100	1	160
mozzarella	4 pcs	170	4	2.0	370	28	1	2	7	0	110	2	130
three cheese	4 pcs	180	5	3.0	360	28	1	3	6	0	100	2	140
Baked beans w/ pork, can	½ cup	150	1	0.0	550	29	7	7	7	0	67	2	391
Beans & rice	1 cup	279	7	1.0	393	43	6	0	11	0	92	4	556
Beef goulash w/ noodles	1 cup	361	14	3.5	130	27	2	2	30	0	45	4	525
Beef stroganoff w/ noodles	1 cup	344	19	7.5	468	23	2	3	20	0	74	2	374
Beefaroni, can	1 cup	260	7	3.0	1070	37	5	5	10	0	31	2	327

COMBINATION FOODS, FROZEN ENTRÉES & MEALS

	Amount	Calories	Fat (g)	Saturated Fat (g)	Sodium (mg)	Carbohydrate (g)	Fiber (g)	Sugar (g)	Protein (g)	Vitamin D (mcg)	Calcium (mg)	Iron (mg)	Potassium (mg)
Burritos, frozen													
bean & cheese	1 (6 oz)	413	11	2.5	941	66	18	6	13	0	97	5	393
beef & bean	1 (6 oz)	352	11	4.0	866	51	6	1	11	0	47	4	307
Casseroles													
chicken w/ cheese sauce	1 cup	368	16	6.5	739	9	0	4	44	1	120	2	284
green bean	1 cup	115	5	1.0	736	16	4	6	4	0	92	1	366
seafood Newburg	1 cup	613	50	29.5	551	10	0	6	30	2	266	1	481
tuna noodle	1 cup	376	16	8.0	571	35	2	5	23	2	146	3	316
Chicken cacciatore w/ pasta	1 cup	320	18	4.5	172	9	1	12	29	0	42	2	586
Chicken cordon bleu	6 oz	281	13	4.0	886	27	3	1	15	0	136	2	356
Chicken divan	6 oz	249	16	7.0	479	10	1	2	16	0	165	1	350
Chicken nuggets, frozen	4 pcs	210	15	3.5	360	9	1	1	11	0	33	1	146
Chicken parmigiana, frozen	1 (6 oz)	364	17	5.5	867	17	2	4	34	0	247	2	477
Chicken tetrazzini	1 cup	290	12	5.0	954	17	1	1	29	0	44	1	317
Chili w/ beans, can													
beef	1 cup	263	7	3.0	1220	34	7	4	16	0	93	9	934
turkey	1 cup	193	3	1.0	1200	26	5	6	17	0	81	3	706
Chimichangas, frozen													
beef	1 (4.5 oz)	360	20	5.0	470	37	3	4	9	0	179	3	337
chicken	1 (4.5 oz)	340	16	4.0	540	39	2	3	11	0	173	3	298
Chipped beef, creamed	1 (6 oz)	187	10	6.0	801	12	1	8	13	2	188	1	295
Chop suey, can													
beef & noodle	1 cup	286	9	2.0	803	27	3	5	23	0	48	4	453
chicken & noodle	1 cup	290	9	1.5	825	27	3	5	23	0	42	2	436
pork & noodle	1 cup	317	12	3.5	799	27	3	5	22	0	48	3	480
Chow mein, can													
beef & noodle	1 cup	286	9	2.0	803	27	3	5	23	0	48	4	453
chicken & noodle	1 cup	290	9	1.5	825	27	3	5	23	0	42	2	436
Corn dogs, frozen	1 (2.7 oz)	180	9	2.5	470	18	1	6	7	0	30	1	130
Egg rolls													
pork	1 (6 oz)	220	11	2.5	390	24	2	3	5	0	21	1	128
shrimp	1 (6 oz)	180	7	1.5	490	25	2	4	5	0	30	1	134
Eggplant parmigiana	1 cup	311	22	8.0	701	17	4	6	13	0	312	1	428
Enchiladas													
beef	1 (6 oz)	211	7	2.0	724	28	4	1	9	0	58	2	236
chicken	1 (6 oz)	213	9	2.5	314	24	3	1	9	0	107	2	140
Fajitas													
beef	1 (6 oz)	305	14	4.0	241	27	2	5	17	0	105	3	413
chicken	1 (6 oz)	277	9	1.5	262	34	4	5	15	0	96	2	340
Frozen breakfasts													
cinnamon French toast w/ sausage	1 (6.5 oz)	414	21	6.5	797	34	1	11	22	2	199	3	372
egg, steak & cheese bagel	1 (8.6 oz)	691	35	13.5	1570	56	0	7	39	1	228	5	355

COMBINATION FOODS, FROZEN ENTRÉES & MEALS

	Amount	Calories	Fat (g)	Saturated Fat (g)	Sodium (mg)	Carbohydrate (g)	Fiber (g)	Sugar (g)	Protein (g)	Vitamin D (mcg)	Calcium (mg)	Iron (mg)	Potassium (mg)
pancakes w/ sausage	1 (6 oz)	459	23	6.0	976	47	1	16	15	1	82	3	291
sausage, egg & cheese biscuit	1 (4.5 oz)	415	28	11.0	756	28	3	4	12	1	174	2	344
scrambled eggs (2) & bacon (2)	1 (5.3 oz)	267	20	6.5	493	3	0	2	17	2	83	2	254
scrambled eggs & sausage w/ hash browns	1 (6.3 oz)	364	27	7.5	779	17	1	2	13	2	60	2	490
Frozen dinners													
baked chicken	1 (8.9 oz)	260	11	5.0	860	18	1	4	21	0	50	1	660
chicken à la king	1 (11.5 oz)	400	15	4.0	950	48	1	4	19	0	120	2	580
chicken fettuccini Alfredo	1 (10.5 oz)	540	31	11.0	940	43	3	5	23	0	220	1	430
chicken Marsala	1 (9 oz)	300	7	3.0	850	40	2	6	20	0	20	1	400
chicken parmesan	1 (12 oz)	490	19	5.0	910	54	4	8	25	3	190	2	650
chicken pot pie	1 (10 oz)	630	37	12.0	920	55	2	7	18	0	140	4	570
fettuccini Alfredo	1 (11.5 oz)	640	37	14.0	970	58	3	6	18	0	310	1	250
fish filet	1 (9 oz)	490	21	5.0	750	49	0	3	26	0	130	2	530
fried chicken	1 (8.9 oz)	380	18	6.0	1040	32	1	2	22	0	50	2	340
green pepper steak	1 (10.5 oz)	290	9	3.0	810	34	1	4	18	0	60	2	840
Healthy Choice													
chicken & noodles	1 (10 oz)	260	7	1.5	480	31	3	3	17	0	50	2	610
chicken margherita w/ balsamic	1 (9.5 oz)	270	6	1.0	360	36	5	7	17	0	0	2	470
crustless chicken pot pie	1 (9.6 oz)	300	6	2.0	600	40	3	6	21	0	40	2	700
grilled chicken pesto w/ vegetables	1 (9.9 oz)	290	7	2.0	590	36	3	2	20	0	90	2	570
lasagna, cheese	1 (10.7 oz)	350	12	6.0	770	43	3	10	18	0	390	2	680
lasagna, meat	1 (10 oz)	420	20	8.0	780	40	3	6	20	0	190	2	720
Lean Cuisine													
chicken fried rice	1 (9 oz)	300	6	1.5	720	44	2	2	17	0	60	2	550
lasagna w/ meat sauce	1 (10.5 oz)	310	7	4.0	600	44	4	8	17	0	210	2	810
glazed turkey tenderloins	1 (9 oz)	300	6	2.0	530	47	3	24	14	0	110	1	510
shrimp scampi	1 (10 oz)	350	9	3.0	660	50	2	4	16	0	90	1	600
meatloaf	1 (9.9 oz)	330	16	7.0	900	25	3	6	22	0	90	2	1020
roast turkey	1 (9.6 oz)	280	10	4.0	770	29	2	3	18	0	60	1	550
Salisbury steak	1 (9.6 oz)	340	16	8.0	1000	26	2	4	23	0	180	2	520
stuffed peppers w/ beef	1 (9.6 oz)	200	8	3.0	770	22	3	7	10	0	50	2	490
Swedish meatballs w/ pasta	1 (11.5 oz)	500	23	10.0	1100	48	3	5	26	1	120	2	530
three cheese ravioli	1 (10 oz)	370	13	6.0	840	43	3	7	21	0	290	3	430
turkey Tetrazzini	1 (12 oz)	470	24	10.0	980	42	2	5	21	0	120	1	610
Hamburger Helper, box, prepared													
beef pasta	1 cup	270	11	4.0	826	25	1	0	24	0	25	3	195
cheeseburger macaroni	1 cup	310	12	5.0	910	27	0	5	22	1	122	2	297
cheesy enchilada	1 cup	352	13	5.5	746	36	1	0	20	0	82	3	260
Italian lasagna	1 cup	280	11	4.0	900	27	0	5	19	0	60	3	284
stroganoff	1 cup	255	10	2.5	834	22	2	3	20	1	81	2	469
Hot Pockets, frozen													
cheeseburger	1 (4.5 oz)	320	15	6.0	660	36	1	5	11	0	210	2	250

COMBINATION FOODS, FROZEN ENTRÉES & MEALS

	Amount	Calories	Fat (g)	Saturated Fat (g)	Sodium (mg)	Carbohydrate (g)	Fiber (g)	Sugar (g)	Protein (g)	Vitamin D (mcg)	Calcium (mg)	Iron (mg)	Potassium (mg)
chicken, broccoli & cheddar	1 (4.5 oz)	270	9	4.0	610	37	1	2	10	0	180	2	140
five cheese pizza	1 (4.5 oz)	290	12	6.0	540	36	1	5	8	0	270	2	200
ham & cheddar	1 (4.5 oz)	270	9	4.5	710	39	1	3	8	0	100	2	170
meatballs & mozzarella	1 (4.5 oz)	290	12	4.0	630	37	2	3	10	1	180	3	270
Philly steak & cheese	1 (4.5 oz)	300	11	5.0	700	40	0	3	9	0	150	2	240
Lasagna													
w/ meat	6 oz	272	11	5.5	272	28	2	6	16	0	139	1	352
w/ vegetables	6 oz	239	7	4.5	284	31	2	4	12	0	458	1	350
Lo mein, pork	6 oz	241	12	2.0	121	18	2	4	17	0	34	2	286
Macaroni & cheese													
frozen	1 (12 oz)	500	24	10.0	1200	51	2	5	21	0	390	1	440
three cheese, box	1 cup	360	12	4.0	750	50	1	8	10	0	180	3	310
Manicotti w/ red sauce	2 large	580	28	12.0	1520	66	6	4	20	1	398	2	564
Meatballs	1 medium	58	3	1.0	83	2	0	0	5	0	10	1	92
Meatloaf	3 oz	169	9	3.5	101	5	0	2	15	0	56	2	236
Moussaka	1 cup	238	13	4.5	460	13	4	6	17	0	118	2	457
Pasta Roni, box													
butter & garlic	1 cup	250	8	2.5	760	39	2	2	8	0	60	2	180
butter & herb Italiano	1 cup	300	12	3.5	860	40	2	2	9	0	100	2	160
cheddar macaroni	1 cup	290	12	3.5	710	38	2	6	8	0	110	2	260
Pepper steak	1 cup	320	20	4.0	563	6	1	4	28	0	37	3	438
Pizza, frozen													
cheese	1 slice (5.2 oz)	341	15	5.5	663	36	2	5	15	0	335	3	296
pepperoni	1 slice (5.2 oz)	378	20	4.5	912	35	2	5	13	0	320	3	300
French bread													
cheese	1 (5.2 oz)	360	16	6.0	700	40	2	5	15	0	290	2	280
pepperoni	1 (5.6 oz)	400	20	7.0	950	40	2	4	15	0	200	3	310
Pot pies, frozen													
beef	½ pie (7 oz)	400	21	9.0	660	40	4	4	13	0	40	3	410
chicken	½ pie (7 oz)	440	26	11.0	650	40	2	2	11	0	30	4	190
Ravioli w/ red sauce													
cheese	6 oz	232	10	4.5	390	26	2	6	10	0	117	1	348
meat	6 oz	268	12	4.0	122	25	2	3	15	0	48	3	364
Salmon loaf	3 oz	168	9	2.5	410	7	0	12	14	7	167	1	243
Salmon patties	1 (4.2 oz)	259	15	3.5	502	14	1	1	16	8	229	1	293
Sandwiches (w/ bread/bun)													
BBQ beef	1 (6 oz)	376	9	3.0	697	44	1	15	28	0	107	4	330
BLT w/ mayonnaise	1 (5 oz)	314	10	3.0	542	41	2	2	15	0	321	3	284
bologna & cheese w/ mayonnaise	1 (4 oz)	336	18	7.0	898	30	1	6	13	2	464	2	228
cheeseburger	1 (6 oz)	459	22	9.0	1068	43	3	9	23	0	209	4	313
chicken, breaded & fried	1 (6 oz)	425	19	4.0	1280	36	2	6	28	0	99	3	417
chicken, roasted/grilled	1 (6 oz)	250	5	1.0	539	25	2	7	23	0	53	2	322
chicken salad w/ mayonnaise	1 (6 oz)	392	17	3.0	599	34	2	4	25	0	112	3	316

COMBINATION FOODS, FROZEN ENTRÉES & MEALS

	Amount	Calories	Fat (g)	Saturated Fat (g)	Sodium (mg)	Carbohydrate (g)	Fiber (g)	Sugar (g)	Protein (g)	Vitamin D (mcg)	Calcium (mg)	Iron (mg)	Potassium (mg)
corned beef	1 (6 oz)	350	12	5.0	1365	34	2	4	24	0	104	4	184
egg salad w/ mayonnaise	1 (6 oz)	503	35	7.0	675	29	2	4	15	2	126	3	178
grilled cheese	1 (4 oz)	386	20	7.0	912	39	2	6	13	2	597	3	195
ham & cheese w/ mustard & mayonnaise	1 (6 oz)	364	18	7.0	1374	29	2	6	20	2	507	3	359
ham salad w/ mayonnaise	1 (6 oz)	376	17	3.5	1240	34	2	5	20	1	111	3	349
hamburger	1 (6 oz)	412	17	6.0	653	45	2	10	22	0	129	5	369
hot dog	1 (3.5 oz)	299	16	5.0	791	27	1	5	10	0	132	2	191
peanut butter & jelly	1 (3 oz)	326	14	3.0	376	42	3	13	10	0	92	2	209
Reuben w/ dressing	1 (6 oz)	485	29	9.5	1214	33	4	7	21	0	281	3	231
roast beef w/ cheese	1 (6 oz)	555	34	14.5	849	29	2	4	31	1	264	4	390
salami & cheese w/ mustard	1 (6 oz)	555	34	15.0	849	29	2	4	31	1	263	4	390
sloppy Joe, beef	1 (6 oz)	396	11	3.5	1202	56	2	28	17	0	116	3	390
tuna salad w/ mayonnaise	1 (6 oz)	340	18	2.5	410	30	5	6	19	0	85	3	191
turkey club w/ bacon	1 (8 oz)	463	24	8.0	1497	33	2	2	25	0	227	3	300
Scalloped potatoes & ham	1 cup	241	7	2.0	956	33	3	5	12	1	107	2	823
Shepherd's pie	1 cup	265	8	2.0	578	34	3	3	15	0	36	2	714
Spaghetti w/ meatballs	1 cup	332	11	2.5	682	43	4	6	14	0	42	3	472
SpaghettiO's, can													
w/ meatballs	1 cup	230	7	2.5	600	31	3	9	11	0	60	2	310
w/o meat	1 cup	170	1	0.5	600	35	3	12	6	0	30	2	270
w/ sliced franks	1 cup	220	6	2.0	600	29	3	10	9	0	30	2	370
w/ tomato & cheese sauce	1 cup	190	1	0.0	950	40	3	14	6	0	30	2	250
Stew													
beef, can	1 cup	200	10	4.0	990	17	1	3	10	0	0	1	281
beef, homemade	1 cup	191	10	5.0	989	17	1	3	9	0	0	0	280
chicken & vegetables	1 cup	170	6	2.0	850	17	2	2	12	0	24	2	168
turkey & vegetables	1 cup	170	6	2.0	850	17	2	2	12	0	24	2	168
Stuffed cabbage rolls	1 (8 oz)	196	7	2.5	818	25	4	10	9	0	44	1	414
Stuffed green peppers w/ rice	1 (6 oz)	274	19	5.0	320	20	2	3	6	0	146	1	218
Stuffed shells w/ red sauce	2 (3 oz)	832	55	32.0	1727	49	2	10	37	0	307	1	83
Suddenly Pasta Salad													
classic	¾ cup	250	7	1.0	390	39	2	3	5	0	0	2	360
creamy Italian	¾ cup	340	16	2.5	350	37	2	3	6	0	0	2	170
creamy Parmesan	¾ cup	350	18	4.0	210	32	2	3	5	0	0	1	110
Sweet & sour pork	1 cup	438	19	3.5	893	41	2	21	26	0	72	2	597
Tacos, soft shell													
beef & bean	1 (4 oz)	299	13	4.5	851	33	5	4	13	0	164	3	368
chicken & bean	1 (4 oz)	226	9	3.0	607	26	4	2	11	0	127	2	271
Tamales, bean & cheese	1 (3 oz)	215	13	3.5	393	18	3	1	8	0	190	1	168
Tortellini w/ red sauce													
cheese	1 cup	373	9	4.0	720	57	4	7	15	0	178	2	403
meat	1 cup	281	10	3.0	1292	33	2	3	14	1	78	3	258

COMBINATION FOODS, FROZEN ENTRÉES & MEALS

	Amount	Calories	Fat (g)	Saturated Fat (g)	Sodium (mg)	Carbohydrate (g)	Fiber (g)	Sugar (g)	Protein (g)	Vitamin D (mcg)	Calcium (mg)	Iron (mg)	Potassium (mg)
Totino's Pizza Rolls, frozen													
cheese	6	190	6	2.0	370	29	1	2	5	0	60	2	70
pepperoni	6	220	8	2.0	380	30	1	2	6	0	20	2	140
Tuna Helper, box													
fettuccine Alfredo	1 cup	195	27	16.0	501	41	2	2	22	1	163	3	191
macaroni & cheese	1 cup	373	15	6.5	430	42	2	6	18	1	115	2	173
tuna Tetrazzini	1 cup	210	7	2.0	724	28	4	1	9	0	58	2	236
Veal Marsala	6 oz	292	15	7.0	245	11	1	1	28	0	17	2	479
Veal parmigiana	6 oz	345	20	7.5	730	14	1	3	26	2	168	2	413
Veal scallopini	6 oz	408	30	8.0	634	3	1	1	31	1	66	2	444
Velveeta Skillets													
chicken & broccoli	1 cup	390	11	3.0	610	40	2	5	33	0	150	3	490
chicken Alfredo	1 cup	340	11	3.0	660	29	1	4	31	0	160	2	340
creamy beef stroganoff	1 cup	390	16	6.0	810	30	1	7	28	1	210	4	570
Ultimate Cheeseburger Mac	1 cup	380	17	6.0	930	27	0	5	28	0	160	4	510
Welsh rarebit, frozen	1 (3 oz)	138	10	4.5	242	5	0	4	6	1	201	0	117
Yorkshire pudding	2 oz	150	5	2.5	169	20	1	2	6	1	67	1	113
Ziti w/ meat sauce	1 cup	361	18	7.0	787	30	2	3	20	0	138	3	385

CONDIMENTS, SAUCES & BAKING INGREDIENTS

Condiments & Sauces

	Amount	Calories	Fat (g)	Saturated Fat (g)	Sodium (mg)	Carbohydrate (g)	Fiber (g)	Sugar (g)	Protein (g)	Vitamin D (mcg)	Calcium (mg)	Iron (mg)	Potassium (mg)
Alfredo sauce	¼ cup	160	14	7.0	780	6	0	2	2	1	60	0	40
BBQ sauce	1 T	20	0	0.0	185	5	0	4	0	0	2	0	7
Béarnaise sauce	2 T	161	17	10.0	124	0	0	0	2	0	15	0	16
Béchamel sauce	2 T	45	4	2.0	130	2	0	1	1	0	20	0	51
Cheese sauce	2 T	55	4	2.0	261	2	0	0	2	0	58	0	9
Chili sauce	2 T	40	0	0.0	460	10	0	6	0	0	2	0	63
Chipotle hot sauce	1 tsp	0	0	0.0	120	0	0	0	0	0	0	0	21
Chipotle salsa	2 T	10	0	0.0	140	14	1	1	0	0	9	0	123
Chutney	2 T	51	0	0.0	81	13	1	11	0	0	13	0	124
Clam sauce													
red	½ cup	70	3	0.0	760	6	1	3	5	0	20	1	70
white	½ cup	160	15	2.0	540	3	0	1	4	0	25	1	115
Cocktail sauce	2 T	37	0	0.0	294	8	1	4	0	0	8	0	93
Cranberry-orange relish	2 T	61	0	0.0	11	16	0	0	0	0	4	0	13
Cranberry sauce	2 T	55	0	0.0	5	13	0	11	0	0	1	0	10
Duck sauce	2 T	81	0	0.0	150	20	0	10	0	0	4	0	29
Enchilada sauce													
green	2 T	13	1	0.0	140	2	0	1	0	0	3	0	124
red	2 T	10	0	0.0	145	2	0	1	0	0	3	0	49
Fish sauce	1 T	6	0	0.0	1413	1	0	1	1	0	8	0	52
Hoisin sauce	1 T	35	1	0.0	258	7	0	4	1	0	5	0	19

Condiments & Sauces

	Amount	Calories	Fat (g)	Saturated Fat (g)	Sodium (mg)	Carbohydrate (g)	Fiber (g)	Sugar (g)	Protein (g)	Vitamin D (mcg)	Calcium (mg)	Iron (mg)	Potassium (mg)
Hollandaise sauce	2 T	161	17	10.5	124	0	0	0	2	0	15	0	16
Horseradish	1 T	7	0	0.0	63	2	1	1	0	0	8	0	37
Horseradish sauce	1 T	75	6	0.0	105	3	0	0	0	0	2	0	7
Ketchup/catsup	1 T	20	0	0.0	160	5	0	4	0	0	3	0	48
Liquid smoke	1 tsp	0	0	0.0	10	0	0	0	0	0	0	0	0
Lobster sauce	1 T	24	2	0.5	131	1	0	0	1	0	3	0	23
Manwich sauce	¼ cup	35	0	0.0	310	8	1	6	0	0	0	0	150
Mole poblano	2 T	47	3	0.5	113	4	1	2	1	0	11	0	75
Mustard													
brown/yellow	1 tsp	0	0	0.0	55	0	0	0	0	0	3	0	8
Dijon	1 tsp	5	0	0.0	120	0	0	0	0	0	3	0	8
honey	1 tsp	10	0	0.0	45	1	0	1	0	0	6	0	15
Olives													
black	5	24	2	0.5	169	1	1	0	0	0	21	1	2
green w/ pimiento	5	25	2	0.5	265	1	1	0	0	0	9	0	7
Oyster sauce	1 T	9	0	0.0	492	2	0	0	0	0	6	0	10
Pasta sauce, red													
arrabbiata, Rao's	½ cup	100	4	1.0	420	6	1	4	2	0	20	0	370
chunky garden combination, Ragú	½ cup	90	3	0.0	460	14	2	10	2	0	26	1	430
four cheese, Classico	½ cup	60	1	0.0	500	10	2	6	2	0	40	1	350
fra diavolo	½ cup	80	4	2.0	460	9	3	6	1	0	20	2	280
marinara													
homemade	½ cup	90	6	1.0	520	5	1	3	1	0	20	1	350
Newman's Own	½ cup	70	1	0.0	490	12	3	7	3	0	30	1	640
meat flavored, Ragú	½ cup	90	4	1.0	480	12	2	7	2	0	22	1	428
primavera, Botticelli	½ cup	95	5	2.0	520	11	2	6	5	0	25	0	250
Sockarooni, Newman's Own	½ cup	70	2	0.0	500	12	3	6	3	0	30	1	590
tomato & basil, Barilla	½ cup	50	1	0.0	460	10	3	5	2	0	84	1	435
traditional													
Barilla	½ cup	50	1	0.0	450	10	3	5	2	0	58	1	428
Prego	½ cup	70	2	0.0	480	13	2	9	2	0	30	1	370
Ragú	½ cup	70	2	0.0	470	13	3	7	2	0	23	1	489
vodka, Classico	½ cup	80	4	1.5	460	9	2	5	2	0	60	1	280
Peanut sauce	2 T	72	5	1.0	374	6	1	5	2	0	6	0	66
Pesto sauce	2 T	171	18	3.0	304	2	0	0	3	0	61	1	60
Pickles													
bread & butter	3 chips	10	0	0.0	170	2	0	2	0	0	14	0	23
dill	1 medium	8	0	0.0	526	2	1	1	0	0	37	0	76
sweet	1 medium	23	0	0.0	114	5	0	5	0	0	15	0	25
Pico de gallo	2 T	10	0	0.0	150	3	0	2	0	0	7	0	94
Pizza sauce	¼ cup	50	0	0.0	360	10	1	8	2	0	0	1	223
Plum sauce	2 T	70	0	0.0	205	16	0	0	0	0	5	1	98

CONDIMENTS, SAUCES & BAKING INGREDIENTS

	Amount	Calories	Fat (g)	Saturated Fat (g)	Sodium (mg)	Carbohydrate (g)	Fiber (g)	Sugar (g)	Protein (g)	Vitamin D (mcg)	Calcium (mg)	Iron (mg)	Potassium (mg)
Condiments & Sauces													
Relish, sweet pickle	1 T	20	0	0.0	95	5	0	3	0	0	0	0	4
Salsa	2 T	10	0	0.0	220	2	1	1	0	0	9	0	82
Salt	1 tsp	0	0	0.0	2325	0	0	0	0	0	1	0	0
Sauerkraut, can	2 T	5	0	0.0	180	1	1	0	0	0	9	0	50
Soy sauce	1 T	10	0	0.0	1250	2	0	1	1	0	0	0	65
light	1 T	20	0	0.0	550	40	0	2	1	0	0	0	600
substitute, liquid aminos	1 tsp	5	0	0.0	310	0	0	0	1	0	0	0	0
Salt substitute	¼ tsp	0	0	0.0	0	0	0	0	0	0	0	0	690
Steak sauce													
A.1.	1 tsp	15	0	0.0	290	3	0	2	0	0	0	0	53
Heinz 57	1 T	20	0	0.0	160	4	0	3	0	0	0	0	0
Stir-fry sauce	1 T	20	0	0.0	520	4	0	3	1	0	6	0	54
Sweet & sour sauce	2 T	60	0	0.0	130	13	0	12	0	0	0	0	31
Szechuan sauce	1 T	15	0	0.0	510	3	0	0	0	0	0	0	30
Tabasco sauce	1 tsp	0	0	0.0	32	0	0	0	0	0	0	0	7
Taco sauce	1 T	8	0	0.0	130	2	0	1	0	0	2	0	18
Tamari sauce	1 T	11	0	0.0	1005	1	0	0	2	0	4	0	38
Tartar sauce	1 T	60	6	1.0	110	2	0	1	0	0	26	0	68
Teriyaki sauce	1 T	16	0	0.0	690	3	0	3	1	0	5	0	41
Tomato sauce, can	½ cup	29	0	0.0	581	7	2	4	2	0	17	1	364
Vinegar													
balsamic	1 T	14	0	0.0	4	3	0	2	0	0	4	0	18
cider/white	1 T	3	0	0.0	1	0	0	0	0	0	1	0	11
raspberry/red wine	1 T	3	0	0.0	1	0	0	0	0	0	1	0	6
Worcestershire sauce	1 tsp	0	0	0.0	60	0	0	0	0	0	6	0	43
Baking Ingredients													
Agave nectar													
amber	1 T	60	0	0.0	0	16	0	16	0	0	0	0	0
light	1 T	60	0	0.0	0	16	0	16	0	0	0	0	0
Baking powder	¼ tsp	0	0	0.0	120	0	0	0	0	0	40	0	0
Baking soda	¼ tsp	0	0	0.0	315	0	0	0	0	0	0	0	0
Bisquick, dry	⅓ cup	150	3	1.0	380	28	1	2	3	0	60	1	0
gluten-free	¼ cup	130	0	0.0	340	29	0	2	2	0	60	0	0
reduced fat	⅓ cup	140	3	0.0	340	27	0	3	3	0	220	2	0
Bread crumbs													
plain	¼ cup	100	1	0.0	150	18	2	2	4	0	50	1	56
seasoned	¼ cup	100	1	0.0	400	18	2	2	4	0	60	1	0
Butterscotch chips	1 T	80	4	3.5	10	9	0	9	0	0	20	0	30
Carob chips, unsweetened	1 T	35	2	1.5	25	4	1	3	1	0	40	0	44
Chocolate, baking													
semisweet	1 oz	70	5	3.0	0	8	1	6	0	0	5	1	61
unsweetened	1 oz	70	7	4.5	0	4	3	0	2	0	0	3	150

Baking Ingredients

	Amount	Calories	Fat (g)	Saturated Fat (g)	Sodium (mg)	Carbohydrate (g)	Fiber (g)	Sugar (g)	Protein (g)	Vitamin D (mcg)	Calcium (mg)	Iron (mg)	Potassium
Chocolate chips													
milk chocolate	1 T	70	5	3.0	10	9	0	8	1	0	20	1	60
semisweet	1 T	70	4	2.5	10	10	0	9	0	0	0	1	40
Cocoa powder	1 T	10	1	0.0	0	3	2	0	1	0	10	1	220
Corn flake crumbs	¼ cup	80	0	0.0	160	19	0	2	2	1	0	6	40
Cornstarch	1 T	30	0	0.0	0	7	0	0	0	0	0	0	0
Corn syrup, dark/light	1 T	60	0	0.0	15	15	0	5	0	0	3	0	0
Cornmeal	2 T	55	1	0.0	5	12	1	0	1	0	1	1	44
Flour													
all-purpose/white	¼ cup	110	0	0.0	0	23	0	0	3	0	0	1	34
bread	¼ cup	110	0	0.0	0	23	0	0	4	0	0	1	34
buckwheat	¼ cup	140	1	0.0	0	29	9	0	4	0	21	1	184
cake	¼ cup	120	0	0.0	0	25	1	0	4	0	0	1	36
carob	¼ cup	57	0	0.0	9	23	10	13	1	0	90	1	213
coconut	¼ cup	120	2	1.0	10	9	5	3	3	0	3	1	309
corn	¼ cup	106	1	0.0	1	22	2	0	2	0	2	1	92
potato	¼ cup	143	0	0.0	22	33	2	1	3	0	26	1	400
rice, white	¼ cup	145	1	0.0	0	32	1	0	2	0	4	0	30
rye, medium	¼ cup	89	0	0.0	1	19	3	0	3	0	6	1	95
soy	¼ cup	130	5	1.0	0	10	4	2	12	0	59	2	579
fat-free	¼ cup	86	0	0.0	5	9	5	4	14	0	63	2	626
white, self-rising	¼ cup	110	0	0.0	390	23	1	0	3	0	80	1	88
whole wheat	¼ cup	102	1	0.0	1	22	3	0	4	0	10	1	109
Graham cracker crumbs	3 T	80	2	0.0	125	14	1	3	1	0	0	1	23
Honey	1 T	64	0	0.0	1	17	0	17	0	0	1	0	11
Matzo meal, unsalted	¼ cup	110	0	0.0	0	23	1	1	3	0	0	1	62
Molasses	1 T	58	0	0.0	7	15	0	15	0	0	41	1	293
Phyllo dough	3 sheets	170	3	1.0	275	30	1	0	4	0	6	2	42
Pie crusts													
graham	⅛ pie	100	5	3.0	115	14	0	6	1	0	5	0	10
chocolate	⅛ pie	100	5	3.0	105	14	0	6	1	0	5	1	20
reduced fat	⅛ pie	100	4	2.5	100	15	0	6	1	0	5	1	10
pastry, homemade	⅛ pie	113	7	2.0	116	10	1	0	1	2	0	1	14
Pie fillings													
apple	⅓ cup	100	0	0.0	5	27	1	23	0	0	0	0	27
blueberry	⅓ cup	80	0	0.0	0	21	0	16	0	0	0	0	99
cherry	⅓ cup	90	0	0.0	20	22	1	18	0	0	0	0	78
lemon	⅓ cup	120	2	0.0	2	27	0	20	0	0	0	0	65
pumpkin	½ cup	140	1	0.0	5	10	3	5	1	0	39	1	187
Shake 'n Bake, box	⅛ pkt	35	0	0.0	190	7	0	0	1	0	0	0	0
Sugar													
brown/raw/white	¼ cup	195	0	0.0	1	50	0	50	0	0	1	0	1
powdered	¼ cup	120	0	0.0	0	30	0	29	0	0	0	0	0

CONDIMENTS, SAUCES & BAKING INGREDIENTS

Baking Ingredients

	Amount	Calories	Fat (g)	Saturated Fat (g)	Sodium (mg)	Carbohydrate (g)	Fiber (g)	Sugar (g)	Protein (g)	Vitamin D (mcg)	Calcium (mg)	Iron (mg)	Potassium (mg)
Sweeteners, artificial													
Equal	1 pkt	0	0	0.0	0	1	0	1	0	0	0	0	0
monk fruit blend	2 tsp	0	0	0.0	0	8	0	0	0	0	0	0	0
Purecane													
baking sweetener	1 tsp	0	0	0.0	0	4	0	0	0	0	0	0	0
brown	1 tsp	0	0	0.0	0	4	0	0	0	0	0	0	0
confectioners' sweetener	1 tsp	0	0	0.0	0	4	0	0	0	0	0	0	0
Splenda	1 pkt	0	0	0.0	0	1	0	1	0	0	0	0	0
Stevia	1 tsp	0	0	0.0	0	1	0	0	0	0	0	0	0
Sugar Twin, brown/white	1 tsp	0	0	0.0	0	0	0	0	0	0	0	0	0
Sweet 'N Low	1 pkt	0	0	0.0	0	1	0	1	0	0	0	0	0
Swerve													
brown	1 tsp	0	0	0.0	0	4	0	0	0	0	0	0	0
confectioners' sweetener	1 tsp	0	0	0.0	0	3	0	0	0	0	0	0	0
granular	1 tsp	0	0	0.0	0	4	0	0	0	0	0	0	0
Truvia	1 pkt	0	0	0.0	0	2	0	0	0	0	0	0	0
Yeast	1 pkt	0	0	0.0	0	0	0	0	0	0	0	0	14

CRACKERS, DIPS & SNACKS

Crackers

	Amount	Calories	Fat (g)	Saturated Fat (g)	Sodium (mg)	Carbohydrate (g)	Fiber (g)	Sugar (g)	Protein (g)	Vitamin D (mcg)	Calcium (mg)	Iron (mg)	Potassium (mg)
Ak-mak	5	110	2	0.0	220	19	3	1	5	0	9	1	102
Animal	16	120	2	0.0	105	25	0	7	2	0	10	1	28
Better Cheddars	18	150	8	1.0	240	17	0	0	3	0	30	1	40
Cheese w/ peanut butter	3	190	9	1.5	310	24	1	4	4	0	20	1	70
Cheez-It	27	150	8	1.5	230	17	0	0	3	0	30	1	30
reduced fat	27	140	6	1.5	250	19	0	0	3	0	30	1	30
white cheddar	26	150	7	1.5	210	18	0	0	3	0	20	1	35
Chicken in a Biskit	12	160	8	0.5	230	19	0	2	2	0	3	1	24
Club	4	70	3	0.0	125	9	0	1	0	0	0	0	10
mini	34	140	6	0.5	300	20	0	3	2	0	10	1	30
multigrain	4	60	3	0.0	140	10	0	2	0	0	0	0	10
reduced fat	5	70	2	0.0	150	12	0	2	1	0	0	1	10
Goldfish													
cheddar	55	140	5	1.0	250	20	0	0	3	0	40	1	50
chocolate brownie grahams	26	90	3	0.5	85	15	1	7	1	0	22	1	0
parmesan	60	140	5	1.0	260	20	0	0	3	0	32	1	40
pizza	55	140	5	0.5	230	20	0	0	3	0	20	1	80
pretzel	43	130	3	0.0	280	24	0	1	3	0	10	1	20
saltine	55	140	6	0.5	230	20	0	0	3	0	20	1	30
Graham	2 sheets	130	3	0.0	160	24	1	8	2	0	13	1	48
reduced fat	2 sheets	140	2	0.0	170	28	2	8	2	0	17	1	62

CRACKERS, DIPS & SNACKS

Crackers

	Amount	Calories	Fat (g)	Saturated Fat (g)	Sodium (mg)	Carbohydrate (g)	Fiber (g)	Sugar (g)	Protein (g)	Vitamin D (mcg)	Calcium (mg)	Iron (mg)	Potassi...
Matzos, lightly salted	1 sheet	110	1	0.0	100	23	1	0	3	0	5	0	38
Oyster	22	60	2	0.0	160	11	0	0	1	0	2	1	16
Popchips, lightly salted	23	130	5	0.0	170	19	1	0	2	0	0	0	240
Rice snacks	18	130	2	0.0	85	26	0	0	2	0	0	0	30
Ritz	5	80	5	1.0	130	10	0	1	1	0	20	1	10
low sodium	5	80	4	1.0	25	10	0	1	0	0	20	1	60
peanut butter sandwiches	6	200	11	2.0	310	22	0	4	4	0	40	1	80
reduced fat	5	70	2	0.0	115	11	0	1	1	0	20	1	10
whole wheat	5	70	3	0.5	120	10	0	2	1	0	20	1	30
Saltines	5	70	2	0.0	135	12	0	0	1	0	3	1	19
reduced sodium	5	70	2	0.0	60	13	0	0	1	0	2	1	17
whole grain	5	70	2	0.0	125	12	1	0	1	0	31	1	54
Sociables	5	70	4	0.5	140	9	0	0	1	0	26	1	23
Table Water	4	50	1	0.0	80	10	0	0	1	0	31	1	29
Teddy Grahams													
chocolate	24	130	4	0.0	95	22	2	8	2	0	130	1	110
cinnamon	24	130	4	1.0	85	22	2	7	2	0	130	1	50
honey	24	130	4	0.0	90	22	1	7	2	0	130	1	49
Toasteds													
Buttercrisp	5	80	4	0.5	180	10	0	1	0	0	0	1	10
Wheat	5	80	4	0.0	140	10	0	1	1	0	0	1	20
Town House	5	80	5	1.0	150	9	0	1	0	0	0	0	10
dipping thins	7	80	4	0.5	160	11	0	0	0	0	20	0	20
flatbread crisps, Italian herb	8	70	2	0.0	120	11	0	0	1	0	0	1	20
FlipSides	5	70	4	0.5	190	10	0	1	1	0	0	1	10
pita, parmesan cheese & basil	6	70	3	0.0	115	11	0	0	1	0	0	0	10
Triscuit	6	120	4	0.0	160	20	3	0	3	0	10	1	120
reduced fat	6	110	3	0.0	150	21	4	0	3	0	10	2	120
Wasa													
Crisp'n Light	3	60	1	0.0	90	13	2	1	2	0	5	0	58
light rye	2	40	0	0.0	70	11	4	0	2	0	9	1	87
sourdough	1	30	0	0.0	50	7	2	0	1	0	4	1	50
whole grain	1	30	0	0.0	50	8	3	0	1	0	7	0	59
Wheat Thins	16	140	5	0.5	200	22	3	5	2	0	30	1	90
low sodium	16	140	5	0.5	55	22	3	4	2	0	10	1	90
multigrain	14	130	4	0.5	190	22	2	3	2	0	9	1	73
ranch	15	140	5	1.0	190	21	2	4	2	0	30	1	86
reduced fat	16	120	3.5	0.0	200	22	3	4	2	0	30	1	90

CRACKERS, DIPS & SNACKS

	Amount	Calories	Fat (g)	Saturated Fat (g)	Sodium (mg)	Carbohydrate (g)	Fiber (g)	Sugar (g)	Protein (g)	Vitamin D (mcg)	Calcium (mg)	Iron (mg)	Potassium (mg)
Dips													
Fritos bean	2 T	35	1	0.0	190	5	2	0	2	0	0	0	94
Good & Gather													
Buffalo-style chicken	2 T	60	5	2.0	250	1	0	1	3	0	26	0	0
spinach	2 T	45	4	2.5	140	2	0	1	1	0	26	0	0
spinach artichoke	2 T	60	5	2.5	160	2	0	1	1	0	26	0	0
Hidden Valley ranch	2 T	60	6	4.0	264	3	0	0	1	0	52	0	0
Lay's French onion	2 T	60	5	0.5	190	2	1	0	1	0	0	0	0
Marzetti													
cream cheese fruit	2 T	60	3	2.0	95	9	0	8	0	0	0	0	0
old fashioned caramel	2 T	130	5	3.0	65	22	0	16	1	0	0	0	47
Sabra classic hummus	2 T	70	5	1.0	130	4	1	0	2	0	0	1	94
Tostitos salsa con queso	2 T	40	3	1.0	280	5	1	1	1	0	26	0	0
Nutrition Bars													
Aloha													
peanut butter chocolate chip	1 bar	240	12	3.0	95	24	10	5	14	0	16	1	173
chocolate chip cookie dough	1 bar	230	10	2.5	80	25	10	5	14	0	17	2	122
coconut chocolate almond	1 bar	260	13	7.0	70	22	6	4	14	0	32	2	186
Atlas protein bar													
almond chocolate chip	1 bar	220	11	2.5	60	22	12	1	15	0	84	4	111
chocolate cacao	1 bar	220	11	2.5	65	22	12	1	15	0	85	3	131
peanut butter chocolate chip	1 bar	230	11	3.0	30	21	10	1	15	0	35	4	146
Balance Bar	1 bar	200	7	3.0	170	21	1	17	15	3	150	4	150
Barebells													
caramel cashew	1 bar	200	8	3.5	50	19	3	2	20	0	0	0	0
cookies & cream	1 bar	190	7	3.5	65	20	3	1	20	0	0	0	0
salty peanut	1 bar	200	8	3.5	105	20	4	1	20	0	0	0	0
Built													
apple almond crisp	1 bar	160	5	2.0	50	19	6	4	18	0	90	1	230
rocky road	1 bar	150	4	1.5	55	19	6	6	17	0	124	1	278
strawberry	1 bar	130	2	1.0	80	12	0	5	17	0	80	0	150
Bulletproof collagen protein													
chocolate chip cookie dough	1 bar	190	12	6.0	85	12	8	2	11	0	22	2	110
fudge brownie	1 bar	180	11	5.0	85	13	8	2	11	0	22	2	123
vanilla shortbread	1 bar	190	12	5.0	90	12	8	2	11	0	21	1	140
CLIF													
Bars													
chocolate brownie & crunchy peanut butter	1 bar	180	5	1.0	150	29	2	11	7	0	34	2	159
chocolate chip	1 bar	260	6	2.0	135	43	5	17	10	0	45	2	250
crunchy peanut butter	1 bar	260	7	1.0	230	40	4	19	11	2	195	2	191
white chocolate macadamia nut	1 bar	260	7	2.0	220	42	4	21	9	2	195	2	191

	Amount	Calories	Fat (g)	Saturated Fat (g)	Sodium (mg)	Carbohydrate (g)	Fiber (g)	Sugar (g)	Protein (g)	Vitamin D (mcg)	Calcium (mg)	Iron (mg)	Potassium (mg)
Builders													
chocolate mint	1 bar	280	9	6.0	200	31	3	17	20	0	42	4	234
crunchy peanut butter	1 bar	300	11	6.0	330	29	2	16	20	0	40	3	198
vanilla almond	1 bar	290	11	6.0	200	29	2	16	20	0	46	3	212
FITCRUNCH													
chocolate peanut butter	1 bar	190	8	4.0	200	14	1	3	16	0	39	1	135
milk & cookies	1 bar	210	11	8.0	130	16	1	3	16	0	65	1	89
peanut butter & jelly	1 bar	190	8	4.0	200	14	1	3	16	0	39	1	135
GoMacro MacroBars													
coconut, almond butter & chocolate chips	1 bar	280	10	3.5	15	36	3	12	11	0	26	1	94
oatmeal chocolate chip	1 bar	270	9	2.0	60	35	3	13	12	0	26	2	188
peanut butter chocolate chip	1 bar	290	11	2.0	10	39	2	14	11	0	26	1	188
KIND													
energy bars													
chocolate chunk	1 bar	230	7	2.0	160	34	5	13	10	0	52	2	188
peanut butter	1 bar	250	10	1.5	190	32	5	13	10	0	52	2	188
nut bars													
caramel almond & sea salt	1 bar	170	15	3.0	125	16	7	5	6	0	72	1	188
cranberry almond	1 bar	160	12	1.0	20	19	5	8	5	0	72	1	188
dark chocolate cherry cashew	1 bar	170	10	3.0	20	22	6	10	4	0	24	1	188
dark chocolate nuts & sea salt	1 bar	180	15	3.0	140	16	7	5	6	0	48	2	188
peanut butter dark chocolate	1 bar	200	14	4.0	20	17	3	9	7	0	24	1	188
protein bars													
crunchy peanut butter	1 bar	250	18	4.0	135	17	6	8	12	0	26	1	188
dark chocolate nut	1 bar	240	17	4.0	125	18	5	8	12	0	52	2	282
Kirkland													
chocolate brownie	1 bar	190	7	2.5	170	23	15	1	21	0	72	2	180
chocolate chip cookie dough	1 bar	190	7	2.5	190	22	10	2	21	0	108	1	117
No Cow													
birthday cake	1 bar	190	5	1.5	150	27	16	1	21	0	6	0	16
chocolate sprinkled donut	1 bar	200	7	3.5	90	25	14	1	20	0	28	4	64
maple	1 bar	200	5	2.0	200	25	14	1	22	0	46	3	25
ONE													
almond bliss	1 bar	240	9	7.0	115	22	3	1	20	0	150	1	125
birthday cake	1 bar	220	8	6.0	140	23	3	1	20	0	110	0	83
maple glazed doughnut	1 bar	230	8	6.0	150	23	3	1	20	0	102	0	80
peanut butter pie	1 bar	220	9	5.0	140	23	8	1	20	0	88	1	124
Pure Protein													
birthday cake	1 bar	200	5	3.5	160	18	0	3	20	0	195	1	80
chewy chcolate chip	1 bar	200	5	3.5	110	18	2	3	20	0	150	1	90
marshmallow crispy treat	1 bar	200	6	3.5	180	19	3	5	20	0	130	1	90

CRACKERS, DIPS & SNACKS

Nutrition Bars

	Amount	Calories	Fat (g)	Saturated Fat (g)	Sodium (mg)	Carbohydrate (g)	Fiber (g)	Sugar (g)	Protein (g)	Vitamin D (mcg)	Calcium (mg)	Iron (mg)	Potassium (mg)
PaleoPro Primal													
cherry cashew	1 bar	260	14	3.5	200	26	12	6	15	0	200	2	100
coconut cacao	1 bar	270	17	5.0	190	23	15	4	15	0	70	2	110
Perfect Bar													
dark chocolate chip peanut butter	1 bar	330	20	4.0	105	24	4	18	15	0	104	1	376
peanut butter	1 bar	340	19	3.0	50	27	3	19	17	0	130	1	470
pumpkin pie	1 bar	310	19	3.0	35	24	3	16	14	0	104	1	470
salted caramel	1 bar	310	19	3.5	130	25	2	17	12	0	120	2	376
Power Crunch													
French vanilla creme	1 bar	220	13	7.0	100	11	0	5	14	0	60	1	100
lemon meringue	1 bar	220	14	7.0	105	11	0	7	13	0	60	0	100
Pro peanut butter fudge	1 bar	300	21	10.0	230	15	2	4	20	0	80	1	230
Pro vanilla creme	1 bar	330	23	11.0	170	13	0	7	20	0	100	1	100
Quest													
birthday cake	1 bar	180	6	3.5	220	24	14	0	21	0	110	0	80
blueberry	1 bar	190	7	2.0	210	22	15	2	21	0	120	0	110
caramel chocolate chunk	1 bar	190	7	3.0	270	23	15	1	20	0	120	1	110
RXBAR													
blueberry	1 bar	210	7	1.0	140	24	4	15	12	0	60	1	460
chocolate sea salt	1 bar	200	9	2.0	260	23	5	13	12	0	60	2	480
peanut butter	1 bar	200	7	1.0	310	25	5	15	12	0	40	1	480
pecan	1 bar	220	9	1.0	180	23	3	18	12	0	30	1	390
snickerdoodle	1 bar	210	8	1.0	180	23	3	17	12	0	50	1	410
Think!													
high protein brownie crunch	1 bar	230	8	3.0	190	23	1	0	20	0	120	2	170
keto protein chocolate peanut butter pie	1 bar	180	14	4.5	95	14	3	2	10	0	70	1	180
vegan high protein peanut butter chocolate chip	1 bar	190	6	3.0	160	24	1	5	13	0	40	2	100
Vega													
chocolate peanut butter	1 bar	290	10	5.0	290	27	4	18	20	0	78	3	0
salted caramel	1 bar	290	10	4.0	270	26	3	16	20	0	130	2	0

Snacks

	Amount	Calories	Fat (g)	Saturated Fat (g)	Sodium (mg)	Carbohydrate (g)	Fiber (g)	Sugar (g)	Protein (g)	Vitamin D (mcg)	Calcium (mg)	Iron (mg)	Potassium (mg)
Bugles	1⅓ cups	150	8	6.0	320	18	0	2	1	0	0	0	0
Cheetos													
crunchy	21	160	10	1.5	250	15	0	0	2	0	15	0	53
puffs	13	160	10	1.5	270	16	0	1	2	0	20	0	60
Cheez Doodles													
crunchy	23	150	8	2.0	320	17	0	2	2	0	195	0	0
puffs	23	150	8	2.0	320	17	0	2	2	0	195	0	0

CRACKERS, DIPS & SNACKS

Snacks	Amount	Calories	Fat (g)	Saturated Fat (g)	Sodium (mg)	Carbohydrate (g)	Fiber (g)	Sugar (g)	Protein (g)	Vitamin D (mcg)	Calcium (mg)	Iron (mg)	Potassium
Cheez-It party mix	½ cup	140	5	1.0	310	20	1	0	3	0	10	1	50
Chex Mix	½ cup	130	4	0.5	230	23	2	2	2	2	0	1	46
Combos, cheddar	9 pcs	140	7	3.0	290	18	0	4	2	0	30	1	0
w/ pretzel	9 pcs	130	5	3.0	280	19	0	4	2	0	40	1	130
Cracker Jack	1 pkg (1 oz)	120	2	0.0	70	23	1	15	2	0	0	1	0
Doritos nacho chips													
cool ranch	12	150	8	1.0	190	18	1	0	2	0	30	0	50
nacho cheese	12	150	8	1.0	210	87	1	0	2	0	40	0	50
spicy sweet chili	12	150	7	1.0	280	18	1	0	2	0	30	0	50
Fritos corn chips	32	160	10	1.5	170	16	1	0	2	0	27	0	35
Funyuns	13	140	6	1.0	280	19	0	0	2	0	10	1	40
Good Sense sesame oat bran sticks	¼ cup	170	12	2.0	340	13	1	0	3	0	52	2	94
Jax	23	150	8	1.0	380	19	1	2	2	0	30	0	20
Mission pork rinds	0.5 oz	80	5	2.0	270	0	0	0	9	0	0	0	0
Popcorn													
Angie's BOOMCHICKAPOP													
cheddar cheese	2⅔ cups	160	10	1.5	310	14	2	3	3	0	60	0	100
kettle corn	2⅓ cups	160	9	1.0	110	19	2	8	2	0	0	1	0
Jiffy Pop	4 cups	140	7	3.5	220	20	3	0	3	0	0	0	0
oil popped, salted	3 cups	165	9	1.5	292	19	3	0	3	0	30	1	74
Old Dutch, air popped	2¾ cups	170	12	1.0	2	14	34	0	2	0	3	0	48
Orville Redenbacher's kettle corn	3 cups	160	8	4.0	160	20	3	0	3	0	0	1	0
Pop Secret, butter	3 cups	130	8	4.0	270	12	2	0	2	0	0	0	0
Skinny Pop, sea salt	3 cups	130	6	1.5	260	17	2	0	2	0	0	1	60
Skinny Pop popcorn mini cakes													
cinnamon sugar	20	120	3	0.0	60	20	4	3	3	0	10	1	40
sea salt	22	120	4	0.0	170	18	4	0	3	0	0	1	50
sharp cheddar	20	120	4	0.0	135	18	4	0	3	0	0	1	50
Smartfood													
caramel & cheddar	1½ cups	140	8	3.0	150	27	1	6	1	0	10	0	0
sweet & salty caramel	3 cups	140	7	1.0	190	17	3	3	3	0	20	1	20
white cheddar	2½ cups	160	10	2.0	240	13	2	2	4	0	60	1	60
SmartPop!, butter	3 cups	120	2	0.5	340	26	4	0	4	0	0	1	0
Potato chips													
Lay's	15	160	10	1.5	170	15	0	0	2	0	10	1	350
BBQ	15	150	90	1.5	150	16	1	2	2	0	10	1	330
Old Dutch, sour cream & onion	15	160	10	1.0	160	15	1	1	2	0	11	0	354
Pringles	16	150	9	2.5	150	16	0	0	1	0	0	0	110
BBQ	15	150	9	2.5	135	16	0	0	1	0	0	0	110
cheddar cheese	15	150	8	2.5	180	16	0	0	1	0	0	0	110
sour cream & onion	16	150	9	2.5	160	16	0	0	1	0	0	0	110
Ruffles, baked	12	120	3	0.0	135	22	1	2	2	0	10	0	330

CRACKERS, DIPS & SNACKS

Snacks	Amount	Calories	Fat (g)	Saturated Fat (g)	Sodium (mg)	Carbohydrate (g)	Fiber (g)	Sugar (g)	Protein (g)	Vitamin D (mcg)	Calcium (mg)	Iron (mg)	Potassium (mg)
Pretzels													
Dot's Homestyle original seasoned	1 oz	130	6	0.0	360	18	0	0	2	0	10	1	52
Snack Factory crisps	11	110	0	0.0	270	24	0	2	2	0	0	1	0
Snyder's													
butter snaps	24	120	1	0.0	270	25	0	0	3	0	0	1	0
mini	20	110	0	0.0	250	25	0	0	3	0	0	1	0
rods	3	120	2	0.0	280	23	1	0	3	0	0	1	0
sourdough, hard	1	110	0	0.0	240	23	0	0	3	0	0	1	0
Quaker rice cakes													
caramel	1	50	0	0.0	25	11	0	3	0	0	0	0	20
chocolate	1	60	1	0.0	35	12	0	4	1	0	0	0	40
plain, lightly salted	1	35	0	0.0	15	7	0	0	0	0	0	0	30
Stacy's Everything Bagel Chips	12	130	4	0.0	330	19	1	2	4	0	10	1	10
Sun Chips	16	140	6	0.5	110	19	2	2	2	0	10	1	70
Tostitos tortilla chips	7	140	7	1.0	115	19	1	0	2	0	30	0	40
bite-size	22	110	7	1.0	115	18	1	0	2	0	20	0	40
crispy rounds	13	150	7	1.0	115	18	1	0	2	0	20	0	40
hint of lime	6	150	7	1.0	130	18	1	0	2	0	30	0	40
organic blue corn	6	140	6	0.5	80	19	1	0	2	0	30	0	40
Scoops!	11	140	7	1.0	115	19	1	0	2	0	30	0	40
strips	11	150	7	1.0	115	19	2	0	2	0	20	0	40
Veggie Straws, sea salt	38	130	7	0.5	210	15	0	0	0	0	80	1	210

DESSERTS, SWEETS & TOPPINGS

Bars	Amount	Calories	Fat (g)	Saturated Fat (g)	Sodium (mg)	Carbohydrate (g)	Fiber (g)	Sugar (g)	Protein (g)	Vitamin D (mcg)	Calcium (mg)	Iron (mg)	Potassium (mg)
Brownies													
w/ nuts	1 (2 in)	210	12	5.0	70	27	2	19	4	0	0	3	200
w/o nuts	1 (2 in)	175	8	3.0	63	28	3	18	2	0	0	3	215
fudge, iced	1 (2 in)	180	6	2.5	120	32	1	22	2	0	7	1	113
Lemon	1 (2 in)	180	7	4.0	60	27	0	20	2	0	30	0	30
Nutty Buddy	2 cookies	470	27	12.0	160	50	2	32	7	0	10	2	160
Rice Krispies Treats													
homemade	1 (2 in)	70	2	1.0	53	14	0	7	1	0	2	4	20
packaged	1	90	2	0.5	105	17	0	8	1	0	0	1	0
strawberry	1	90	2	0.5	105	17	0	8	0	0	0	1	0
Seven layer	1 (2 in)	257	15	8.0	103	21	1	17	2	0	10	1	84
Cakes, Pastries & Sweet Breads													
Angel food cake	1/14 cake	159	0	0.0	72	34	0	26	6	0	5	1	152
Apple dumplings	1 (6 oz)	504	24	5.5	354	72	6	40	4	0	17	2	189
Apple fritters	1 (3 oz)	248	9	3.0	243	40	2	23	3	0	62	1	110
Baklava	1 (2 in)	213	15	5.5	48	21	1	15	2	0	14	1	54
Banana bread	1/12 loaf	172	1	0.5	170	37	2	18	4	0	23	1	175

DESSERTS, SWEETS & TOPPINGS

Cakes, Pastries & Sweet Breads

	Amount	Calories	Fat (g)	Saturated Fat (g)	Sodium (mg)	Carbohydrate (g)	Fiber (g)	Sugar (g)	Protein (g)	Vitamin D (mcg)	Calcium (mg)	Iron (mg)	Potassium (mg)
Black forest cake	1/10 cake	447	14	3.0	441	78	3	41	6	0	73	2	247
Caramel rolls	1/12 recipe	251	12	6.0	178	34	1	14	4	0	30	1	72
Carrot cake, iced	1/12 cake	569	36	7.0	470	59	3	40	6	0	69	2	470
Cheesecake													
amaretto	1/12 cake	417	26	15.5	314	37	0	29	7	0	86	1	314
chocolate	1/12 cake	527	37	21.5	342	43	2	32	10	0	74	3	149
regular, New York–style	1/12 cake	556	37	22.0	408	47	1	33	11	0	114	2	194
Chocolate cake, iced	1/12 cake	528	19	7.0	491	84	3	64	6	0	76	2	77
Cinnamon rolls	1/12 recipe	376	19	12.0	437	46	1	21	6	0	52	2	105
Cobbler, fruit	1/4 recipe	384	13	8.0	371	65	1	47	4	0	136	1	119
Coffee cake													
apple crumble	1/8 recipe	631	34	13.0	435	76	3	34	10	0	122	3	254
regular w/ crumb topping	1/24 recipe	255	14	2.0	220	31	1	22	3	0	60	1	79
Cream puffs	1/8 recipe	257	16	7.5	91	26	1	14	4	0	18	1	44
Crepes	1/8 recipe	163	8	3.5	235	17	0	5	6	0	66	1	115
Cupcakes, iced													
chocolate	1	220	10	2.5	180	32	2	19	3	0	14	1	76
chocolate filled	1	284	16	3.0	193	35	1	24	3	0	33	1	59
vanilla lemon filled	1	379	19	9.0	237	50	0	43	3	0	37	1	48
Danish													
cheese	1/10 recipe	498	29	14.0	582	51	0	32	8	0	40	2	60
kringle	1/18 recipe	411	30	15.0	157	35	1	23	4	0	46	1	104
Devil Dogs	1 cake	180	7	3.0	130	26	1	17	2	0	10	1	80
Ding Dongs	2 cakes	310	18	11.0	310	43	1	31	2	0	0	2	120
Donuts													
cake	1 medium	200	11	6.0	220	23	0	11	2	0	0	1	30
holes, glazed	4 medium	220	10	5.0	170	31	0	17	2	0	70	1	40
raised, glazed	1 medium	190	11	4.5	90	21	1	10	2	0	78	1	46
Eclairs, chocolate	1 (5 in)	210	12	11.0	120	25	0	20	2	0	52	1	33
Funnel cake	1 (6 in)	278	14	2.5	117	29	1	14	7	1	124	2	148
Funny Bones	2 cakes	330	16	10.0	250	41	1	29	5	0	0	1	220
Gingerbread cake	1/12 cake	359	14	2.0	353	56	4	31	6	0	90	1	374
Ho Hos	3 cakes	380	20	13.0	300	52	1	40	2	0	0	2	120
Honey buns, iced	1 (1.8 oz)	220	12	6.0	170	26	0	14	3	0	90	1	50
Lemon cake, iced	1/12 cake	335	13	8.0	161	53	0	41	3	0	47	1	39
Marble cake	1/12 cake	276	11	2.0	398	41	1	25	4	0	10	0	24
Pecan caramel roll	1/12 recipe	327	13	5.0	293	47	2	18	6	0	72	2	120
Pineapple upside down cake	1/12 cake	506	25	8.0	384	69	2	53	4	0	116	2	207
Pop Tarts													
frosted raspberry	1 pkg	370	9	3.0	320	70	1	30	3	0	0	2	40
unfrosted blueberry	1 pkg	380	10	3.0	360	69	1	24	4	0	0	1	40

Cakes, Pastries & Sweet Breads	Amount	Calories	Fat (g)	Saturated Fat (g)	Sodium (mg)	Carbohydrate (g)	Fiber (g)	Sugar (g)	Protein (g)	Vitamin D (mcg)	Calcium (mg)	Iron (mg)	Potassium (mg)
Pound cake	1/12 cake	580	26	16.0	172	79	1	55	8	0	65	2	115
Pumpkin bread	1/12 loaf	257	9	2.0	274	42	2	23	4	0	86	2	171
Ring Dings	1 cake	180	9	6.0	130	24	1	17	1	0	0	1	90
Snoballs	1 cake	160	5	3.0	180	29	1	20	1	0	10	1	55
Spice cake, iced	1/16 cake	275	13	8.0	222	36	1	19	4	0	115	1	90
Sponge cake	1/14 cake	148	3	1.0	37	28	0	22	4	0	16	1	53
Strudel w/ fruit	1/6 recipe	501	17	4.0	130	88	4	62	6	0	70	2	406
Toaster Strudel, strawberry	2 pastries	350	13	5.0	300	53	1	19	5	0	0	2	0
Turnovers w/ fruit	1 (3 oz)	380	25	7.0	210	34	1	10	4	0	26	1	70
Twinkies	2 cakes	280	9	4.0	370	47	0	32	2	0	0	1	0
Yankee Doodles	1 cake	140	5	2.5	150	22	1	13	2	0	0	1	90
Yellow cake, iced	1/12 cake	253	10	3.0	285	37	1	22	4	0	99	1	69
Yodels	2 cakes	280	15	10.0	130	35	1	25	2	0	0	2	160
Zingers	2 cakes	290	10	4.5	230	49	0	39	1	0	23	1	41
Cookies													
Animal	7	77	2	0.5	70	13	0	2	1	0	0	0	21
iced	7	150	8	7.0	50	20	0	12	1	0	10	1	20
Arrowroot biscuit	1	20	1	0.0	5	3	0	1	0	0	0	1	5
Biscotti													
almond, mini	2	120	5	2.0	50	16	0	9	2	0	20	1	40
chocolate dipped, mini	2	150	7	3.0	55	21	0	12	3	0.1	30	1	60
dark chocolate almond	1	170	7	3.0	35	26	1	14	3	0	26	1	40
toffee almond dipped	1	110	5	2.0	80	17	0	10	2	0.1	20	1	40
Chocolate chip													
Chips Ahoy!	3	160	8	2.5	110	22	0	11	1	0	10	1	40
chewy	2	140	6	3.0	95	21	0	12	1	0	0	1	30
chunky	2	160	8	3.0	75	21	0	11	1	0	10	1	50
reduced fat	3	150	6	2.0	140	24	1	11	2	0	0	1	40
homemade	1	170	9	4.0	150	21	0	11	2	0	6	2	51
Chocolate wafers	5	140	5	1.0	180	23	0	9	2	0	0	2	70
E. L. Fudge	2	180	9	3.5	95	24	0	13	2	0	0	1	50
Fig Newtons	2	100	2	0.0	95	21	1	12	1	0	20	1	70
strawberry	2	100	2	0.0	95	21	1	12	0	0	10	1	50
Fudge Stripes	2	140	7	4.0	75	19	1	9	1	0	10	1	60
Ginger snaps	4	120	4	1.5	120	22	1	10	1	0	10	1	30
Girl Scout cookies													
Caramel deLites	2	140	6	5.0	50	19	0	12	0	0	0	1	0
Lemonades	2	150	7	4.5	70	20	0	9	1	0	0	1	0
Peanut Butter Patties	2	130	7	4.0	90	15	0	8	2	0	0	1	0
Peanut Butter Sandwiches	3	170	8	2.5	105	22	1	9	3	0	0	1	0
S'mores	2	150	7	3.5	110	21	1	10	2	0	0	1	50
Thin Mints	4	160	7	5.0	105	22	0	10	1	0	0	2	0
Trefoils	4	120	5	2.0	110	19	0	6	1	0	0	1	0

DESSERTS, SWEETS & TOPPINGS

Cookies	Amount	Calories	Fat (g)	Saturated Fat (g)	Sodium (mg)	Carbohydrate (g)	Fiber (g)	Sugar (g)	Protein (g)	Vitamin D (mcg)	Calcium (mg)	Iron (mg)	Potassium (mg)
Ladyfingers	4	110	1	0.0	30	23	0	13	3	0	0	0	0
Lorna Doone shortbread	4 (1 pkg)	140	7	1.5	150	20	0	5	1	0	0	1	20
LU Le Pim's milk chocolate biscuits	2	130	6	3.5	60	17	1	10	2	0	20	1	50
Macaroons	2	100	4	1.0	10	13	1	12	2	0	16	0	51
Mallomars	2	110	5	2.5	35	18	0	12	1	0	10	1	50
Milano, dark chocolate	3	180	9	4.0	60	22	1	11	2	0	10	1	70
Iced molasses	3	120	2	0.0	180	25	0	13	1	0	0	1	90
Nutter Butter	4 (1 pkg)	260	11	2.5	200	39	1	16	4	0	20	1	80
Oatmeal raisin	1	150	5	2.0	80	24	1	13	2	0	11	1	43
Oreo	3	160	7	2.0	135	25	1	14	1	0	10	1	50
Doublestuf	2	140	7	2.0	90	21	0	13	1	0	10	1	40
golden	3	170	7	2.0	120	25	0	12	1	0	0	1	20
thins	4	140	6	2.0	95	21	0	12	1	0	0	1	40
Peanut butter	2	120	4	1.0	150	20	0	12	2	0	0	0	25
Sandies													
classic shortbread	2	160	9	4.0	90	19	0	7	2	0	0	1	15
pecan shortbread	2	170	10	3.0	110	18	1	7	2	0	0	1	20
SnackWell's													
devil's food	2	120	3	2.5	45	24	1	14	1	0	10	1	70
vanilla creme sandwich	2	110	3	1.0	95	18	0	9	1	0	10	1	20
Social Tea biscuits	7	140	4	1.0	120	24	1	7	2	0	0	1	20
Sugar	2	160	7	2.5	95	24	0	13	1	0	11	1	26
Sugar wafers	3	150	7	1.5	30	22	0	16	0	0	2	0	8
Vanilla wafers	8	140	6	1.5	115	21	0	11	1	0	0	1	30
Vienna Fingers, creme filled	2	150	6	2.0	95	22	0	10	1	0	0	1	15
Frozen Yogurt													
Chocolate	½ cup	111	3	2.0	55	19	2	17	3	0	87	0	204
Flavored	½ cup	111	3	2.0	55	19	0	17	3	0	87	0	136
fat-free	½ cup	110	0	0.0	60	23	0	15	3	0	150	0	230
Premium	½ cup	136	32	1.0	50	27	0	6	4	0	95	1	136
Soft serve													
chocolate	½ cup	115	4	2.5	71	18	2	16	3	0	106	1	188
vanilla	½ cup	115	4	2.5	63	17	0	17	3	0	103	0	152
Ice Cream													
Butter pecan	½ cup	122	7	3.0	112	15	1	4	3	0	88	0	130
Cherry Garcia	½ cup	255	15	10.0	41	27	0	23	4	1	113	2	180
Cookie dough	½ cup	181	9	5.0	73	23	0	16	3	0	69	0	120
Chocolate fudge brownie	½ cup	172	7	4.0	60	25	1	18	3	0	78	1	224
Chocolate/strawberry/vanilla	½ cup	140	7	4.5	50	19	1	17	3	0	72	1	164
fat-free, 98%	½ cup	94	2	1.0	51	21	4	14	3	0	86	1	162
light	½ cup	140	5	3.5	53	19	1	19	4	0	119	1	128

DESSERTS, SWEETS & TOPPINGS

Ice Cream

	Amount	Calories	Fat (g)	Saturated Fat (g)	Sodium (mg)	Carbohydrate (g)	Fiber (g)	Sugar (g)	Protein (g)	Vitamin D (mcg)	Calcium (mg)	Iron (mg)	Potassium (mg)
no added sugar	½ cup	130	4	3.0	56	20	1	4	3	0	91	0	147
premium	½ cup	186	13	7.5	42	15	1	13	4	0	105	1	176
Gelato	½ cup	170	10	7.0	50	18	0	17	3	0	99	0	138
Italian ice	½ cup	130	0	0.0	25	32	0	22	0	0	3	0	4
Mint chocolate chip	½ cup	133	5	3.0	46	19	0	17	3	0	109	0	55
Rocky road	½ cup	160	6	3.0	58	24	1	15	3	0	83	1	183
Sherbet	½ cup	107	2	1.0	34	23	1	18	1	0	40	0	71
Sorbet	½ cup	100	0	0.0	0	25	1	24	0	0	3	0	28
Ice Cream Cones													
Cake/wafer	1	20	0	0.0	5	4	0	0	0	0	0	0	10
Sugar	1	60	1	0.0	20	13	0	4	1	0	10	1	20
Waffle	1	60	1	0.0	20	12	0	4	0	0	0	1	10
Ice Cream Novelties													
Chocolate eclair bars	1 (3 oz)	150	7	3.5	65	21	1	12	2	0	30	0	0
Creamsicle													
regular/low-fat	1 (2.5 oz)	100	2	1.0	30	20	0	12	1	0	50	0	113
no sugar added	1 (1.5 oz)	32	0	0.0	18	6	2	1	2	0	60	0	26
Crunch bars	2 (1 oz)	170	11	7.0	50	19	0	13	1	0	40	1	50
Dove													
bar	1 (2.5 oz)	250	16	11.0	40	24	1	22	3	0	100	0	150
minis	1 (0.6 oz)	70	5	3.0	10	7	0	6	0	0	0	0	0
Drumstick crunch	1 (3 oz)	280	12	10.0	115	41	1	29	2	0	50	1	85
Fruit juice bars	1 (2 oz)	45	0	0.0	3	10	0	8	0	0	2	0	22
Fudgesicle	2 (2.8 oz)	80	2	1.0	90	18	4	5	3	0	200	1	0
Ice cream sandwiches	1 (2.3 oz)	180	6	3.5	150	29	1	14	3	0	60	1	152
Klondike bars	1 (3 oz)	250	14	11.0	65	29	1	23	3	0	90	0	180
cookies & creme	1 (2.6 oz)	240	13	10.0	110	29	0	19	2	0	70	1	140
Heath	1 (2.6 oz)	220	13	10.0	70	25	1	14	2	0	70	0	140
no sugar added	1 (2.6 oz)	170	9	8.0	65	22	0	5	3	0	100	0	190
M&M's sandwich cookies	1 (3 oz)	230	10	6.0	150	37	1	23	3	0	80	1	110
Nondairy, vanilla													
almond milk	⅔ cup (3.6 oz)	210	10	7.0	85	28	0	21	2	0	10	0	20
cashew milk	⅔ cup (3.6 oz)	190	9	5.0	130	26	0	19	2	0	10	1	90
coconut milk	⅔ cup (3.6 oz)	200	12	11.0	5	23	0	18	0	0	0	0	50
oat milk	⅔ cup (3.6 oz)	220	13	8.0	40	24	1	19	1	0	0	0	0
soy milk	⅔ cup (3.6 oz)	160	4	0.5	10	31	4	16	2	1	10	0	80
Popsicle	1 (1.7 oz)	40	0	0.0	0	10	0	7	0	0	0	0	5
sugar-free	1 (1.7 oz)	15	0	0.0	0	4	0	0	0	0	0	0	3
Push-Ups, sherbet	1 (2.5 oz)	90	1	0.0	25	22	0	14	1	0	33	0	15
Snickers bars	1 (1.7 oz)	180	11	6.0	50	18	0	15	3	0	60	0	120
Snow cones	1 (6 oz)	30	0	0.0	5	8	0	5	0	0	0	0	0
Tofutti	½ cup (2.5 oz)	210	13	2.0	130	21	0	16	2	0	0	0	0
Yasso Greek yogurt bars	1 (2 oz)	80	0	0.0	45	15	1	12	6	0	150	1	200

DESSERTS, SWEETS & TOPPINGS

Other Sweets	Amount	Calories	Fat (g)	Saturated Fat (g)	Sodium (mg)	Carbohydrate (g)	Fiber (g)	Sugar (g)	Protein (g)	Vitamin D (mcg)	Calcium (mg)	Iron (mg)	Potassium (mg)
Caramel apples	1	424	7	2.0	198	95	6	77	4	0	125	0	429
Chocolate mousse	½ cup	247	15	8.0	437	28	0	21	3	0	73	1	271
Crepes, dessert	1 (2.5 oz)	164	8	3.5	235	17	0	5	6	0	66	1	115
Custard	½ cup	147	7	3.0	86	16	0	16	7	0	151	1	209
Flan w/ caramel													
homemade	½ cup	222	6	3.0	81	35	0	35	7	0	127	1	181
mix	½ cup	117	2	1.0	129	22	0	22	3	1	129	0	186
Gelatin	½ cup	84	0	0.0	101	19	0	18	2	0	4	0	1
sugar-free	½ cup	23	0	0.0	56	5	0	0	1	0	4	0	1
Marshmallows	4 large	100	0	0.0	25	24	0	17	1	0	1	0	1
Pudding													
bread, homemade	½ cup	189	4	2.0	95	36	1	28	4	0	104	1	190
chocolate													
instant, sugar-free, w/ skim	½ cup	70	0	0.0	173	15	0	6	4	5	150	1	125
instant, w/ 2%	½ cup	160	3	1.5	490	31	0	25	5	2	150	1	220
regular, ready-to-eat	1 (4 oz)	153	5	1.5	164	25	0	19	2	0	55	1	199
rice, regular, ready-to-eat	½ cup	122	2	1.5	110	21	0	13	4	0	107	0	141
tapioca, ready-to-eat	½ cup	143	4	1.0	160	24	0	16	2	0	78	0	101
vanilla													
instant, sugar-free, w/ skim	½ cup	65	0	0.0	58	18	0	6	4	5	150	0	125
instant, w/ 2%	½ cup	229	4	2.0	361	42	0	25	7	0	245	0	311
regular, ready-to-eat	1 (4 oz)	126	4	1.0	138	22	0	17	1	0	48	0	63

Pies*	Amount	Calories	Fat (g)	Saturated Fat (g)	Sodium (mg)	Carbohydrate (g)	Fiber (g)	Sugar (g)	Protein (g)	Vitamin D (mcg)	Calcium (mg)	Iron (mg)	Potassium (mg)
Apple/cherry	1 slice	413	19	4.5	327	58	1	27	4	0	11	2	123
Banana cream	1 slice	387	20	5.0	346	47	1	17	6	1	108	2	238
Boston cream	⅙ pie (8 in)	231	8	2.0	234	40	1	33	2	0	21	0	36
Chocolate creme	1 slice	360	13	7.0	302	58	2	45	6	0	127	1	159
Coconut cream	1 slice	259	17	8.0	309	27	1	10	4	0	68	0	133
Grasshopper	1 slice	270	17	7.0	211	28	0	15	2	0	32	1	76
Hostess fruit	1 (4.5 oz)	480	20	10.0	380	69	1	39	4	0	7	1	35
Key lime	1 slice	345	13	4.5	237	52	1	43	7	0	158	1	249
Lemon meringue	1 slice	382	12	5.0	387	67	0	51	4	0	20	1	73
Pecan	1 slice	582	38	10.5	383	57	3	37	6	0	57	2	214
Pumpkin	1 slice	323	13	3.0	318	46	2	25	5	0	85	1	222
Rhubarb	1 slice	315	13	5.5	177	47	2	27	3	0	63	2	199
Shoofly	1 slice	376	11	4.0	323	66	1	36	4	0	104	4	659
Strawberry cream	1 slice	353	21	12.0	203	37	2	26	3	0	47	1	175
Sweet potato	1 slice	530	22	10.5	348	80	2	57	6	0	89	1	227

* Based on a 10-in pie (8 slices) unless indicated.

DESSERTS, SWEETS & TOPPINGS

Syrups & Toppings

	Amount	Calories	Fat (g)	Saturated Fat (g)	Sodium (mg)	Carbohydrate (g)	Fiber (g)	Sugar (g)	Protein (g)	Vitamin D (mcg)	Calcium (mg)	Iron (mg)	Potassium (mg)
Agave	1 T	60	0	0.0	0	16	0	16	0	0	0	0	0
Apple butter	1 T	29	0	0.0	3	7	0	6	0	0	2	0	16
Butterscotch/caramel	2 T	103	0	0.0	143	27	0	27	1	0	22	0	34
Chocolate syrup	2 T	112	0	0.0	29	26	1	20	1	0	6	1	90
light	2 T	54	0	0.0	35	12	0	10	1	0	4	0	66
Coffee syrup	2 T	80	0	0.0	0	20	0	20	0	0	0	0	0
Frosting/icing													
chocolate	2 T	159	7	2.0	73	25	0	23	0	0	3	1	78
sugar-free	2 T	100	6	3.0	85	16	1	0	0	0	0	1	97
vanilla	2 T	140	5	2.5	70	23	0	19	0	0	0	0	15
sugar-free	2 T	100	6	3.0	60	17	0	0	0	0	0	0	0
Fruit spread	1 T	45	0	0.0	0	11	0	10	0	0	2	0	13
Grenadine syrup	1 T	54	0	0.0	5	13	0	9	0	0	1	0	6
Honey	1 T	64	0	0.0	1	17	0	17	0	0	1	0	11
Hot fudge	2 T	133	3	1.5	132	24	1	13	2	0	19	1	108
sugar-free	2 T	90	1	0.0	40	24	1	0	1	0	0	1	0
Jam/jelly/marmalade	1 T	56	0	0.0	6	14	0	10	0	0	4	0	15
Maple syrup	1 T	52	0	0.0	2	13	0	12	0	0	20	0	42
Marshmallow crème	2 T	81	0	0.0	20	20	0	12	0	0	1	0	1
Pancake syrup	1 T	47	0	0.0	16	12	0	4	0	0	1	0	3
low-calorie	1 T	25	0	0.0	27	7	0	5	0	0	2	0	1
Sugar, brown/raw/white	1 tsp	16	0	0.0	0	4	0	4	0	0	0	0	0
Whipped cream, homemade	2 T	116	11	7.0	11	4	0	3	1	0	19	0	23
Whipped toppings													
Cool Whip	2 T	20	1	1.0	0	3	0	1	0	0	0	0	0
pressurized	2 T	15	1	1.0	1	1	0	1	0	0	6	0	9
Reddi Wip	2 T	15	1	0.5	0	1	0	0	0	0	0	0	0
fat-free	2 T	5	0	0.0	0	1	0	1	0	0	0	0	0

EGGS, EGG DISHES & EGG SUBSTITUES

Eggs

	Amount	Calories	Fat (g)	Saturated Fat (g)	Sodium (mg)	Carbohydrate (g)	Fiber (g)	Sugar (g)	Protein (g)	Vitamin D (mcg)	Calcium (mg)	Iron (mg)	Potassium (mg)
Chicken													
boiled/poached	1 large	73	5	1.5	147	0	0	0	6	1	27	0	67
deviled w/ filling	½ egg	60	5	1.0	166	1	0	0	3	0	17	1	36
Eggland's Best	1 large	60	4	1.0	65	0	0	0	6	6	28	1	69
fried w/ ½ tsp fat	1 large	90	7	2.0	95	0	0	0	6	1	29	1	70
powdered, whites	2 T	20	0	0.0	120	0	0	0	8	0	0	0	120
powdered, whole	2 T	89	7	2.0	71	0	0	0	7	1	36	1	81
scrambled w/ 1 tsp fat	2 large	182	13	4.0	178	2	0	2	12	2	81	1	161
whites	1	21	0	0.0	66	0	0	0	4	0	3	0	65
yolk	1	55	5	1.5	8	1	0	0	3	1	22	1	19

EGGS, EGG DISHES & EGG SUBSTITUTES

Eggs	Amount	Calories	Fat (g)	Saturated Fat (g)	Sodium (mg)	Carbohydrate (g)	Fiber (g)	Sugar (g)	Protein (g)	Vitamin D (mcg)	Calcium (mg)	Iron (mg)	Potassium (mg)
Duck	1	130	10	3.0	102	1	0	1	9	0	44	3	155
Goose	1	266	19	5.0	199	2	0	1	20	2	86	5	302
Quail	1	14	1	0.5	13	0	0	0	1	0	6	0	12
Turkey	1	135	9	3.0	119	1	0	0	11	0	78	3	112
Egg Dishes													
Frittatas, plain (10 in)													
carmelized onion sausage	¼ pie	367	29	12.0	690	6	1	3	19	2	71	2	341
egg white	¼ pie	170	11	4.0	879	7	2	4	11	0	124	1	350
Omelets													
cheese	1 (2 egg)	299	24	9.0	325	1	0	0	19	2	247	2	160
egg white	1 (4 egg white)	171	12	7.0	376	1	0	1	15	0	13	0	220
ham & cheese	1 (2 egg)	531	39	15.0	2380	6	2	1	38	0	328	3	492
vegetable & cheese	1 (2 egg)	536	14	14.0	938	11	2	6	36	0	717	4	593
Quiche (9 in)													
ham & cheese	⅛ pie	327	23	10.0	538	16	1	2	14	0	219	2	167
Lorraine	⅙ pie	761	68	30.5	1022	19	1	1	19	0	224	2	285
spinach	⅙ pie	613	48	27.0	1155	24	3	6	23	0	563	3	393
Soufflés													
cheese	1 cup	439	33	19.0	721	23	0	20	14	0	191	2	130
spinach	1 cup	440	29	17.0	661	14	4	2	34	0	774	4	591
Egg Substitutes													
Egg Beaters	3 T	25	0	0.0	90	0	0	0	5	0	0	1	70
Liquid egg whites	3 T	25	0	0.0	75	0	0	0	5	0	0	0	75

FATS, OILS, CREAM & GRAVY

	Amount	Calories	Fat (g)	Saturated Fat (g)	Sodium (mg)	Carbohydrate (g)	Fiber (g)	Sugar (g)	Protein (g)	Vitamin D (mcg)	Calcium (mg)	Iron (mg)	Potassium (mg)
Bacon fat	1 T	116	13	5.0	19	0	0	0	0	0	0	0	0
Beef fat/tallow	1 T	116	13	6.5	0	0	0	0	0	0	0	0	0
Benecol spread	1 T	70	8	1.0	105	0	0	0	0	0	0	0	0
light	1 T	50	5	1.0	95	0	0	0	0	0	0	0	0
Butter													
stick	1 tsp	34	4	2.5	30	0	0	0	0	0	1	0	1
	1 T	102	12	7.0	91	0	0	0	0	0	3	0	3
stick, unsalted	1 tsp	34	4	2.5	1	0	0	0	0	0	1	0	1
whipped	1 tsp	23	3	1.5	21	0	0	0	0	0	1	0	1
Butter flavored sprinkles	1 tsp	5	0	0.0	180	1	0	0	0	0	0	0	0
Chicken fat	1 T	115	13	4.0	0	0	0	0	0	1	0	0	0
Coconut milk creamer	1 T	30	1	1.0	15	4	0	4	0	0	0	0	0
Coffee-Mate	1 T	20	1	0.0	5	2	0	0	0	0	0	0	0
liquid, flavored	1 T	35	2	0.0	5	5	0	5	0	0	0	0	0
fat-free	1 T	25	0	0.0	5	5	0	5	0	0	0	0	0
sugar-free	1 T	15	1	1.0	5	0	0	0	0	0	0	0	0
powder	1 tsp	10	1	1.0	5	1	0	0	0	0	0	0	0

FATS, OILS, CREAM & GRAVY	Amount	Calories	Fat (g)	Saturated Fat (g)	Sodium (mg)	Carbohydrate (g)	Fiber (g)	Sugar (g)	Protein (g)	Vitamin D (mcg)	Calcium (mg)	Iron (mg)	Potassium (mg)
fat-free	1 tsp	10	0	0.0	0	2	0	0	0	0	0	0	0
regular, flavored	1 tsp	15	1	1.0	5	2	0	2	0	0	0	0	0
sugar-free, flavored	1 tsp	15	1	1.0	5	0	0	0	0	0	0	0	0
Coffee Rich	1 T	10	1	1.0	0	1	0	0	0	0	0	0	20
Cooking spray	⅓ second	2	0	0.0	0	0	0	0	0	0	0	0	0
	2 seconds	14	1	0.0	1	0	0	0	0	0	0	0	0
Cream													
heavy	1 T	52	6	3.5	6	0	0	0	0	0	10	0	11
light	1 T	44	5	3.0	5	0	0	0	0	0	10	0	15
Gravy, beef													
au jus, jar	¼ cup	5	0	0.0	230	0	0	0	1	0	0	0	0
brown, mix	¼ cup	20	0	0.0	251	4	0	0	1	0	16	0	16
fat-free, can	¼ cup	20	0	0.0	300	3	0	0	1	0	0	0	0
homemade	¼ cup	51	1	0.0	740	10	1	1	2	0	21	0	40
regular, can	¼ cup	31	1	0.5	326	3	0	0	2	0	4	0	47
Gravy, chicken													
dry	1 T	31	1	0.0	332	5	0	0	1	0	12	0	32
fat-free, can	¼ cup	15	0	0.0	310	3	0	0	1	0	0	0	0
giblet, homemade	¼ cup	49	3	0.5	341	3	0	0	3	0	12	2	117
regular, can	¼ cup	47	3	1.0	252	3	0	1	1	0	12	0	65
Gravy, other													
mushroom, can	¼ cup	30	2	0.0	339	3	0	0	1	0	4	0	63
onion, mix	¼ cup	19	0	0.0	251	4	0	0	1	0	17	0	16
pork, can	¼ cup	45	3	1.5	310	3	0	1	1	0	0	0	0
sausage, can	¼ cup	70	56	1.5	270	3	0	1	2	0	0	0	120
turkey, can	¼ cup	30	1	0.5	344	3	0	0	2	0	2	0	65
turkey, mix	¼ cup	24	1	0.0	274	4	0	0	1	0	8	0	221
Half & half	1 T	20	2	1.0	6	1	0	1	0	0	16	0	20
fat-free	1 T	9	0	0.0	15	1	0	1	0	0	14	0	31
Lard/pork fat	1 T	116	13	5.0	0	0	0	0	0	0	0	0	0
Margarine													
fat-free	1 tsp	2	0	0.0	42	0	0	0	0	0	2	0	3
	1 T	7	0	0.0	125	0	0	0	0	0	6	0	8
light	1 tsp	16	2	0.5	27	0	0	0	0	0	0	0	2
	1 T	47	5	1.0	81	0	0	0	0	0	0	0	5
regular, soft/tub	1 tsp	33	4	1.0	31	0	0	0	0	0	0	0	1
	1 T	101	11	2.0	93	0	0	0	0	0	0	0	2
regular, soft/tub, unsalted	1 T	101	11	2.0	4	0	0	0	0	0	0	0	2
regular, stick	1 tsp	33	4	1.0	38	0	0	0	0	0	0	0	1
	1 T	100	11	2.0	105	0	0	0	0	0	0	0	3
regular, stick, unsalted	1 T	102	12	2.0	0	0	0	0	0	0	0	0	3

FATS, OILS, CREAM & GRAVY

	Amount	Calories	Fat (g)	Saturated Fat (g)	Sodium (mg)	Carbohydrate (g)	Fiber (g)	Sugar (g)	Protein (g)	Vitamin D (mcg)	Calcium (mg)	Iron (mg)	Potassium (mg)
Mayonnaise	1 T	94	10	1.5	88	0	0	0	0	0	1	0	3
light	1 T	36	3	0.5	124	1	0	0	0	0	1	0	5
low-fat	1 T	15	1	0.0	130	2	0	0	0	0	0	0	0
vegan	1 T	47	8	1.0	100	0	0	0	0	0	0	0	0
Miracle Whip	1 T	40	4	0.5	95	2	0	1	0	0	1	0	5
light	1 T	23	1	0.0	121	2	0	1	0	0	1	0	5
Mocha Mix	1 T	20	2	0.0	5	1	0	0	0	0	0	0	0
fat-free	1 T	10	0	0.0	5	1	0	0	0	0	0	0	0
Oils													
avocado	1 T	124	14	1.5	0	0	0	0	0	0	0	0	0
canola	1 T	124	14	1.0	0	0	0	0	0	0	0	0	0
chili, flavored	1 T	130	14	3.0	0	0	0	0	0	0	0	0	0
coconut	1 T	117	14	12.0	0	0	0	0	0	0	0	0	0
cod liver/fish	1 T	123	14	3.0	0	0	0	0	0	34	0	0	0
corn	1 T	122	14	2.0	0	0	0	0	0	0	0	0	0
cottonseed	1 T	120	14	3.5	0	0	0	0	0	0	0	0	0
flaxseed/linseed	1 T	120	14	1.0	0	0	0	0	0	0	0	0	0
grapeseed	1 T	120	14	1.5	0	0	0	0	0	0	0	0	0
olive	1 T	119	14	2.0	0	0	0	0	0	0	0	0	0
palm	1 T	120	14	6.5	0	0	0	0	0	0	0	0	0
palm kernel	1 T	116	14	11.0	0	0	0	0	0	0	0	0	0
peanut	1 T	119	14	2.5	0	0	0	0	0	0	0	0	0
safflower	1 T	120	14	1.0	0	0	0	0	0	0	0	0	0
sesame	1 T	120	14	2.0	0	0	0	0	0	0	0	0	0
soybean	1 T	120	14	2.0	0	0	0	0	0	0	0	0	0
sunflower	1 T	120	14	1.5	0	0	0	0	0	0	0	0	0
walnut	1 T	120	14	1.0	0	0	0	0	0	0	0	0	0
wheat germ	1 T	120	14	2.5	0	0	0	0	0	0	0	0	0
Popcorn topping	1 T	120	14	2.0	0	0	0	0	0	0	0	0	0
Silk creamer													
vanilla almond	1 T	25	1	0.0	20	4	0	4	0	0	0	0	0
vanilla one oat	1 T	25	1	0.0	15	4	0	4	0	0	0	0	0
original soy	1 T	20	2	0.5	0	2	0	1	0	0	0	0	0
vanilla soy	1 T	30	2	0.5	0	4	0	3	0	0	0	0	0
Sour cream	1 T	23	2	1.0	6	0	0	0	0	0	13	0	17
fat-free	1 T	11	0	0.0	21	2	0	0	1	0	19	0	19
imitation, soy	1 T	31	3	3.0	15	1	0	1	0	0	1	0	24
light	1 T	20	2	1.0	13	1	0	0	1	0	21	0	32
Vegetable shortening	1 T	110	12	3.0	0	0	0	0	0	0	0	0	0
Yogurt spread	1 T	46	5	1.0	88	0	0	0	0	0	7	0	9

FISH & SEAFOOD

	Amount	Calories	Fat (g)	Saturated Fat (g)	Sodium (mg)	Carbohydrate (g)	Fiber (g)	Sugar (g)	Protein (g)	Vitamin D (mcg)	Calcium (mg)	Iron (mg)	Potassium (mg)
Abalone													
baked/broiled	3 oz	119	1	0.0	341	7	0	0	19	0	27	3	213
flour fried	3 oz	161	6	1.5	503	9	0	0	17	0	32	3	241
Anchovies, oil pack, can	3	25	1	0.5	440	0	0	0	4	0	28	1	65
Anchovy paste	1 T	25	2	0.5	1130	0	0	0	3	4	20	2	33
Bass, freshwater	3 oz	124	4	1.0	77	0	0	0	21	3	88	2	388
Bluefish	3 oz	135	5	1.0	66	0	0	0	22	11	23	1	406
Burbot	3 oz	98	1	0.0	105	0	0	0	21	1	54	1	440
Butterfish	3 oz	159	9	2.5	97	0	0	0	19	11	24	1	409
Calamari/squid													
baked/broiled	3 oz	78	1	0.0	37	3	0	0	16	0	28	1	209
flour fried	3 oz	149	6	1.5	260	7	0	0	15	0	33	1	237
Carp													
baked/broiled	3 oz	138	6	1.0	54	0	0	0	19	26	44	1	363
flour fried	3 oz	239	13	3.0	175	11	0	0	18	26	46	1	370
Catfish, farmed													
baked/broiled	3 oz	122	6	1.5	101	0	0	0	16	8	8	0	311
flour fried	3 oz	195	11	3.0	238	7	1	1	15	8	37	1	289
Catfish, wild	3 oz	89	2	0.5	43	0	0	0	16	11	9	0	356
Caviar, black/red	1 T	42	3	0.5	240	1	0	0	4	1	44	2	29
Chilean sea bass, grilled	3 oz	105	2	0.5	74	0	0	0	20	6	11	0	279
Cisco, smoked	3 oz	151	10	1.5	409	0	0	0	14	11	22	0	249
Clams													
breaded & fried	10 small	190	11	2.5	342	10	0	0	13	0	59	13	306
raw	6 large	103	1	0.0	721	4	0	0	18	0	47	2	55
stuffed, frozen	3 oz	142	5	0.0	467	13	0	3	7	0	33	1	0
Cod, Atlantic/Pacific													
baked/broiled	3 oz	89	1	0.0	66	0	0	0	19	1	12	0	208
breaded & fried	3 oz	150	7	1.5	320	12	1	2	10	1	0	1	260
dried & salted	3 oz	247	2	0.5	5976	0	0	0	53	3	136	2	1239
Crab													
Alaska king	3 oz	83	1	0.0	912	0	0	0	16	0	50	1	223
blue, can	1 cup	112	1	0.5	760	0	0	0	24	0	123	1	350
blue, fresh	3 oz	74	1	0.0	249	0	0	0	15	0	75	1	280
dungeness	3 oz	94	1	0.0	322	1	0	0	19	0	50	0	347
imitation	3 oz	24	0	0.0	132	4	0	2	2	0	3	0	23
snow	3 oz	100	2	0.0	590	0	0	0	20	0	20	0	170
soft shell, flour fried	1 crab	358	24	3.5	76	25	1	2	9	0	64	2	149
Crab cakes	1 (2 oz)	160	10	2.0	491	5	0	0	11	0	202	1	162
Crawdads/crayfish	3 oz	70	1	0.0	80	0	0	0	14	0	51	1	252
Croaker, breaded & fried	3 oz	188	11	3.0	296	6	0	0	16	1	27	1	289

FISH & SEAFOOD

	Amount	Calories	Fat (g)	Saturated Fat (g)	Sodium (mg)	Carbohydrate (g)	Fiber (g)	Sugar (g)	Protein (g)	Vitamin D (mcg)	Calcium (mg)	Iron (mg)	Potassium (mg)
Cusk	3 oz	95	1	0.0	34	0	0	0	21	1	11	1	428
Cuttlefish	3 oz	134	1	0.0	633	1	0	0	28	0	153	9	541
Dolphinfish/mahi mahi	3 oz	93	1	0.0	96	0	0	0	20	12	16	1	453
Drum, freshwater	3 oz	130	5	1.0	82	0	0	0	19	1	66	1	300
Eel	3 oz	201	13	2.5	55	0	0	0	20	25	22	1	297
Escargot/snails	3 oz	77	1	0.0	59	2	0	0	14	0	9	3	325
Fish cakes, breaded, pan fried	1 (3 oz)	75	3	3.0	263	15	1	0	6	1	30	1	71
Fish fillets, frozen	1 (3.5 oz)	156	7	2.0	311	9	0	1	9	0	58	0	212
Fish sticks, frozen	3 oz	223	9	1.0	516	24	2	2	9	0	41	1	200
Flounder													
baked/broiled	3 oz	73	2	0.5	309	0	0	0	21	3	21	0	168
breaded & fried	3 oz	200	12	2.5	347	14	0	3	10	3	17	1	150
Gefilte fish	3 oz	71	2	0.5	445	6	0	0	8	8	20	2	77
Grouper	3 oz	100	1	0.5	45	0	0	0	21	6	18	1	404
Haddock													
baked/broiled	3 oz	77	1	0.0	222	0	0	0	17	1	12	0	298
breaded & fried	3 oz	108	4	1.0	126	10	0	1	8	1	24	1	200
smoked	3 oz	99	1	0.0	649	0	0	0	21	1	42	1	353
Halibut													
Atlantic/Pacific	3 oz	94	1	0.5	70	0	0	0	19	5	8	0	449
Greenland	3 oz	203	15	2.5	88	0	0	0	16	3	3	1	292
Herring, Atlantic													
baked/broiled	3 oz	173	10	2.0	98	0	0	0	20	5	63	1	356
pickled	3 oz	223	15	2.0	740	8	0	7	12	2	66	1	59
Herring, Pacific	3 oz	213	15	3.5	81	0	0	0	18	5	90	1	461
Ling/lingcod	3 oz	93	1	0.0	65	0	0	0	19	1	15	0	476
Lobster													
tail	3 oz	98	1	0.0	399	2	0	0	21	0	75	0	170
Northern, broiled/steamed	3 oz	76	1	0.0	413	0	0	0	16	0	82	0	196
spiny, steamed	3 oz	122	2	0.5	193	3	0	0	23	0	54	1	177
Lox/smoked salmon	3 oz	150	9	1.5	810	0	0	0	15	15	0	0	149
Mackerel													
Atlantic	3 oz	223	15	3.5	71	0	0	0	20	17	13	1	341
Jack/Pacific	3 oz	171	9	2.5	94	0	0	0	22	17	25	1	443
king	3 oz	114	2	0.5	173	0	0	0	22	17	34	2	474
Spanish	3 oz	134	5	1.5	56	0	0	0	20	17	11	1	471
Milkfish	3 oz	162	7	2.0	78	0	0	0	22	5	55	0	318
Monkfish	3 oz	83	2	0.5	20	0	0	0	16	1	9	0	436
Mullet, striped	3 oz	128	4	1.0	60	0	0	0	21	2	26	1	389
Mussels	3 oz	146	4	0.5	314	6	0	0	20	0	28	6	228
Octopus	3 oz	139	2	0.5	391	4	0	0	25	0	90	8	536
Orange roughy	3 oz	89	1	0.0	59	0	0	0	19	1	9	1	154

FISH & SEAFOOD

	Amount	Calories	Fat (g)	Saturated Fat (g)	Sodium (mg)	Carbohydrate (g)	Fiber (g)	Sugar (g)	Protein (g)	Vitamin D (mcg)	Calcium (mg)	Iron (mg)	Potassium (mg)
Oysters													
Eastern, breaded & fried	6 (3 oz)	175	11	3.0	367	10	0	0	8	0	55	6	215
Eastern, raw	6 (3 oz)	43	1	0.5	71	5	0	0	5	0	50	4	131
Pacific, raw	3 (3 oz)	69	2	0.5	90	4	0	0	8	0	7	4	143
smoked, oil pack, can	3 oz	320	29	14.0	192	3	0	0	11	0	32	7	230
Perch													
baked/broiled	3 oz	100	1	0.0	67	0	0	0	21	4	87	1	292
breaded & fried	3 oz	226	15	2.0	465	11	0	0	21	3	83	1	250
Pollock, Atlantic	3 oz	100	1	0.0	94	0	0	0	21	1	66	1	388
Pompano, Florida	3 oz	179	10	4.0	65	0	0	0	20	12	37	1	541
Rockfish, Pacific	3 oz	93	1	0.5	76	0	0	0	19	4	15	0	397
Roe	3 oz	174	7	1.5	100	2	0	0	24	12	24	1	241
Sablefish	3 oz	213	17	3.5	61	0	0	0	15	12	38	1	390
Salmon													
Atlantic	3 oz	155	7	1.0	48	0	0	0	22	14	13	1	534
Chinook	3 oz	197	11	2.5	51	0	0	0	22	14	24	1	429
coho	3 oz	156	6	1.5	45	0	0	0	23	14	39	1	387
pink, can	3 oz	109	4	0.5	342	0	0	0	17	12	183	1	293
sockeye, can	3 oz	142	6	1.0	347	0	0	0	20	18	197	1	267
Sardines, oil pack, can	2	50	3	0.5	74	0	0	0	6	1	92	1	95
Scallops													
bay and sea, steamed	3 oz	94	1	0.0	567	5	0	0	18	0	9	1	267
imitation	3 oz	84	0	0.0	676	9	0	0	11	0	7	0	88
sea, breaded & fried	6 large	201	10	2.5	432	9	0	0	17	0	39	1	310
Scup	3 oz	115	3	1.0	46	0	0	0	21	1	43	1	313
Shad	3 oz	214	15	4.0	55	0	0	0	19	4	51	1	418
Shad roe	3 oz	173	7	1.5	100	2	0	0	24	13	24	1	241
Shark	3 oz	194	12	2.5	104	5	0	0	16	1	43	1	132
Shrimp													
baked/broiled/raw	10 large	66	1	0.5	521	1	0	0	13	0	50	2	94
breaded & fried	10 large	376	23	4.0	1373	27	1	1	16	0	51	2	132
Smelt, rainbow													
baked/broiled	3 oz	105	3	0.5	66	0	0	0	0	1	1	1	316
flour fried	3 oz	217	11	2.5	188	11	0	0	18	1	1	1	340
Snapper	3 oz	109	2	0.5	49	0	0	0	22	1	34	0	444
Sole													
baked/broiled	3 oz	67	1	0.5	236	11	1	3	5	3	28	0	45
breaded & fried	3 oz	189	9	0.5	411	21	2	0	8	3	13	1	154
Sturgeon													
baked/broiled	3 oz	115	4	1.0	59	0	0	0	18	11	15	1	309
smoked	3 oz	147	4	1.0	629	0	0	0	27	14	15	1	322
Sucker, white	3 oz	101	3	0.5	43	0	0	0	18	18	77	1	414
Sunfish	3 oz	97	1	0.0	88	0	0	0	21	2	88	1	382

FISH & SEAFOOD

	Amount	Calories	Fat (g)	Saturated Fat (g)	Sodium (mg)	Carbohydrate (g)	Fiber (g)	Sugar (g)	Protein (g)	Vitamin D (mcg)	Calcium (mg)	Iron (mg)	Potassium (mg)
Swordfish	3 oz	146	7	1.5	83	0	0	0	20	14	5	0	424
Tilefish	3 oz	125	4	0.5	50	0	0	0	21	11	22	0	435
Trout, rainbow													
baked/broiled	3 oz	128	5	1.5	48	0	0	0	20	20	73	0	381
parmesan crusted	3 oz	263	13	2.5	253	2	0	1	33	20	90	2	578
Tuna, can													
light, oil pack	3 oz	168	7	1.5	354	0	0	0	25	6	11	1	176
light, water pack	3 oz	73	1	0.0	210	0	0	0	17	1	15	1	152
low sodium, water pack	3 oz	109	3	0.5	43	0	0	0	20	3	12	1	202
white, oil pack	3 oz	158	7	1.0	337	0	0	0	23	1	3	1	283
white, water pack	¼ cup	108	3	0.5	321	0	0	0	22	2	12	1	202
Tuna, fresh													
bluefin	3 oz	156	5	1.5	43	0	0	0	25	5	9	1	275
yellowfin	3 oz	111	1	0.0	46	0	0	0	25	3	3	1	448
Turbot	3 oz	104	3	0.5	163	0	0	0	18	3	20	0	259
Walleye	3 oz	94	1	0.0	356	0	0	0	20	1	61	1	366
Whitefish	3 oz	146	6	1.0	55	0	0	0	21	17	28	0	345
Whiting	3 oz	99	1	0.5	112	0	0	0	20	2	53	0	369
Yellowtail	3 oz	159	6	1.0	43	0	0	0	25	11	25	1	457

FRUIT & VEGETABLE JUICES

Fruit Juices & Nectars

	Amount	Calories	Fat (g)	Saturated Fat (g)	Sodium (mg)	Carbohydrate (g)	Fiber (g)	Sugar (g)	Protein (g)	Vitamin D (mcg)	Calcium (mg)	Iron (mg)	Potassium (mg)
Apple cider/juice	1 cup	120	0	0.0	30	20	0	30	0	0	0	0	240
Ceres 100% juice blend													
peach	1 cup	120	0	0.0	5	21	0	20	0	0	10	0	360
pear	1 cup	110	0	0.0	5	19	0	18	0	0	10	0	290
Dole pineapple, unsweetened	6 oz	100	0	0.0	0	24	0	22	1	0	0	1	240
Grapefruit													
100%, regular	1 cup	100	0	0.0	10	25	0	21	0	0	20	0	300
white, regular	1 cup	90	0	0.0	15	24	0	17	0	0	0	0	315
Jumex apricot nectar	11.3 oz	170	0	0.0	55	42	2	40	0	0	26	0	0
Iberia guava nectar	1 cup	150	0	0.0	10	43	0	41	0	0	0	0	0
Lemon	1 tsp	0	0	0.0	0	0	0	0	0	0	0	0	0
Lime	1 tsp	0	0	0.0	0	0	0	0	0	0	0	0	0
Mango	1 cup	140	0	0.0	10	33	0	32	0	0	0	0	166
Mott's apple-cherry	1 cup	120	0	0.0	30	29	0	28	0	0	0	1	300
Naked													
Blue Machine	15.2 oz	320	0	0.0	20	76	3	55	2	0	50	1	700
Green Machine	15.2 oz	270	0	0.0	25	63	0	53	4	0	40	1	760
Mighty Mango	15.2 oz	290	0	0.0	20	68	0	57	2	0	40	1	650
strawberry banana	15.2 oz	250	0	0.0	10	59	0	44	2	0	40	1	870
Ocean Spray													
cranberry cocktail													
red, diet	1 cup	5	0	0.0	40	2	0	1	0	0	0	0	0

FRUIT & VEGETABLE JUICES

Fruit Juices & Nectars	Amount	Calories	Fat (g)	Saturated Fat (g)	Sodium (mg)	Carbohydrate (g)	Fiber (g)	Sugar (g)	Protein (g)	Vitamin D (mcg)	Calcium (mg)	Iron (mg)	Potassium (mg)
red, regular	1 cup	100	0	0.0	55	28	0	25	0	0	0	0	0
white, regular	1 cup	100	0	0.0	40	26	0	25	0	0	0	0	0
Cran-Apple	1 cup	120	0	0.0	45	31	0	31	0	0	0	0	0
Cran-Pomegranate	1 cup	120	0	0.0	20	32	0	26	0	0	0	1	0
Cran-Raspberry	1 cup	100	0	0.0	40	27	0	26	0	0	0	0	0
diet	1 cup	5	0	0.0	35	2	0	1	0	0	0	0	0
White Cran-Peach	1 cup	100	0	0.0	40	26	0	26	0	0	0	0	0
Orange	1 cup	110	0	0.0	0	26	0	22	2	0	20	0	450
Pom Wonderful													
100%, pomegranate	1 cup	160	0	0.0	5	39	0	34	0	0	20	0	550
100%, pomegranate cherry	1 cup	160	0	0.0	10	38	0	32	1	0	27	0	570
Sunsweet prune	1 cup	180	0	0.0	50	42	3	25	3	0	26	1	706
Welch's grape													
100%, regular	1 cup	140	0	0.0	10	37	0	35	1	0	30	0	140
100% white, regular	1 cup	140	0	0.0	15	37	0	36	1	0	30	0	140
purple, light	1 cup	45	0	0.0	80	12	0	11	0	0	0	0	110
white, sparkling, regular	1 cup	160	0	0.0	45	39	0	38	0	0	0	0	95

Vegetable Juices

	Amount	Calories	Fat (g)	Saturated Fat (g)	Sodium (mg)	Carbohydrate (g)	Fiber (g)	Sugar (g)	Protein (g)	Vitamin D (mcg)	Calcium (mg)	Iron (mg)	Potassium (mg)
Bolthouse carrot	1 cup	70	0	0.0	150	15	1	13	2	0	50	0	540
Clamato tomato cocktail	1 cup	60	0	0.0	800	12	0	11	1	0	0	1	170
Tomato	1 cup	50	0	0.0	600	10	1	6	2	0	26	1	430
V-8	1 cup	45	0	0.0	640	9	2	7	2	0	40	1	470
fruit & vegetable blends													
Caribbean greens	1 cup	60	0	0.0	110	15	0	14	1	0	20	0	320
healthy greens	1 cup	60	0	0.0	180	15	0	13	1	0	30	1	300
sweet greens	1 cup	80	0	0.0	70	18	0	16	1	0	20	0	230
Fusion													
peach mango	1 cup	110	0	0.0	80	27	0	23	0	0	30	1	200
strawberry banana	1 cup	110	0	0.0	80	27	0	23	0	0	40	1	340
low sodium	1 cup	45	0	0.0	140	9	1	7	2	0	30	1	850

FRUITS

	Amount	Calories	Fat (g)	Saturated Fat (g)	Sodium (mg)	Carbohydrate (g)	Fiber (g)	Sugar (g)	Protein (g)	Vitamin D (mcg)	Calcium (mg)	Iron (mg)	Potassium (mg)
Apples													
dried	12 pcs	130	0	0.0	0	32	3	28	0	0	7	7	310
fresh	1 medium	80	0	0.0	0	22	4	15	0	0	11	0	195
Applesauce													
natural/unsweetened	½ cup	50	0	0.0	10	12	1	11	0	0	5	0	110
sweetened	½ cup	90	0	0.0	10	23	1	20	0	0	5	0	90
Apricots													
dried	5	100	0	0.0	0	25	3	21	1	0	20	1	460
fresh	1	17	0	0.0	0	4	1	4	0	0	0	1	427
heavy syrup, can	½ cup	100	0	0.0	5	25	1	21	0	0	0	1	181
light syrup, can	½ cup	70	0	0.0	10	17	1	15	1	0	0	1	175

FRUITS

	Amount	Calories	Fat (g)	Saturated Fat (g)	Sodium (mg)	Carbohydrate (g)	Fiber (g)	Sugar (g)	Protein (g)	Vitamin D (mcg)	Calcium (mg)	Iron (mg)	Potassium
Avocados	⅓ medium	80	8	1.0	0	4	3	0	1	0	10	0	250
Banana chips, sweetened	¼ cup	200	11	10.0	0	27	1	12	0	0	0	0	350
Bananas, fresh	1 medium	105	0	0.0	2	27	3	14	1	0	13	0	422
Blackberries, fresh	1 cup	60	1	0.0	1	12	6	6	1	0	52	1	233
Blueberries, fresh/frozen	1 cup	70	1	0.0	0	17	4	12	0	0	0	0	80
Boysenberries, fresh	1 cup	62	1	0.0	1	14	8	7	2	0	42	1	233
Cantaloupe, fresh	1 cup	53	0	0.0	25	13	1	12	1	0	14	0	417
Cherries													
maraschino	1 medium	5	0	0.0	0	2	0	2	0	0	3	0	1
red	½ cup	43	0	0.0	0	11	1	9	1	0	9	0	153
sweet, heavy syrup, can	⅓ cup	100	0	0.0	15	24	0	20	0	0	0	0	100
tart, juice packed, jar	5	10	0	0.0	4	2	0	2	0	0	3	0	30
Coconut, shredded													
fresh	1 cup	283	27	24.0	16	12	7	5	3	0	11	2	285
sweetened, dried	2 T	70	5	4.0	45	7	1	5	0	0	2	0	39
unsweetened, dried	2½ T	100	10	9.0	5	4	2	1	1	0	4	0	80
Cranberries													
Craisins/sweetened, dried	¼ cup	100	0	0.0	0	33	10	12	0	0	4	0	20
fresh/frozen	1 cup	90	8	0.0	0	22	3	18	1	0	20	1	310
Currants, fresh	1 cup	63	0	0.0	1	15	5	8	1	0	37	1	308
Dates, dried	2	110	0	0.0	0	30	3	25	1	0	20	0	270
Figs													
dried	3	110	0	0.0	0	26	5	20	1	0	60	1	240
fresh	1 medium	111	0.5	0.0	1	29	4	24	1	0	53	1	348
Fruit cocktail													
100% juice, can	½ cup	60	0	0.0	5	15	1	12	1	0	8	0	170
heavy syrup, can	½ cup	100	0	0.0	5	25	1	21	0	0	0	0	100
Gooseberries, fresh	1 cup	70	1	0.0	2	15	6	0	1	0	40	0	270
Grapefruit													
light syrup, can	½ cup	90	0	0.0	0	21	1	17	1	0	26	3	164
whole, fresh	½ medium	52	0	0.0	0	13	2	8	1	0	27	0	166
Grapes, fresh	1 cup	52	0	0.0	2	14	1	12	1	0	8	0	144
Guavas, fresh	1 medium	38	1	0.0	1	8	3	5	1	0	0.2	0	229
Honeydew melon, fresh	1 cup	61	0	0.0	31	15	1	13	1	0	10	0	388
Kiwifruit, fresh	1 medium	42	0	0.0	2	10	2	6	1	0	23	0	215
Kumquats, fresh	1 medium	13	0	0.0	2	3	1	2	0	0	13	0	35
Lemons, fresh	1	17	0	0.0	1	5	2	1	1	0	15	0	80
Limes, fresh	1	20	0	0.0	1	7	2	1	0	0	22	0	68
Loganberries, fresh	1 cup	80	1	0.0	2	19	8	11	2	0	38	1	213
Mandarin oranges, can	½ cup	80	0	0.0	0	19	2	17	1	0	30	0	140
Mangoes, fresh	½ cup	50	0	0.0	1	12	1	11	1	0	9	0	139

FRUITS	Amount	Calories	Fat (g)	Saturated Fat (g)	Sodium (mg)	Carbohydrate (g)	Fiber (g)	Sugar (g)	Protein (g)	Vitamin D (mcg)	Calcium (mg)	Iron (mg)	Potassium (mg)
Melon balls, frozen	1 cup	40	0	0.0	15	10	0	8	2	0	40	0	242
Mixed fruit													
dried	¼ cup	110	0	0.0	95	27	4	18	1	0	16	1	330
no sugar added, frozen	1 cup	60	0	0.0	0	16	2	12	1	0	20	1	200
Mulberries, fresh	1 cup	60	2	0.0	14	14	2	11	2	0	54	3	218
Nectarines, fresh	1 medium	62	0	0.0	0	15	2	11	2	0	9	0	285
Oranges, fresh	1 medium	69	0	0.0	0	18	3	12	1	0	60	0	232
Papayas, fresh	½ cup	31	0	0.0	6	8	1	6	0	0	15	0	132
Passion fruit, fresh	1 cup	18	0	0.0	5	4	2	2	0	0	2	0	63
Peaches													
100% juice, can	½ cup	70	0	0.0	10	17	1	13	0	0	26	0	210
fresh	1 medium	60	0	0.0	0	14	2	13	1	0	9	0	292
heavy syrup, can	½ cup	100	0	0.0	5	25	1	21	0	0	0	0	100
Pears													
100% juice, can	½ cup	60	0	0.0	5	15	2	11	0	0	26	0	115
fresh	1 medium	112	0	0.0	2	27	5	17	1	0	16	0	179
heavy syrup, can	½ cup	100	0	0.0	5	25	2	20	0	0	0	0	60
Persimmons, fresh	1 medium	32	0	0.0	0	8	0	8	0	0	7	1	78
Pineapple chunks													
100% juice, can	2 slices	60	0	0.0	10	16	1	14	0	0	18	0	186
fresh	1 cup	83	0	0.0	2	22	2	16	1	0	21	1	180
heavy syrup, can	½ cup	90	0	0.0	10	24	1	22	0	0	18	0	146
Plantains, cooked	½ cup	170	7	1.0	150	29	2	13	1	0	3	1	447
Plums, fresh	1 medium	30	0	0.0	0	8	1	7	0	0	4	0	104
Pomegranates, fresh	½ medium	72	1	0.0	3	16	4	12	1	0	13	0	205
seeds	½ cup	100	1	0.0	0	20	5	14	2	0	0	0	188
Prickly pears, fresh	1 medium	61	1	0.0	8	14	5	9	1	0	83	0	328
Prunes, dried	6	110	0	0.0	5	26	2	13	1	0	0	1	330
Quince, fresh	1 medium	52	0	0.0	4	14	2	12	0	0	10	1	181
Raisins	¼ cup	140	0	0.0	10	33	1	26	1	0	20	1	310
Raspberries, fresh	1 cup	64	1	0.0	1	15	8	5	1	0	31	1	186
Rhubarb													
fresh	1 cup	11	0	0.0	2	2	1	1	1	0	44	0	147
sweetened, cooked	1 cup	278	0	0.0	2	75	5	69	1	0	348	1	230
Starfruit, fresh	1 medium	41	0	0.0	3	9	4	5	1	0	4	0	176
Strawberries													
fresh	1 cup	23	0	0.0	1	6	1	4	0	0	12	0	110
sweetened, frozen	23	50	0	0.0	0	13	3	6	1	0	20	1	200
Tangerines, fresh	1 medium	50	0	0.0	0	13	2	9	1	0	52	0	146
Tropical fruit, light, can	½ cup	90	0	0.0	0	21	1	20	0	0	0	0	140
Watermelon, fresh	1 cup	45	0	0.0	2	11	1	9	1	0	11	0	170

MEATS*

Beef & Veal

Beef & Veal	Amount	Calories	Fat (g)	Saturated Fat (g)	Sodium (mg)	Carbohydrate (g)	Fiber (g)	Sugar (g)	Protein (g)	Vitamin D (mcg)	Calcium (mg)	Iron (mg)	Potassium (mg)
Bottom round, roasted	3 oz	190	11	4.0	29	0	0	0	22	0	5	2	179
Chuck roast													
arm, braised	3 oz	174	5	2.0	49	0	0	0	29	0	15	3	239
blade, braised	3 oz	215	11	4.5	60	0	0	0	26	0	11	3	224
Corned brisket, roasted	3 oz	214	16	5.5	828	0	0	0	16	0	7	2	123
Eye of round, roasted	3 oz	177	8	3.0	32	0	0	0	24	0	6	2	193
Filet mignon, broiled	3 oz	185	8	3.5	49	0	0	0	26	0	12	3	303
Flank steak, broiled	3 oz	165	7	3.0	48	0	0	0	24	0	13	3	288
Ground													
extra lean, 5% fat, pan-browned	3 oz	164	6	3.0	72	0	0	0	22	0	8	3	390
lean, 10% fat	3 oz	196	10	4.0	74	0	0	2	24	0	14	3	368
lean, 15% fat	3 oz	218	13	5.0	78	0	0	0	24	0	19	3	346
regular, 20% fat	3 oz	231	15	5.5	77	0	0	0	23	0	24	2	323
London broil	3 oz	165	7	3.0	48	0	0	0	24	0	13	2	288
New York Strip, boneless	3 oz	125	6	2.0	37	0	0	0	18	2	12	2	242
Porterhouse steak	3 oz	173	7	3.0	57	0	0	0	25	0	17	3	248
Pot roast, chuck	3 oz	207	15	6.0	53	0	0	0	16	0	14	1	247
Prime rib	3 oz	349	30	12.5	55	0	0	0	19	0	11	2	275
Rib eye steak	3 oz	153	9	3.5	75	1	0	0	17	0	5	2	303
Round steak, top, grilled	3 oz	134	4	1.0	59	0	0	0	26	0	14	3	324
Rump roast	3 oz	204	10	3.5	37	0	0	0	28	0	7	2	229
Short ribs, bone in	3 oz	204	12	3.0	89	0	0	0	25	0	12	3	235
Sirloin steak, grilled	3 oz	154	6	2.5	53	0	0	0	24	0	15	2	315
Sirloin tips	3 oz	155	7	2.5	47	0	0	0	23	0	15	1	289
Stew meat	3 oz	164	6	2.5	55	0	0	0	28	0	15	3	268
T-bone steak	3 oz	210	14	5.0	57	0	0	0	21	0	4	3	257
Tenderloin, lean	3 oz	179	8	3.0	48	0	0	0	25	0	11	3	298
Top round	3 oz	164	5	2.0	36	0	0	0	27	0	6	2	234
Top sirloin	3 oz	171	11	4.0	44	0	0	0	17	0	20	1	268
Tri tip roast	3 oz	179	9	3.0	45	0	0	0	22	0	16	1	275
Veal													
chops, grilled	3 oz	135	4	1.5	72	0	0	0	25	1	11	1	203
chops, breaded & fried	3 oz	190	13	5.0	370	10	2	2	12	0	26	1	297
cutlets/loin chops, braised	3 oz	190	10	4.0	95	0	0	0	21	0	20	1	243
ground	3 oz	196	15	7.0	60	0	0	0	16	0	9	1	298
loin, braised	3 oz	241	15	5.5	68	0	0	0	26	0	24	1	238
patties, breaded & fried	3 oz	190	13	5.0	370	10	2	2	12	0	20	0	240
shoulder, roasted	3 oz	139	5	2.0	77	0	0	0	22	0	23	1	303
sirloin, braised	3 oz	214	11	4.5	67	0	0	0	27	0	15	4	273

* Cooked w/o fat unless indicated.

MEATS

Game	Amount	Calories	Fat (g)	Saturated Fat (g)	Sodium (mg)	Carbohydrate (g)	Fiber (g)	Sugar (g)	Protein (g)	Vitamin D (mcg)	Calcium (mg)	Iron (mg)	Potassium (mg)
Beefalo, roasted	3 oz	160	5	2.5	70	0	0	0	26	0	20	3	390
Bison/buffalo, roasted	3 oz	122	2	1.0	49	0	0	0	24	0	7	3	307
Rabbit													
domestic, roasted	3 oz	168	7	2.0	40	0	0	0	25	0	16	2	326
wild, stewed	3 oz	147	3	1.0	38	0	0	0	28	0	15	4	292
Venison, roasted	3 oz	134	3	1.0	46	0	0	0	26	0	6	4	285
Lamb													
Chops	3 oz	253	22	9.5	54	0	0	0	13	0	12	1	223
Leg	3 oz	183	10	4.5	55	0	0	0	22	0	12	2	291
Shoulder	3 oz	202	9	3.5	66	0	0	0	29	0	23	2	244
Pork													
Chops													
broiled	3 oz	172	10	3.0	50	1	0	0	21	1	7	1	346
fried	3 oz	166	7	2.0	84	1	0	0	25	0	43	1	322
Ground, 96% lean	3 oz	157	5	1.5	75	0	0	0	27	0	17	1	353
Ham													
cured, lean	3 oz	90	3	1.0	882	0	0	0	16	0	3	1	271
hocks	2 oz	118	7	2.0	41	0	0	0	13	0	8	1	176
leg, fresh	3 oz	208	16	5.5	40	0	0	0	15	0	4	1	268
picnic/shoulder roast	3 oz	194	11	3.5	68	0	0	0	23	1	8	1	298
Loin	3 oz	196	11	4.0	71	0	0	0	23	1	28	1	298
Spareribs, lean & fat, braised	3 oz	338	26	9.5	79	0	0	0	25	2	40	2	272
Tenderloin, lean, broiled	3 oz	122	3	1.0	49	0	0	0	22	0	5	1	358
Processed & Luncheon Meats													
Bacon	1 oz	118	11	4.0	188	0	0	0	4	0	1	0	56
Bacon bits	1 T	25	2	1.0	210	0	0	0	3	0	7	0	10
imitation	1 T	33	2	0.5	124	2	1	0	2	0	65	1	10
Beef jerky	1 oz	90	1	0.0	330	1	0	0	20	0	6	2	179
Beef sticks/Slim Jim	1	79	6	3.0	406	1	0	0	6	0	0	1	69
Bologna													
beef/beef & pork	1 oz	87	7	2.5	272	2	0	2	4	0	24	0	89
turkey	1 oz	59	5	1.0	300	1	0	1	3	0	3	1	38
Braunschweiger	1 oz	93	8	2.5	277	1	0	0	4	0	3	3	56
Canadian bacon	1 slice	45	2	0.5	371	0	0	0	6	0	2	0	94
Corned beef, can	2 oz	142	9	3.5	509	0	0	0	15	0	7	1	77
Corned beef hash, can	1 cup	372	23	10.0	934	21	3	1	20	0	43	2	390
Deviled ham spread	¼ cup	180	15	5.0	480	1	0	0	8	0	26	0	0
Ham, chopped, can	1 oz	68	5	2.0	363	0	0	0	5	0	2	0	81
Ham, deli, extra lean	1 slice	23	1	0.0	294	0	0	0	4	0	13	1	113
Headcheese	1 oz	71	5	1.5	424	0	0	0	4	0	7	1	14

MEATS*

Processed & Luncheon Meats	Amount	Calories	Fat (g)	Saturated Fat (g)	Sodium (mg)	Carbohydrate (g)	Fiber (g)	Sugar (g)	Protein (g)	Vitamin D (mcg)	Calcium (mg)	Iron (mg)	Potass.
Hot dogs													
beef	1	180	20	5.0	820	4	2	0	10	0	20	1	121
bun length	1	340	31	12.0	1250	4	0	1	11	0	20	2	170
w/ cheese	1	190	16	6.0	627	4	0	2	7	0	234	1	198
chicken/pork	1	150	13	4.5	550	4	0	3	4	0	26	0	60
Liverwurst	1 oz	90	8	3.0	285	1	0	0	5	0	0	0	48
Mortadella	1 oz	76	7	2.5	248	0	0	0	5	0	0	0	46
Olive loaf	1 oz	67	5	2.0	274	3	0	0	3	0	31	0	85
Pastrami, beef	1 oz	42	2	1.0	306	0	0	0	6	0	3	1	60
Pepperoni	1 oz	138	12	4.0	493	0	0	0	6	0	6	1	78
Roast beef, deli	1 oz	33	1	0.5	242	0	0	0	5	0	1	1	183
Salami													
beef	1 oz	74	6	3.0	323	1	0	0	4	0	2	1	53
beef & pork	1 oz	95	7	3.0	493	1	0	0	6	0	4	0	90
Sandwich steaks, frozen	1 (2 oz)	120	10	4.0	35	0	0	0	8	0	0	0	169
Sausages													
bockwurst	1 (1.5 oz)	100	9	3.0	280	0	0	0	5	0	0	0	118
bratwurst	1 (2 oz)	196	17	4.0	560	1	0	0	8	0	5	1	187
breakfast	2 (1.5 oz)	150	13	4.0	374	1	0	1	9	0	0	1	157
chorizo	1 (2 oz)	258	22	8.0	700	1	0	0	14	1	5	1	226
Italian	1 (2 oz)	195	16	5.5	684	2	0	1	11	1	12	1	172
kielbasa	1 (2 oz)	110	8	2.5	520	1	0	0	8	0	39	1	213
knockwurst	1 (2 oz)	155	14	6.0	475	1	0	0	8	0	1	1	90
Polish	1 (2 oz)	185	16	6.0	497	1	0	0	8	0	6	1	134
smoked, beef	1 (2 oz)	177	15	6.5	641	1	0	0	8	0	4	1	100
smoked, pork	1 (2 oz)	175	16	5.0	469	1	0	1	13	1	6	0	274
summer	1 (1 oz)	120	11	3.0	420	1	0	0	6	0	23	1	58
Vienna	1 (1 oz)	65	6	2.0	249	1	0	0	3	0	3	0	29
Spam, can	2 oz	180	16	6.0	790	1	0	0	7	0	0	0	229
light	2 oz	110	8	3.0	580	1	0	0	9	0	0	0	258
reduced sodium	2 oz	180	16	6.0	580	1	0	1	7	0	0	0	140
Specialty & Organ Meats													
Brains, beef, pan fried	3 oz	167	14	3.0	134	0	0	0	11	0	8	2	301
Chitterlings, pork, stewed	3 oz	198	17	8.0	15	0	0	0	11	0	21	1	12
Frog legs	3 oz	73	0	0.0	58	0	0	0	16	0	18	2	285
Hearts, beef	3 oz	140	4	1.0	50	0	0	0	24	0	4	5	186
Liver, beef, pan fried	3 oz	142	4	2.0	62	4	0	0	22	1	5	5	284
Oxtail, beef	3 oz	207	12	5.0	48	0	0	0	23	0	39	2	285
Pigs' feet, pickled	3 oz	80	6	2.0	620	0	0	0	7	0	20	0	11
Sweetbreads	3 oz	122	6	2.0	44	0	0	0	18	0	5	1	301
Tongue, beef	3 oz	241	19	7.0	55	0	0	0	16	0	4	2	156
Tripe, beef	3 oz	80	3	1.0	58	2	0	0	10	0	69	1	36

MILK & YOGURT

Milk & Alternatives

	Amount	Calories	Fat (g)	Saturated Fat (g)	Sodium (mg)	Carbohydrate (g)	Fiber (g)	Sugar (g)	Protein (g)	Vitamin D (mcg)	Calcium (mg)	Iron (mg)	Potassium (mg)
Acidophilus milk, low-fat	1 cup	105	3	1.5	95	13	0	12	8	3	307	0	388
Almond milk	1 cup	60	3	0.0	150	8	0	7	1	5	450	1	170
unsweetened	1 cup	30	3	0.0	170	1	0	0	1	5	450	1	160
chocolate	1 cup	100	3	0.0	150	21	0	19	1	5	450	1	220
vanilla	1 cup	80	3	0.0	150	14	0	13	1	5	450	1	170
unsweetened	1 cup	30	3	0.0	170	1	0	0	1	5	450	1	160
Buttermilk													
dried	2 T	60	1	0.5	70	8	0	7	5	3	132	0	266
low-fat	1 cup	90	0	0.0	260	14	0	12	9	3	315	0	422
Carnation Breakfast Essentials													
chocolate	8 oz	220	6	1.0	210	26	1	12	15	10	350	4	450
vanilla	8 oz	220	6	1.0	200	26	1	12	15	10	350	4	400
Chocolate milk													
low-fat	1 cup	150	3	1.5	200	22	0	21	8	3	260	1	470
ultra-filtered	1 cup	140	5	3.0	280	13	1	12	13	5	390	1	550
Coconut milk	1 cup	70	5	4.0	10	9	1	7	0	3	130	0	40
can	⅓ cup	120	13	11.0	15	2	0	1	0	0	40	0	30
lite	⅓ cup	40	4	3.5	15	1	0	0	0	0	40	0	20
unsweetened	1 cup	50	5	4.5	105	1	0	0	1	3	350	0	60
Condensed milk, sweetened, can													
fat-free	2 T	110	0	0.0	55	25	0	25	4	0	195	0	90
whole	2 T	130	3	2.0	35	22	0	22	3	0	130	0	90
Eggnog, nonalcoholic													
low-fat	1 cup	140	3	1.5	85	23	0	22	6	0	260	0	175
whole	½ cup	190	9	5.0	130	24	0	20	4	0	131	0	175
Evaporated milk, can													
low-fat	2 T	25	1	0.0	30	3	0	3	2	1	70	0	120
whole	2 T	40	2	1.0	25	3	0	3	2	1	78	0	94
Filled milk	2 T	120	3	1.5	45	21	0	21	3	0	130	0	42
Goat milk	1 cup	140	10	4.0	115	11	0	11	8	2	300	0	420
Human breast milk	½ cup	86	5	2.5	21	9	0	8	1	0	79	0	125
Instant Breakfast, prepared, w/ skim													
chocolate	1 cup	220	1	1.0	190	39	0	31	13	10	500	4	660
light	1 cup	150	1	1.0	190	23	2	19	13	10	500	4	660
vanilla	1 cup	220	0	0.0	210	39	0	30	13	10	500	4	600
Kefir													
flavored, low-fat	1 cup	140	2	1.5	125	20	3	20	11	5	390	0	376
plain, low-fat	1 cup	110	2	1.5	125	12	3	12	11	5	390	0	376
plain, non-fat	1 cup	90	0	0.0	120	12	0	12	11	5	390	0	376
Lactaid milk													
1%	1 cup	110	3	1.5	125	13	0	12	8	3	300	0	410
2%	1 cup	130	5	3.0	125	13	0	12	8	3	300	0	410
fat-free	1 cup	90	0	0.0	125	13	0	12	8	3	310	0	420
whole	1 cup	160	8	5.0	125	12	0	12	8	3	300	0	400

MILK & YOGURT

Milk & Alternatives

	Amount	Calories	Fat (g)	Saturated Fat (g)	Sodium (mg)	Carbohydrate (g)	Fiber (g)	Sugar (g)	Protein (g)	Vitamin D (mcg)	Calcium (mg)	Iron (mg)	Potass.
Low-fat milk													
1%	1 cup	110	3	1.5	135	13	0	12	8	5	310	0	420
protein fortified	1 cup	100	3	1.5	120	6	0	6	13	5	390	0	420
2%	1 cup	130	5	3.0	135	13	0	12	8	5	320	0	420
Malted milk powder	3 T	90	2	1.0	100	16	0	12	2	0	50	0	130
Oat milk	1 cup	120	5	0.5	100	16	2	7	3	4	350	0	390
Ovaltine, low-fat													
chocolate malt	1 cup	140	3	1.5	160	22	0	22	8	4	410	3	450
chocolate rich	1 cup	140	3	1.5	125	22	0	22	8	4	410	3	420
Powdered milk, dry													
nonfat	¼ cup	90	0	0.0	100	13	1	11	8	0	310	0	410
whole	¼ cup	140	8	4.5	105	11	0	10	8	3	480	0	370
Rice Dream rice drink	1 cup	120	3	0.0	100	23	0	10	1	5	390	1	525
vanilla	1 cup	130	3	0.0	105	26	0	12	1	5	390	0	525
Silk soy milk													
chocolate	1 cup	150	5	1.0	85	19	3	15	9	3	450	3	520
plain	1 cup	110	5	0.5	90	9	2	6	8	3	450	1	380
unsweetened	1 cup	80	4	0.5	75	3	2	1	7	3	300	1	350
vanilla	1 cup	100	4	0.5	85	11	1	9	6	3	450	1	300
light	1 cup	80	4	0.5	70	4	2	1	7	3	210	1	350
Skim/nonfat milk	1 cup	80	0	—	135	13	0	12	8	5	300	0	430
Strawberry milk, Nesquik, 1%	1 cup	160	3	1.5	120	26	0	26	8	3	300	0	360
Whole milk	1 cup	160	8	5.0	135	12	0	12	8	5	310	0	410

Yogurt & Alternatives

	Amount	Calories	Fat (g)	Saturated Fat (g)	Sodium (mg)	Carbohydrate (g)	Fiber (g)	Sugar (g)	Protein (g)	Vitamin D (mcg)	Calcium (mg)	Iron (mg)	Potass.
Almond	1 cup	120	3	0.0	30	22	1	11	5	0	150	1	90
Silk, mixed berry acai	1 (5 oz)	180	11	1.0	75	19	3	14	5	2	130	1	210
Greek													
Chobani Complete, mixed berry	1 (5 oz)	120	3	1.5	55	12	3	7	15	0	130	0	188
Chobani Less Sugar, Clingstone peach	1 (5 oz)	110	3	1.5	50	9	0	9	12	0	130	0	188
Stonyfield, vanilla	1 (7 oz)	170	5	3.5	55	16	0	14	14	1	150	0	180
Yoplait, Greek 100	1 (5 oz)	100	0	0.0	55	10	0	7	14	3	130	0	188
Light													
Yoplait, strawberry	1 (6 oz)	80	0	0.0	75	15	0	7	5	3	210	0	260
Low-fat													
Dannon, vanilla	1 (5 oz)	140	2	1.5	90	24	0	22	7	0	325	0	310
Oat													
Chobani, blueberry	1 (5 oz)	130	3	1.0	25	22	1	15	6	0	10	0	140
Original, flavored													
Dannon, blended strawberry	1 (5 oz)	120	1	0.5	70	23	0	19	4	1	130	0	188
Dannon, fruit on the bottom strawberry	1 (5 oz)	130	2	1.0	90	25	0	21	5	2	195	0	282
Yoplait original, vanilla	1 (6 oz)	150	2	1.5	90	28	0	20	6	3	260	0	180

MILK & YOGURT

Yogurt & Alternatives

	Amount	Calories	Fat (g)	Saturated Fat (g)	Sodium (mg)	Carbohydrate (g)	Fiber (g)	Sugar (g)	Protein (g)	Vitamin D (mcg)	Calcium (mg)	Iron (mg)	Potassium (mg)
Plain													
Dannon, low-fat	1 (6 oz)	110	3	1.5	110	12	0	10	8	0	310	0	380
Dannon, nonfat	1 (6 oz)	80	0	0.0	115	13	0	10	8	0	320	0	390
Dannon, whole milk	1 (6 oz)	110	6	4.0	85	7	0	7	6	0	230	0	290
Soy													
Silk, peach mango	1 (5 oz)	120	4	0.0	85	17	2	12	6	2	200	1	370

Yogurt Drinks & Squeeze Yogurts

	Amount	Calories	Fat (g)	Saturated Fat (g)	Sodium (mg)	Carbohydrate (g)	Fiber (g)	Sugar (g)	Protein (g)	Vitamin D (mcg)	Calcium (mg)	Iron (mg)	Potassium (mg)
Drinkable yogurt													
Activia probiotic yogurt drink, strawberry	7 oz	160	4	2.0	115	25	2	22	7	4	260	0	376
Chobani Greek yogurt, stawberry banana	7 oz	140	4	2.5	85	18	1	15	10	0	260	0	340
Stonyfield probiotic smoothie, wild berry	6 oz	110	2	1.0	85	17	0	15	6	2	210	0	280
Yogurt tubes													
Stonyfield, berry	1 tube	50	1	0.5	35	8	0	6	2	1	80	0	110
Yoplait GoGurt, berry & cherry	3 tubes	150	1	0.5	75	29	0	22	6	3	430	0	240
Yoplait GoGurt, simply berry & strawberry banana	3 tubes	140	2	1.0	90	23	0	16	7	4	350	0	290
Yoplait smoothies													
peach mango/strawberry	7 oz	150	3	2.0	85	23	0	18	5	3.4	200	0	260
Trix	7 oz	150	3	2.0	115	27	0	22	5	3.4	190	0	260

NUTS, SEEDS & NUT/SEED BUTTERS

	Amount	Calories	Fat (g)	Saturated Fat (g)	Sodium (mg)	Carbohydrate (g)	Fiber (g)	Sugar (g)	Protein (g)	Vitamin D (mcg)	Calcium (mg)	Iron (mg)	Potassium (mg)
Almond butter	1 T	98	9	1.0	36	3	2	1	3	0	56	1	120
Almond paste	1 T	65	4	0.5	1	7	1	5	1	0	24	0	45
Almonds	23	160	14	1.0	1	6	3	1	6	0	74	1	202
Brazil nuts	8	264	27	6.5	1	5	3	1	6	0	64	1	264
Cashew butter	1 T	97	8	1.5	47	5	0	1	2	0	10	1	72
Cashews, salted	23	5	16	3.0	138	11	1	2	5	0	15	2	187
Chestnuts	3	59	1	0.0	0	13	1	3	1	0	7	0	142
Filberts/hazelnuts	20	188	18	1.0	0	5	3	1	4	0	34	1	204
Flax seeds	2 T	112	9	1.0	6	6	6	0	4	0	54	1	171
Macadamias	11	197	21	3.5	97	4	2	1	2	0	19	1	100
Mixed nuts, salted													
w/ peanuts	¼ cup	215	19	2.5	111	7	3	2	7	0	33	1	214
w/o peanuts	¼ cup	217	20	2.5	114	8	3	2	6	0	48	1	218
Nutella	2 T	200	11	3.5	15	22	1	21	3	0	40	2	151
Peanut butter													
chunky	2 T	190	17	2.5	117	6	2	3	8	0	14	6	238
creamy	2 T	195	17	3.0	114	5	2	1	8	0	14	1	250
natural	2 T	190	16	3.0	110	7	3	2	8	0	18	1	201
reduced fat	2 T	187	12	2.0	194	13	2	3	9	0	13	1	241

NUTS, SEEDS & NUT/SEED BUTTERS

	Amount	Calories	Fat (g)	Saturated Fat (g)	Sodium (mg)	Carbohydrate (g)	Fiber (g)	Sugar (g)	Protein (g)	Vitamin D (mcg)	Calcium (mg)	Iron (mg)	Potassium (mg)
Peanuts													
Beer Nuts original peanuts, can	1 oz	160	10	2.5	110	9	2	1	7	0	16	1	185
dry roasted, salted	1 oz	170	15	2.5	91	4	3	1	8	0	17	0	206
honey roasted	1 oz	223	18	3.0	136	12	3	6	8	0	19	1	210
Pecans	20	104	11	1.0	0	2	1	1	1	0	10	0	62
Pine nuts	¼ cup	227	23	2.0	1	4	1	1	5	0	5	2	201
Pistachio nuts, salted	32	92	8	1.0	62	4	2	1	3	0	16	1	155
Poppy seeds	1 T	45	4	0.5	2	2	2	0	2	0	127	1	63
Pumpkin/squash seeds	2 T	103	9	2.0	3	3	1	0	5	0	9	1	141
Sesame butter/tahini	1 T	89	8	1.0	17	3	1	0	3	0	64	1	62
Sesame seeds	2 T	101	10	1.5	8	2	2	0	3	0	10	1	59
Soynut butter	2 T	170	11	1.5	140	10	3	3	7	0	60	0	324
Soynuts, salted	3 T	160	9	1.5	55	11	6	1	12	0	40	1	508
Sunflower seeds, salted	2 T	104	9	1.0	83	4	2	0	3	0	13	1	151
Trail mix													
w/ chocolate chips	¼ cup	175	11	2.0	51	17	2	12	4	0	28	1	172
w/ fruit, tropical	¼ cup	158	9	1.0	47	18	2	13	4	0	22	1	183
w/ seeds	¼ cup	177	12	2.0	44	16	2	8	5	0	40	1	237
Walnuts, chopped	2 T	98	10	1.0	0	2	1	0	2	0	15	0	66

PASTA, RICE & OTHER GRAINS

Pasta*

	Amount	Calories	Fat (g)	Saturated Fat (g)	Sodium (mg)	Carbohydrate (g)	Fiber (g)	Sugar (g)	Protein (g)	Vitamin D (mcg)	Calcium (mg)	Iron (mg)	Potassium (mg)
Cellophane noodles, dry	1 cup	176	0	0.0	4	44	2	9	0	0	30	0	0
Chow mein noodles, can	1 cup	292	18	3.0	212	29	1	0	6	0	12	1	50
Couscous	1 cup	178	0	0.0	302	37	2	0	6	0	13	1	93
Egg noodles	1 cup	221	3	1.0	264	40	2	1	8	0	19	2	61
Gnocchi, potato	1 cup	250	12	7.0	541	32	2	2	4	0	41	1	256
Macaroni/pasta	1 cup	308	1	0.0	36	63	4	1	11	0	29	4	239
whole wheat	1 cup	207	2	0.0	329	42	5	1	8	0	18	2	133
Pastina	1 cup	219	3	0.0	378	40	2	1	7	0	19	2	61
Pierogi, potato, frozen													
w/ cheese	3 (1.4 oz)	222	7	1.5	540	34	1	2	6	0	40	1	122
w/o cheese	3 (1.4 oz)	225	5	2.0	651	37	2	1	7	0	72	2	182
Ramen noodles w/ seasoning	1 cup	67	3	1.5	790	26	0	0	2	0	0	0	28
Ravioli w/o sauce													
beef	9 (2 in)	257	10	4.0	1053	24	1	0	17	0	43	3	193
cheese	9 (2 in)	232	8	4.0	875	29	1	0	10	0	132	2	165
Rice noodles	1 cup	187	0	0.0	438	42	2	0	3	0	7	0	7
Soba noodles	1 cup	113	0	0.0	68	24	1	1	6	0	5	1	40
Spaghetti	1 cup	207	2	0.0	329	42	5	1	8	0	18	2	133
Tortellini w/o sauce													
beef	1 cup	280	5	2.0	350	47	3	1	11	0	20	4	245
cheese	1 cup	354	8	4.0	234	54	2	1	16	0	166	1	32

* Cooked unless indicated.

PASTA, RICE & OTHER GRAINS

	Amount	Calories	Fat (g)	Saturated Fat (g)	Sodium (mg)	Carbohydrate (g)	Fiber (g)	Sugar (g)	Protein (g)	Vitamin D (mcg)	Calcium (mg)	Iron (mg)	Potassium (mg)
Rice													
Basmati	1 cup	204	0	0.0	387	44	1	0	4	0	16	2	55
Brown	1 cup	238	2	0.5	394	50	3	0	5	0	6	1	168
instant	1 cup	360	4	0.0	0	78	4	0	8	0	0	0	140
Pilaf	1 cup	280	6	1.0	853	50	1	1	7	0	60	2	115
Rice-A-Roni, chicken	1 cup	218	7	2.0	308	34	1	1	5	0	39	2	118
reduced sodium	1 cup	245	7	1.0	530	40	1	0	5	0	15	1	77
Risotto w/ cream sauce	1 cup	440	19	8.0	795	37	3	1	14	1	259	1	282
Spanish	1 cup	245	2	0.5	765	48	3	4	7	0	51	3	306
White	1 cup	204	0	0.0	387	44	1	0	4	0	16	2	55
instant	1 cup	340	0	0.0	0	76	0	0	8	0	0	2	30
Wild	1 cup	164	0	0.0	238	21	2	1	4	0	3	1	100
Other Grains													
Barley													
pearled	½ cup	97	0	0.0	2	22	3	0	2	0	9	3	280
whole	½ cup	104	0	0.0	159	24	3	0	2	0	9	1	79
Buckwheat/kasha	½ cup	78	0	0.0	123	17	2.5	1	3	0	6	1	75
Bulgur	½ cup	58	0	0.0	154	13	3	0	2	0	7	1	48
Millet	½ cup	101	1	0.0	143	1	1	0	3	0	3	1	53
Polenta													
fried, slice, w/ oil	1 (4 oz)	199	14	2.0	300	16	0	1	2	0	0	2	57
fried, slice, w/o oil	1 (4 oz)	80	0	0.0	300	16	0	1	2	0	0	2	57
w/ water	1 cup	140	0	0.0	0	32	4	1	3	0	10	2	50
Quinoa, dry	¼ cup	157	3	0.5	4	27	3	1	6	0	20	2	239
Semolina, dry	1 T	38	0	0.0	0	8	0	0	1	0	2	0	19

POULTRY

	Amount	Calories	Fat (g)	Saturated Fat (g)	Sodium (mg)	Carbohydrate (g)	Fiber (g)	Sugar (g)	Protein (g)	Vitamin D (mcg)	Calcium (mg)	Iron (mg)	Potassium (mg)
Chicken													
Breasts													
BBQ w/ skin	3 oz	149	7	2.0	280	0	0	0	22	0	14	0	235
breaded & fried w/ skin	3 oz	221	11	3.0	234	8	0	0	21	0	11	1	207
deli	1 oz	50	2	0.5	93	0	0	0	7	0	5	0	78
fried w/ skin & flour	3 oz	222	9	2.0	76	2	0	0	32	0	16	1	259
fried w/o skin	3 oz	188	4	1.0	435	9	0	0	28	0	19	1	345
roasted w/ skin	3 oz	197	8	2.0	60	0	0	0	30	0	14	1	245
roasted w/o skin	3 oz	165	4	1.0	63	0	0	0	31	0	15	1	256
Capon, roasted, w/ skin	3 oz	229	12	3.0	42	0	0	0	29	0	14	1	255
Cornish hens													
roasted w/ skin	3 oz	220	16	4.5	54	0	0	0	19	0	11	1	208
roasted w/o skin	3 oz	114	3	1.0	54	0	0	0	20	0	11	1	212
Giblets, fried	3 oz	277	13	4.0	96	4	0	0	33	0	18	10	330
Gizzards, simmered	3 oz	154	3	1.0	56	0	0	0	30	0	17	3	179
Hearts, simmered	3 oz	185	8	2.0	48	0	0	0	26	0	19	9	132

POULTRY

Chicken

	Amount	Calories	Fat (g)	Saturated Fat (g)	Sodium (mg)	Carbohydrate (g)	Fiber (g)	Sugar (g)	Protein (g)	Vitamin D (mcg)	Calcium (mg)	Iron (mg)	Potassium
Hot dogs, chicken	1 (1.6 oz)	134	10	2.0	519	2	0	1	7	0	89	1	223
Legs													
breaded & fried w/ skin	3 oz	273	16	4.0	237	9	0	0	22	0	18	1	189
fried w/ skin & flour	3 oz	254	14	4.0	75	3	0	0	27	0	13	1	233
fried w/o skin	3 oz	247	13	2.5	82	8	0	0	24	0	21	1	233
roasted w/ skin	3 oz	184	9	2.5	74	0	0	0	24	0	12	1	264
roasted w/o skin	3 oz	162	7	2.0	81	0	0	0	24	0	10	1	259
Livers, simmered	3 oz	167	7	2.0	76	1	0	0	24	0	11	12	263
Pâté, chicken liver, can	1 oz	201	13	4.0	109	7	0	0	13	0	10	9	95
Patties, breaded & fried	1 (3 oz)	220	9	2.0	300	16	1	1	18	0	0	1	222
Strips, breaded & fried	4 (1.6 oz)	511	28	5.5	1432	31	2	1	34	1	31	1	659
Thighs													
breaded & fried w/ skin	3 oz	277	17	4.5	288	9	1	0	22	0	18	1	192
fried w/ skin & flour	3 oz	262	15	4.0	88	3	0	0	27	0	14	1	237
fried w/o skin	3 oz	190	6	1.5	463	9	0	0	25	0	22	1	256
roasted w/ skin	3 oz	232	15	4.0	102	0	0	0	23	0	9	1	253
roasted w/o skin	3 oz	179	8	2.5	106	0	0	0	25	0	9	1	269
Wings													
fried w/ skin & flour	1 (1 oz)	321	22	6.0	22	2	0	0	7	0	15	1	177
roasted w/ skin	1 (1 oz)	254	17	5.0	98	0	0	0	23	0	18	1	212

Game

	Amount	Calories	Fat (g)	Saturated Fat (g)	Sodium (mg)	Carbohydrate (g)	Fiber (g)	Sugar (g)	Protein (g)	Vitamin D (mcg)	Calcium (mg)	Iron (mg)	Potassium
Duck, roasted													
w/ skin	3 oz	336	28	10.0	221	0	0	0	19	0	11	3	203
w/o skin	3 oz	200	11	4.0	227	0	0	0	23	0	12	3	251
Goose, roasted													
w/ skin	3 oz	305	21	7.0	70	0	0	0	25	0	13	3	329
w/o skin	3 oz	238	13	4.5	76	0	0	0	29	0	14	3	388
Ostrich													
ground	3 oz	165	9	2.0	72	0	0	0	20	0	7	3	291
tenderloin	3 oz	123	3	1.0	86	0	0	0	22	0	6	5	320
Pheasant, roasted													
w/ skin	3 oz	205	11	3.0	45	0	0	0	26	0	14	1	230
w/o skin	3 oz	151	4	1.5	42	0	0	0	27	0	3	0	223
Quail, roasted													
w/ skin	3 oz	218	14	4.0	60	0	0	0	22	0	13	4	183
w/o skin	3 oz	152	5	1.5	58	0	0	0	25	0	15	5	268

Turkey

	Amount	Calories	Fat (g)	Saturated Fat (g)	Sodium (mg)	Carbohydrate (g)	Fiber (g)	Sugar (g)	Protein (g)	Vitamin D (mcg)	Calcium (mg)	Iron (mg)	Potassium
Bacon	2 slices (1 oz)	104	7	2.0	573	1	0	1	8	0	46	1	189
Bologna	1 oz	59	4	1.0	300	1	0	1	3	0	34	1	38
Breast, deli	1 oz	100	2	0.5	922	0	0	2	16	0	7	0	401
Dark meat, roasted													
w/ skin	3 oz	206	10	3.0	105	0	0	0	27	0	17	1	228
w/o skin	3 oz	173	6	2.0	104	0	0	0	28	0	17	1	227

POULTRY

Turkey

	Amount	Calories	Fat (g)	Saturated Fat (g)	Sodium (mg)	Carbohydrate (g)	Fiber (g)	Sugar (g)	Protein (g)	Vitamin D (mcg)	Calcium (mg)	Iron (mg)	Potassium (mg)
Ground													
extra lean	3 oz	120	2	0.5	65	0	0	0	28	0	5	1	303
lean	3 oz	128	7	2.0	59	0	0	0	16	0	18	1	181
Ham, deli	1 oz	124	4	1.0	1038	3	0	0	20	0	5	1	299
Hot dogs	1 (1.6 oz)	140	12	0.0	560	1	0	1	7	0	89	1	223
Light meat, roasted													
w/ skin	3 oz	177	6	1.5	101	0	0	0	30	0	11	1	248
w/o skin	3 oz	147	2	0.5	99	0	0	0	30	0	9	1	249
Pastrami, deli	1 oz	41	2	1.0	302	1	0	0	6	0	3	1	59
Patties, breaded & fried	1 (3 oz)	241	15	4.0	680	13	0	0	12	0	13	2	259
Sausages	1 (2 oz)	93	6	1.5	470	0	0	0	11	0	11	0	103

RESTAURANT FAVORITES

Appetizers

	Amount	Calories	Fat (g)	Saturated Fat (g)	Sodium (mg)	Carbohydrate (g)	Fiber (g)	Sugar (g)	Protein (g)	Vitamin D (mcg)	Calcium (mg)	Iron (mg)	Potassium (mg)
Breadsticks	1 medium	147	6	1.5	264	19	1	0	5	0	37	2	57
Bruschetta	1 (4 in)	73	3	0.5	113	9	1	1	2	0	21	1	80
Buffalo wings	4	353	27	9.0	1044	4	0	3	25	0	38	1	310
Clams casino	6	211	9	2.0	587	18	2	4	35	0	16	2	286
Crab cakes, fried	1 (4 oz)	290	19	4.0	893	20	0	1	9	0	88	1	243
Focaccia bread	1 slice (6 in)	284	9	1.0	640	41	2	2	10	0	40	4	130
Garlic bread	1 slice (4 in)	136	6	2.0	242	16	0	1	3	0	10	1	40
Jalapeño poppers	6	360	22	10.0	810	32	3	6	7	1	186	3	349
Mozzarella sticks	4	572	32	12.0	1516	44	4	4	26	0	588	1	190
Mushrooms, fried	8	346	20	0.0	507	38	2	3	7	0	40	2	298
Nachos, deluxe	1 order	1133	66	19.0	1881	87	8	6	52	0	702	3	908
Oysters Rockefeller	6	186	10	4.5	624	13	3	2	11	0	152	5	364
Pork dumplings, fried	1 (3.5 oz)	263	17	4.0	463	22	1	6	7	0	31	3	214
Potato skins	6	416	26	9.0	876	34	3	2	13	0	296	1	792
Shrimp cocktail w/ sauce	5	141	2	0.5	585	12	1	5	2	0	80	1	251
Spring rolls w/ meat	1 (2.5 oz)	111	3	0.5	389	17	1	4	6	0	35	1	219
Stuffed mushrooms	3	211	11	3.0	480	20	2	3	4	1	8	2	292
Wontons w/ meat	1 (0.7 oz)	190	11	2.5	464	14	0	3	9	0	29	1	299

Desserts

	Amount	Calories	Fat (g)	Saturated Fat (g)	Sodium (mg)	Carbohydrate (g)	Fiber (g)	Sugar (g)	Protein (g)	Vitamin D (mcg)	Calcium (mg)	Iron (mg)	Potassium (mg)
Apple pie à la mode	1 (6 oz)	418	20	9.0	366	56	2	14	5	0	100	1	211
Caramel apple bars	1 (4 oz)	395	22	14.0	210	51	3	39	2	0	35	1	131
Carrot cake w/ icing	1 (4 oz)	428	27	9.0	234	46	2	34	4	0	33	1	122
Cheesecake	1 (3 oz)	321	23	10.0	438	26	0	22	6	1	51	1	90
Chocolate chip cookies	1 (2 oz)	419	19	6.0	290	65	2	32	3	0	13	3	106
Chocolate mousse cake	1 (3 oz)	299	20	10.0	130	30	2	21	3	0	60	1	110
Chocolate peanut butter pie	1 (6 oz)	650	49	25.0	330	43	3	30	9	0	40	2	118
Crème brûlée	¾ cup	215	5	3.0	146	35	0	35	8	2	227	0	295
Fortune cookies	1	30	0	0.0	2	7	0	4	0	0	1	0	3

RESTAURANT FAVORITES

Desserts	Amount	Calories	Fat (g)	Saturated Fat (g)	Sodium (mg)	Carbohydrate (g)	Fiber (g)	Sugar (g)	Protein (g)	Vitamin D (mcg)	Calcium (mg)	Iron (mg)	Potassium (mg)
Fudge brownie sundae	1 (8 oz)	706	42	23.0	229	84	4	65	8	0	193	1	485
Key lime pie	1 (4.5 oz)	352	17	13.0	242	45	1	34	5	0	138	1	188
Smoothie	1 (16 fl oz)	272	5	2.0	121	50	5	36	10	3	350	1	778
Tiramisu	1 (5 oz)	354	24	14.0	155	30	0	19	6	1	66	1	156

Entrées

American

	Amount	Calories	Fat (g)	Saturated Fat (g)	Sodium (mg)	Carbohydrate (g)	Fiber (g)	Sugar (g)	Protein (g)	Vitamin D (mcg)	Calcium (mg)	Iron (mg)	Potassium (mg)
Baked potato w/ broccoli & cheese	1 (11 oz)	444	20	12.0	734	56	6	3	13	0	227	3	1420
BBQ beef sandwich	1 (6.5 oz)	600	35	11.0	1310	50	2	20	26	0	200	4	601
BBQ pork sandwich	1 (6.5 oz)	209	4	1.0	582	30	1	16	12	0	57	1	244
BBQ ribs	8 oz	776	50	18.0	879	29	1	23	48	1	102	4	691
Chicken fried steak	8 oz	612	35	12.0	887	27	1	0	48	1	61	5	488
Eggs Benedict	2 eggs	878	67	35.0	1526	27	2	4	43	4	189	5	1014
Filet mignon	8 oz	734	56	22.0	129	0	0	0	54	1	20	7	749
Fried shrimp	12 large	432	24	4.0	914	22	1	2	31	1	161	2	289
Grilled salmon	8 oz	468	28	5.5	138	0	0	0	50	26	260	1	872
King crab legs	9 oz	248	4	0.0	2735	0	0	0	50	0	150	2	668
Lobster Newburg	2 cups	1186	98	54.0	2320	12	0	12	57	5	542	2	986
Prime rib	12 oz	1160	92	37.0	216	0	0	0	76	0	34	8	1100
Shrimp Creole w/ rice	2 cups	598	18	3.0	2120	58	4	5	50	0	374	8	554
Shrimp jambalaya	2 cups	768	36	9.0	2524	73	2	4	35	0	90	3	831
Stuffed shrimp	2 cups	488	25	6.0	1510	17	1	1	46	1	222	2	554
T-bone steak	10 oz	453	21	8.0	99	0	0	0	63	0	59	5	743
Turkey & cheese bagel	1 (11 oz)	478	14	7.0	1636	61	2	4	26	1	309	2	418

Asian

	Amount	Calories	Fat (g)	Saturated Fat (g)	Sodium (mg)	Carbohydrate (g)	Fiber (g)	Sugar (g)	Protein (g)	Vitamin D (mcg)	Calcium (mg)	Iron (mg)	Potassium (mg)
Beef & broccoli	2 cups	682	46	8.0	1906	23	6	6	46	0	148	5	1332
Cashew chicken	2 cups	947	48	9.0	1774	41	4	13	88	0	113	6	1689
Chicken curry	2 cups	508	31	7.5	1804	31	7	12	31	0	96	4	1344
Egg rolls, meatless	1 (2.5 oz)	172	9	1.5	296	19	2	4	4	0	30	1	134
Kung pao chicken	2 cups	418	23	4.0	1302	22	5	10	32	0	65	2	706
Pork chow mein w/ noodles	2 cups	630	28	9.0	1430	49	7	7	46	0	88	6	950
Shrimp & snow peas	2 cups	488	19	3.5	1223	19	4	6	60	0	243	5	1005
Stir-fry chicken & fried rice	2 cups	686	15	2.5	1422	109	4	2	29	0	48	2	396
Sushi w/ fish & vegetables	1 cup	140	1	0.0	642	28	2	3	4	0	9	0	71
Sushi rolls w/ rice													
fish	1 small	29	0	0.0	103	5	0	0	2	0	1	0	36
vegetarian	1 small	20	0	0.0	79	4	0	0	0	0	1	0	15
Sweet & sour pork w/ rice	2 cups	898	35	6.5	1634	96	4	36	49	1	137	5	1098
Tofu & vegetable stir-fry	2 cups	293	14	2.0	445	34	10	2	15	0	279	7	524

Italian/Mediterranean

	Amount	Calories	Fat (g)	Saturated Fat (g)	Sodium (mg)	Carbohydrate (g)	Fiber (g)	Sugar (g)	Protein (g)	Vitamin D (mcg)	Calcium (mg)	Iron (mg)	Potassium (mg)
Calzones w/ pepperoni	1 (6 oz)	1450	74	24.5	1840	131	6	3	62	1	746	10	670
Chicken cacciatore	2 cups	850	52	12.5	3240	34	5	8	64	0	204	5	1416

RESTAURANT FAVORITES

Entrées

	Amount	Calories	Fat (g)	Saturated Fat (g)	Sodium (mg)	Carbohydrate (g)	Fiber (g)	Sugar (g)	Protein (g)	Vitamin D (mcg)	Calcium (mg)	Iron (mg)	Potassium (mg)
Chicken cordon bleu	8 oz	229	10	3.5	478	10	1	1	25	0	95	1	299
Chicken Marsala	8 oz	346	15	4.0	1330	5	0	1	49	0	64	1	571
Chicken/veal parmigiana	8 oz	395	19	6.0	941	19	2	4	37	0	268	2	517
Fettuccini Alfredo	2 cups	1186	73	44.0	884	106	6	4	28	1	290	4	268
Gyros	½ pita	326	9	0.5	92	9	1	1	6	0	23	1	102
Linguini w/ pesto sauce	2 cups	735	57	9.0	771	43	4	2	17	0	207	4	329
Moussaka	2 cups	390	22	8.0	730	19	6	12	29	1	236	4	914
Pasta carbonara	2 cups	764	25	8.0	724	100	6	2	33	1	285	5	290
Pasta marinara	2 cups	520	6	1.0	1010	99	9	15	18	0	85	5	880
Seafood Alfredo	2 cups	1033	47	16.0	1399	104	4	17	45	2	180	3	307
Shrimp scampi	2 cups	538	33	5.0	262	5	0	0	53	2	224	2	430
Spanakopita	8 oz	305	23	7.0	573	17	2	2	8	1	200	3	344
Stuffed grape leaves	4	372	27	4.0	372	31	7	6	5	0	199	3	340
Veal scallopini	8 oz	670	49	13.5	1042	4	1	2	52	1	109	2	754
Vegetarian lasagna	2 cups	930	47	25.0	1916	73	6	12	56	1	1344	4	1030

Mexican & Tex-Mex

	Amount	Calories	Fat (g)	Saturated Fat (g)	Sodium (mg)	Carbohydrate (g)	Fiber (g)	Sugar (g)	Protein (g)	Vitamin D (mcg)	Calcium (mg)	Iron (mg)	Potassium (mg)
Chimichangas, beef & cheese	1 (6.5 oz)	454	21	7.0	1172	49	5	5	16	0	225	4	424
Enchiladas													
cheese	2 (6 in)	420	28	12.0	538	28	5	5	17	0	466	1	372
seafood	2 (6 in)	734	36	20.0	1174	56	3	9	38	0	500	4	576
Fajitas w/ tortillas													
chicken	1 (9 oz)	370	17	5.5	980	34	3	6	22	0	129	3	455
steak	1 (9 oz)	380	16	6.0	807	34	3	6	24	0	131	3	513
Huevos rancheros	1 order	280	15	4.0	988	21	4	5	16	2	113	3	516
Quesadillas	1 (2 oz)	486	25	11.5	959	46	3	4	18	0	453	3	155
Rice & beans	2 cups	558	14	2.0	786	86	13	1	22	0	184	9	1112

Salads*

	Amount	Calories	Fat (g)	Saturated Fat (g)	Sodium (mg)	Carbohydrate (g)	Fiber (g)	Sugar (g)	Protein (g)	Vitamin D (mcg)	Calcium (mg)	Iron (mg)	Potassium (mg)
Caesar	3 cups	481	40	8.0	1152	23	6	5	10	0	250	3	613
Chicken Caesar	4 cups	618	34	8.0	952	16	4	4	58	0	200	4	860
Greek	14 oz	448	38	14.0	925	19	4	11	13	0	325	2	595
Niçoise	12 oz	398	19	3.0	455	39	9	3	23	4	122	6	1277
Oriental chicken	9 oz	197	17	2.0	207	9	2	3	4	0	45	1	220
Tossed w/ gorgonzola	4 cups	398	29	6.0	325	33	4	26	7	0	138	1	293

Side Dishes

	Amount	Calories	Fat (g)	Saturated Fat (g)	Sodium (mg)	Carbohydrate (g)	Fiber (g)	Sugar (g)	Protein (g)	Vitamin D (mcg)	Calcium (mg)	Iron (mg)	Potassium (mg)
Garlic mashed potatoes	1 cup	252	10	6.0	1599	34	3	3	9	0	190	1	643
Grilled vegetables	1½ cups	78	5	0.5	84	8	2	0	1	0	21	0	398
Oven roasted potatoes	1½ cups	224	0	0.0	381	51	4	4	5	0	12	1	933
Polenta	½ cup	70	0	0.0	85	15	1	0	1	0	5	1	25
Ratatouille	1 cup	140	10	1.5	327	12	4	7	2	0	45	1	471
Risotto	½ cup	281	15	9.0	851	29	1	0	7	0	112	1	72
Soft pretzels	1 large	493	6	2.0	1110	99	2	0	12	0	33	5	123

* Dressing included.

RESTAURANT FAVORITES

Soups

	Amount	Calories	Fat (g)	Saturated Fat (g)	Sodium (mg)	Carbohydrate (g)	Fiber (g)	Sugar (g)	Protein (g)	Vitamin D (mcg)	Calcium (mg)	Iron (mg)	Potassium
Borscht	1 cup	93	4	2.5	348	11	2	7	3	0	56	1	299
Cheese	1 cup	166	7	5.0	926	20	3	11	5	1	201	0	241
Chicken chili	1 cup	143	2	0.0	578	18	5	3	15	0	50	2	417
Chilled fruit	1 cup	68	0	0.0	19	17	2	14	1	0	22	1	257
Clam chowder	1 cup	134	3	2.0	1000	19	3	4	7	0	67	3	384
Egg drop	1 cup	66	2	0.5	903	11	1	0	3	0	17	1	54
French onion	1 cup	369	16	7.5	1030	39	2	6	17	0	328	3	374
Gazpacho	1 cup	95	6	1.0	625	10	3	6	2	0	34	1	508
Hot & sour	1 cup	95	3	0.5	917	11	1	1	6	0	46	2	134
Minestrone	1 cup	143	3	0.5	611	23	4	3	8	0	63	3	479
Seafood stew	1 cup	225	9	2.0	506	5	1	1	31	7	75	2	638
Shrimp gumbo	1 cup	149	5	2.0	922	11	2	4	16	0	161	3	471
Tomato Florentine	1 cup	140	2	0.0	1600	26	2	9	5	0	100	2	504
Vichyssoise	1 cup	62	2	1.0	324	9	1	3	2	1	68	0	153
Wonton	1 cup	77	1	0.0	978	13	0	1	5	0	12	1	77

RESTAURANT & FAST FOOD CHAINS

A&W

Entrées

	Amount	Calories	Fat (g)	Saturated Fat (g)	Sodium (mg)	Carbohydrate (g)	Fiber (g)	Sugar (g)	Protein (g)	Vitamin D (mcg)	Calcium (mg)	Iron (mg)	Potassium
Burger patty	1	130	9	3.5	80	0	0	0	13	n/a	12	1	n/a
Cheeseburger	1	400	16	6.0	890	42	0	10	22	n/a	117	4	n/a
Chicken club sandwich													
hand-breaded	1	490	20	5.0	1390	42	0	7	36	n/a	103	3	n/a
grilled	1	470	17	4.0	1170	39	0	7	22	n/a	103	3	n/a
Chicken sandwich													
hand-breaded	1	440	15	2.5	1150	42	0	7	33	n/a	15	3	n/a
grilled	1	410	12	1.5	930	38	0	7	19	n/a	15	3	n/a
Chicken tenders													
freezer-to-fryer	3 pcs	370	18	2.5	1190	29	2	8	21	n/a	0	2	n/a
hand-breaded	3 pcs	260	9	2.5	1100	5	1	0	40	n/a	0	2	n/a
Coney cheese dog	1	360	22	8.0	1160	29	0	4	13	n/a	75	0	n/a
footlong	1	700	42	17.0	2230	54	2	7	26	n/a	125	2	n/a
Coney dog	1	320	19	7.0	960	26	0	4	12	n/a	61	0	n/a
footlong	1	630	37	15.0	1810	48	0	7	25	n/a	96	2	n/a
Corn dog nuggets	5 pcs	270	13	2.5	330	30	6	6	8	n/a	87	2	n/a
Crispy chicken club	1	540	25	5.0	1510	52	2	12	26	n/a	8	3	n/a
Fish sandwich	1	440	21	4.5	810	61	1	9	12	n/a	114	2	n/a
Hamburger	1	350	11	3.5	650	41	0	9	20	n/a	28	4	n/a
Hot dog	1	310	18	6.0	860	28	0	6	10	n/a	56	0	n/a
footlong	1	610	34	14.0	1610	52	1	12	21	n/a	96	2	n/a

RESTAURANT & FAST FOOD CHAINS

A&W

	Amount	Calories	Fat (g)	Saturated Fat (g)	Sodium (mg)	Carbohydrate (g)	Fiber (g)	Sugar (g)	Protein (g)	Vitamin D (mcg)	Calcium (mg)	Iron (mg)	Potassium (mg)
Mushroom onion melt													
burger	1	400	17	6.0	960	38	0	7	23	n/a	129	4	n/a
chicken, hand-breaded	1	430	14	4.0	1610	42	0	7	36	n/a	117	3	n/a
chicken, grilled	1	410	11	3.0	1300	38	0	7	23	n/a	117	3	n/a
Texas toast	1	380	18	6.0	1060	34	0	3	23	n/a	210	4	n/a
Original bacon cheeseburger	1	460	23	7.0	840	40	1	8	23	n/a	118	4	n/a
Papa Burger	1	450	22	7.0	890	42	1	10	22	n/a	118	4	n/a
Pork tenderloin sandwich	1	520	17	2.5	1180	65	3	7	21	n/a	44	4	n/a
Shrimp	16 pcs	480	26	6.0	1010	45	3	1	18	n/a	125	3	n/a
Sides													
Cheese curds	1 order	570	40	21.0	1220	27	2	3	27	n/a	80	10	n/a
Coleslaw	1 order	100	6	1.5	200	7	2	5	1	n/a	42	0	n/a
Fries	1 order	310	13	3.0	460	45	4	0	3	n/a	0	0	n/a
cheese	1 order	390	17	4.5	880	50	1	0	5	n/a	28	0	n/a
chili	1 order	380	16	4.5	840	49	1	2	7	n/a	15	1	n/a
chili cheese	1 order	410	18	5.0	1040	51	1	2	8	n/a	29	1	n/a
Mott's applesauce	1 order	70	0	0.0	5	18	1	17	0	n/a	0	0	n/a
Onion rings	1 order	280	4	0.0	930	53	2	5	6	n/a	0	6	n/a
Sauces													
BBQ	1 cup	40	0	0.0	370	10	0	9	0	n/a	0	0	n/a
Buttermilk ranch	1 cup	130	14	2.5	220	1	0	0.5	0	n/a	0	0	n/a
Honey mustard	1 cup	45	0	0.0	160	10	0	9	0	n/a	0	0	n/a
Spicy Papa	1 cup	130	12	2.0	340	6	0	5	0	n/a	0	0	n/a
Root Beer													
Diet	regular	0	0	0.0	180	0	0	0	0	n/a	0	0	n/a
Regular	regular	290	0	0.0	135	78	0	75	0	n/a	30	0	n/a
Sweets & Treats													
Cones													
chocolate	1 (5.5 oz)	290	7	4.5	210	51	0.5	40	6	n/a	223	0	n/a
root beer	1 (5.5 oz)	260	8	4.5	210	41	0	32	6	n/a	245	0	n/a
vanilla	1 (5.5 oz)	270	8	5.0	220	42	0	33	7	n/a	260	0	n/a
Floats													
orange	regular	330	5	3.0	1010	71	0	67	4	n/a	165	0	n/a
root beer	regular	340	5	3.0	190	68	0	66	4	n/a	165	0	n/a
diet	regular	160	5	3.0	200	24	0	21	4	n/a	165	0	n/a
Freezes													
orange	regular	500	12	7.0	1050	94	0	87	10	n/a	377	0	n/a
root beer	regular	520	12	7.0	350	92	0	86	10	n/a	377	0	n/a
diet	regular	360	12	7.0	360	54	0	48	0	n/a	377	0	n/a
Shakes													
chocolate	regular	770	23	14.0	540	129	0	109	17	n/a	615	0	n/a
strawberry	regular	730	22	14.0	510	115	0	98	16	n/a	615	0	n/a
vanilla	regular	690	22	14.0	510	110	0	94	16	n/a	615	0	n/a

RESTAURANT & FAST FOOD CHAINS

A&W	Amount	Calories	Fat (g)	Saturated Fat (g)	Sodium (mg)	Carbohydrate (g)	Fiber (g)	Sugar (g)	Protein (g)	Vitamin D (mcg)	Calcium (mg)	Iron (mg)	Potassium (mg)
Polar swirls													
cookie dough	regular	740	26	15.0	500	111	0	88	17	n/a	580	1	n/a
M&M's	regular	900	32	19.0	500	137	2	122	19	n/a	657	1	n/a
Oreo	regular	750	20	11.0	620	114	0	90	17	n/a	585	2	n/a
Reese's	regular	780	32	16.0	620	109	2	97	20	n/a	610	1	n/a
Sundaes													
chocolate	1	360	11	8.0	240	61	0	50	7	n/a	259	0	n/a
hot caramel	1	380	11	7.0	270	65	0	51	7	n/a	259	0	n/a
strawberry	1	340	11	7.0	220	54	0	44	7	n/a	259	1	n/a
Arby's													
Breakfast													
Bacon biscuit	1	340	17	10.0	1180	36	1	3	10	n/a	n/a	n/a	n/a
Bacon & cheese croissant	1	330	19	10.0	670	27	1	3	13	n/a	n/a	n/a	n/a
Bacon, egg & cheese													
biscuit	1	480	29	15.0	1720	38	1	5	18	n/a	n/a	n/a	n/a
croissant	1	440	27	13.0	1010	29	1	5	18	n/a	n/a	n/a	n/a
sourdough	1	490	23	8.0	1260	46	2	6	23	n/a	n/a	n/a	n/a
wrap	1	500	27	10.0	1370	42	4	5	20	n/a	n/a	n/a	n/a
Chicken biscuit	1	390	18	9.0	1250	44	2	2	13	n/a	n/a	n/a	n/a
Ham biscuit	1	340	16	9.0	1420	37	1	4	13	n/a	n/a	n/a	n/a
Ham & Swiss croissant	1	340	17	10.0	910	29	1	4	16	n/a	n/a	n/a	n/a
Ham, egg & cheese													
biscuit	1	470	25	12.0	1830	39	1	5	21	n/a	n/a	n/a	n/a
croissant	1	420	23	11.0	1120	30	1	5	21	n/a	n/a	n/a	n/a
sourdough	1	470	19	6.0	1370	47	2	6	26	n/a	n/a	n/a	n/a
wrap	1	440	22	8.0	1280	42	4	5	17	n/a	n/a	n/a	n/a
Sausage biscuit	1	500	33	15.0	1450	36	1	3	12	n/a	n/a	n/a	n/a
Sausage & cheese croissant	1	490	35	16.0	940	28	1	3	15	n/a	n/a	n/a	n/a
Sausage, egg & cheese													
biscuit	1	640	45	20.0	1990	39	1	5	20	n/a	n/a	n/a	n/a
croissant	1	590	44	19.0	1280	30	1	5	20	n/a	n/a	n/a	n/a
sourdough	1	640	39	13.0	1530	47	2	6	25	n/a	n/a	n/a	n/a
wrap	1	630	41	15.0	1550	42	4	5	20	n/a	n/a	n/a	n/a
Sausage gravy biscuit	1	480	28	13.0	1770	48	1	3	9	n/a	n/a	n/a	n/a
double	1	970	56	27.0	3540	96	3	5	18	n/a	n/a	n/a	n/a
French toast sticks	1 order	350	10	1.5	250	57	5	13	7	n/a	n/a	n/a	n/a
Platters													
bacon & egg w/ biscuit	1	590	32	13.0	1620	49	3	4	23	n/a	n/a	n/a	n/a
ham & egg w/ biscuit	1	570	29	12.0	1830	50	2	5	23	n/a	n/a	n/a	n/a
sausage & egg w/ biscuit	1	720	46	18.0	1860	50	3	4	22	n/a	n/a	n/a	n/a
Chicken													
Bacon & Swiss	1	610	30	9.0	1510	51	5	10	35	n/a	n/a	n/a	n/a
Buffalo	1	500	23	4.5	1860	49	4	7	24	n/a	n/a	n/a	n/a

RESTAURANT & FAST FOOD CHAINS

Arby's

	Amount	Calories	Fat (g)	Saturated Fat (g)	Sodium (mg)	Carbohydrate (g)	Fiber (g)	Sugar (g)	Protein (g)	Vitamin D (mcg)	Calcium (mg)	Iron (mg)	Potassium (mg)
Classic crispy	1	510	25	5.0	1230	48	4	7	24	n/a	n/a	n/a	n/a
Roasts	1	370	16	3.5	860	35	3	7	24	n/a	n/a	n/a	n/a
bacon & Swiss	1	480	21	8.0	1140	39	3	10	34	n/a	n/a	n/a	n/a
Buffalo	1	360	14	3.5	1490	36	3	7	24	n/a	n/a	n/a	n/a
Tenders	5 pcs	610	30	4.5	1990	47	3	0	39	n/a	n/a	n/a	n/a
dipping sauces													
Buffalo	1 pkt	10	1	0.0	720	2	0	0	0	n/a	n/a	n/a	n/a
honey mustard	1 pkt	140	13	2.0	130	5	0	4	0	n/a	n/a	n/a	n/a
ranch	1 pkt	100	11	2.5	190	2	0	1	1	n/a	n/a	n/a	n/a
tangy barbeque	1 pkt	40	0	0.0	350	9	0	8	0	n/a	n/a	n/a	n/a
Roast Beef													
Beef 'n Cheddar	1	450	20	6.0	1280	45	2	9	23	n/a	n/a	n/a	n/a
double	1	630	32	11.0	2100	48	2	9	39	n/a	n/a	n/a	n/a
half pound	1	740	39	14.0	2530	48	2	9	49	n/a	n/a	n/a	n/a
Fire-Roasted Philly	1	630	35	13.0	1890	45	3	3	34	n/a	n/a	n/a	n/a
French dip & Swiss/au jus	1	540	22	10.0	2550	51	2	3	34	n/a	n/a	n/a	n/a
half pound	1	740	35	16.0	3400	52	2	3	55	n/a	n/a	n/a	n/a
Roast beef	1	360	14	5.0	970	37	2	5	23	n/a	n/a	n/a	n/a
double	1	510	24	9.0	1610	38	2	5	23	n/a	n/a	n/a	n/a
half pound	1	610	30	12.0	2040	38	2	5	48	n/a	n/a	n/a	n/a
three cheese	1	700	43	17.0	1870	42	3	6	38	n/a	n/a	n/a	n/a
Sauces													
Arby's	1 pkt	15	0	0.0	180	3	0	2	0	n/a	n/a	n/a	n/a
Horsey	1 pkt	60	5	1.0	150	3	0	2	0	n/a	n/a	n/a	n/a
Signature													
Gyros													
roast beef	1	550	29	7.0	1290	48	3	5	24	n/a	n/a	n/a	n/a
traditional Greek	1	710	44	13.0	1360	55	4	6	23	n/a	n/a	n/a	n/a
turkey	1	470	20	3.5	1520	48	3	5	25	n/a	n/a	n/a	n/a
Sandwiches													
loaded Italian	1	680	40	14.0	2270	49	3	7	32	n/a	n/a	n/a	n/a
reuben	1	680	31	8.0	2420	62	4	5	37	n/a	n/a	n/a	n/a
Smokehouse brisket	1	600	35	12.0	1240	42	2	7	33	n/a	n/a	n/a	n/a
Turkey													
Grand turkey club	1	480	24	7.0	1610	37	2	9	30	n/a	n/a	n/a	n/a
Roast turkey													
ranch & bacon													
sandwich	1	800	34	10.0	2420	79	5	16	45	n/a	n/a	n/a	n/a
wrap	1	620	34	11.0	2130	39	4	6	37	n/a	n/a	n/a	n/a
ranch & Swiss													
sandwich	1	710	28	7.0	1930	79	5	15	38	n/a	n/a	n/a	n/a
wrap	1	520	27	9.0	1640	39	4	6	30	n/a	n/a	n/a	n/a

Arby's

	Amount	Calories	Fat (g)	Saturated Fat (g)	Sodium (mg)	Carbohydrate (g)	Fiber (g)	Sugar (g)	Protein (g)	Vitamin D (mcg)	Calcium (mg)	Iron (mg)	Potassium
Salads													
Chopped farmhouse													
crispy chicken	1	430	25	8.0	1170	27	4	4	28	n/a	n/a	n/a	n/a
roast chicken	1	250	14	7.0	690	8	3	4	25	n/a	n/a	n/a	n/a
roast turkey	1	230	24	8.0	870	8	2	5	22	n/a	n/a	n/a	n/a
Chopped side	1	70	5	2.5	100	4	1	2	5	n/a	n/a	n/a	n/a
Dressing													
balsamic vinaigrette	1 pkt	130	12	2.0	470	4	0	4	0	n/a	n/a	n/a	n/a
buttermilk ranch	1 pkt	210	22	3.5	330	2	0	1	0	n/a	n/a	n/a	n/a
Dijon honey mustard	1 pkt	180	16	2.5	230	8	0	7	0	n/a	n/a	n/a	n/a
light Italian	1 pkt	20	1	0.0	720	2	0	2	0	n/a	n/a	n/a	n/a
Sides													
Curly fries	medium	550	29	4.0	1250	65	6	0	6	n/a	n/a	n/a	n/a
loaded	1 order	700	46	9.0	1990	57	5	2	14	n/a	n/a	n/a	n/a
add ketchup	1 pkt	10	0	0.0	85	3	0	2	0	n/a	n/a	n/a	n/a
Jalapeño bites	8 pcs	470	27	10.0	1060	50	3	4	8	n/a	n/a	n/a	n/a
add Bronco Berry Sauce	1 pkt	60	0	0.0	25	15	0	15	0	n/a	n/a	n/a	n/a
Mozzarella sticks	6 pcs	650	35	14.0	2110	56	3	4	29	n/a	n/a	n/a	n/a
add marinara sauce	1 pkt	20	0	0.0	170	4	1	3	1	n/a	n/a	n/a	n/a
Potato cakes	3	370	21	3.0	650	35	4	0	3	n/a	n/a	n/a	n/a
Steakhouse onion rings	5 pcs	420	21	3.0	1740	52	3	4	6	n/a	n/a	n/a	n/a
Sliders													
Buffalo chicken	1	300	14	2.0	940	31	1	2	12	n/a	n/a	n/a	n/a
Chicken tender 'n cheese	1	290	12	3.5	720	30	1	1	15	n/a	n/a	n/a	n/a
Ham 'n cheese	1	230	9	3.5	750	22	1	3	13	n/a	n/a	n/a	n/a
Jalapeño roast beef 'n cheese	1	240	11	4.5	670	21	1	1	14	n/a	n/a	n/a	n/a
Pizza	1	300	17	6.0	930	23	1	2	13	n/a	n/a	n/a	n/a
Roast beef 'n cheese	1	240	11	4.5	670	21	1	1	14	n/a	n/a	n/a	n/a
Turkey 'n cheese	1	200	7	2.5	760	21	1	2	14	n/a	n/a	n/a	n/a
Desserts													
Salted caramel & chocolate cookie	1	430	18	10.0	360	63	1	33	4	n/a	n/a	n/a	n/a
Shakes													
Jamocha handcrafted chocolate	medium	750	23	15.0	550	124	1	112	18	n/a	n/a	n/a	n/a
orange cream	medium	750	22	15.0	490	124	1	103	18	n/a	n/a	n/a	n/a
ultimate chocolate	medium	760	24	15.0	540	126	2	111	18	n/a	n/a	n/a	n/a
vanilla handcrafted	medium	630	23	15.0	480	95	1	88	18	n/a	n/a	n/a	n/a
Triple chocolate cookie	1	450	21	13.0	370	60	2	31	5	n/a	n/a	n/a	n/a
Turnovers													
apple	1	430	18	9.0	210	65	2	39	4	n/a	n/a	n/a	n/a
cherry	1	390	13	6.0	200	65	2	40	4	n/a	n/a	n/a	n/a

RESTAURANT & FAST FOOD CHAINS

	Amount	Calories	Fat (g)	Saturated Fat (g)	Sodium (mg)	Carbohydrate (g)	Fiber (g)	Sugar (g)	Protein (g)	Vitamin D (mcg)	Calcium (mg)	Iron (mg)	Potassium (mg)
Meals (w/o sides or bread)													
Dark chicken (2 drumsticks, 1 thigh)													
creamy garlic	1 order	350	20	7.0	1120	5	0	2	39	n/a	130	3	n/a
honey balsamic basil	1 order	460	30	6.0	850	11	0	7	38	n/a	104	2	n/a
Parmesan rotisserie	1 order	400	21	7.0	1340	12	0	2	41	n/a	130	1	n/a
roasted garlic	1 order	450	27	12.0	1330	13	0	2	40	n/a	130	2	n/a
rotisserie	1 order	300	16	5.0	780	0	0	0	37	n/a	52	1	n/a
sesame	1 order	430	23	6.0	1230	18	0	0	38	n/a	78	2	n/a
Meatloaf	1 order	470	33	14.0	910	17	2	5	26	n/a	52	3	n/a
Quarter white chicken													
creamy garlic	1 order	320	14	5.0	930	5	0	1	45	n/a	130	1	n/a
honey balsamic basil	1 order	430	24	4.5	660	11	0	7	44	n/a	104	2	n/a
Parmesan rotisserie	1 order	370	15	6.0	1150	12	0	2	46	n/a	130	1	n/a
roasted garlic	1 order	420	22	10.0	1140	12	0	2	45	n/a	78	1	n/a
rotisserie	1 order	270	11	3.5	590	0	0	0	43	n/a	52	1	n/a
skinless	1 order	210	5	1.5	480	1	0	1	40	n/a	52	1	n/a
sesame	1 order	400	17	4.0	1040	18	0	3	43	n/a	78	1	n/a
Rotisserie chicken pot pie	1 order	750	42	19.0	1780	64	3	10	28	n/a	195	5	n/a
Rotisserie prime rib	1 order	630	47	12.0	770	0	1	1	55	n/a	26	12	n/a
Turkey breast	1 order	160	5	2.0	440	0	0	0	30	n/a	26	2	n/a
Turkey pot pie	1 order	710	38	18.0	1670	64	3	10	28	n/a	130	4	n/a
Market Bowls													
BBQ chicken	1 order	580	21	8.0	1290	76	6	17	20	n/a	52	3	n/a
Cheeseburger mac & cheese	1 order	510	23	12.0	1790	54	2	20	22	n/a	520	2	n/a
Home style meatloaf	1 order	680	36	14.0	1460	61	7	17	25	n/a	104	5	n/a
Rotisserie chicken	1 order	510	18	7.0	1020	51	8	10	34	n/a	26	5	n/a
Rotisserie turkey breast	1 order	330	13	2.5	870	28	0	5	25	n/a	78	3	n/a
Southwest chicken & cilantro lime rice	1 order	520	15	2.5	790	58	1	3	26	n/a	130	5	n/a
Vegetarian	1 order	470	14	5.0	640	64	4	5	9	n/a	195	3	n/a
Ribs													
½ order baby back ribs	1 order	1020	60	21.0	2170	260	0	29	70	n/a	130	5	n/a
w/ ¼ rotisserie chicken	1 order	1280	71	24.0	2760	51	0	29	113	n/a	195	6	n/a
Full order baby back ribs	1 order	1870	117	40.0	4130	70	0	46	138	n/a	195	6	n/a
Sandwiches													
Chicken avocado club	1	1110	66	19.0	2130	75	7	4	56	n/a	390	6	n/a
Chicken salad carver	1	870	51	10.0	1430	63	7	5	38	n/a	130	5	n/a

RESTAURANT & FAST FOOD CHAINS

	Amount	Calories	Fat (g)	Saturated Fat (g)	Sodium (mg)	Carbohydrate (g)	Fiber (g)	Sugar (g)	Protein (g)	Vitamin D (mcg)	Calcium (mg)	Iron (mg)	Potassium
Boston Market													
Roasted turkey carver	1	970	55	16.0	1930	73	5	4	46	n/a	390	6	n/a
Rotisserie chicken carver	1	980	53	15.0	1880	73	5	4	52	n/a	390	6	n/a
Southwest chicken carver	1	1110	65	19.0	2330	76	7	5	17	n/a	390	5	n/a
Salads & Soups													
Southwest Cobb	1	760	53	10.0	1390	30	8	10	43	n/a	130	5	n/a
Caesar side salad	1	310	24	6.0	870	16	2	3	9	n/a	260	2	n/a
House side salad	1	200	16	3.0	350	10	2	3	4	n/a	104	1	n/a
Chicken noodle soup	1	240	9	3.0	1100	20	2	3	16	n/a	26	2	n/a
Sides													
Bacon brussels sprouts	1 order	240	15	2.5	530	20	6	6	7	n/a	52	1	n/a
Cinnamon apples	1 order	250	4	5.0	270	55	4	49	0	n/a	26	1	n/a
Cornbread	1 order	160	3	1.5	220	31	0	12	2	n/a	26	1	n/a
Creamed spinach	1 order	240	17	11.0	640	12	3	3	11	n/a	325	4	n/a
Fresh steamed vegetables	1 order	60	4	0.0	40	7	3	3	2	n/a	52	1	n/a
Fresh vegetable stuffing	1 order	220	10	1.0	520	28	1	5	4	n/a	52	2	n/a
Garlic dill new potatoes	1 order	100	2	0.5	75	20	2	2	2	n/a	26	1	n/a
Macaroni & cheese	1 order	310	10	6.0	1270	41	1	10	14	n/a	325	2	n/a
Mashed potatoes	1 order	270	11	5.0	620	37	4	2	5	n/a	26	2	n/a
Steamed broccoli	1 order	60	4	0.0	260	6	4	2	4	n/a	52	1	n/a
Sweet corn	1 order	160	7	2.0	135	20	5	10	3	n/a	0	1	n/a
Sweet potato casserole	1 order	460	12	3.0	220	87	4	56	3	n/a	52	2	n/a
Sauces													
Beef gravy	1 order	10	0	0.0	180	2	0	0	0	n/a	0	0	n/a
Cranberry walnut relish	1 order	140	2	0.0	5	31	2	27	1	n/a	260	1	n/a
Horseradish	1 order	60	3	0.0	115	6	0	0	0	n/a	0	0	n/a
Zesty barbecue, mild	1 order	40	0	0.0	230	10	0	9	0	n/a	0	0	n/a
Desserts													
Cake													
carrot	1 slice	730	35	13.0	520	99	1	79	5	n/a	52	1	n/a
chocolate	1 slice	570	33	11.0	360	66	3	46	5	n/a	52	1	n/a
Chocolate chip fudge brownie	1	340	14	3.5	180	53	3	39	5	n/a	26	4	n/a
Chocolate chunk cookie	1	370	18	9.0	200	53	2	32	4	n/a	26	4	n/a
Pie													
apple	1 slice	560	32	15.0	290	66	3	47	4	n/a	26	2	n/a
pecan	1 slice	720	42	15.0	550	80	2	76	7	n/a	26	3	n/a
Burger King													
Breakfast													
Bacon, egg & cheese													
biscuit	1	400	26	13.0	1270	29	1	3	13	n/a	n/a	n/a	n/a
Croissan'wich	1	370	21	9.0	760	30	1	4	14	n/a	n/a	n/a	n/a

Burger King	Amount	Calories	Fat (g)	Saturated Fat (g)	Sodium (mg)	Carbohydrate (g)	Fiber (g)	Sugar (g)	Protein (g)	Vitamin D (mcg)	Calcium (mg)	Iron (mg)	Potassium (mg)
Egg & cheese Croissan'wich	1	340	18	8.0	610	29	1	4	12	n/a	n/a	n/a	n/a
Egg-Normous burrito	1	780	42	15.0	1960	68	3	4	32	n/a	n/a	n/a	n/a
French toast sticks	5 pcs	380	18	3.0	430	49	2	13	5	n/a	n/a	n/a	n/a
Fully loaded													
biscuit	1	640	45	20.0	2190	31	1	4	28	n/a	n/a	n/a	n/a
Croissan'wich	1	610	40	17.0	1680	31	1	5	28	n/a	n/a	n/a	n/a
Ham, egg & cheese													
biscuit	1	400	24	12.0	1550	29	1	3	17	n/a	n/a	n/a	n/a
Croissan'wich	1	370	19	8.0	1030	30	1	5	17	n/a	n/a	n/a	n/a
Ham & sausage Croissan'wich	1	580	38	16.0	1530	31	1	5	27	n/a	n/a	n/a	n/a
Hash browns	medium	500	33	7.0	1140	48	7	0	4	n/a	n/a	n/a	n/a
Sausage													
biscuit	1	420	28	6.0	1050	28	1	2	12	n/a	n/a	n/a	n/a
Croissan'wich	1	710	52	20.0	1420	31	1	5	29	n/a	n/a	n/a	n/a
Platters													
BK Ultimate Breakfast	1	930	44	11.0	2230	110	4	40	24	n/a	n/a	n/a	n/a
pancake & sausage	1	610	31	9.0	1010	72	1	30	12	n/a	n/a	n/a	n/a
Sausage, egg & cheese													
biscuit	1	530	38	17.0	1440	29	1	3	19	n/a	n/a	n/a	n/a
Croissan'wich	1	500	33	13.0	930	30	1	4	19	n/a	n/a	n/a	n/a
Sausage & bacon double Croissan'wich	1	580	40	16.0	1260	31	1	5	23	n/a	n/a	n/a	n/a
Burgers													
Bacon King	1	1150	79	31.0	2150	49	2	10	61	n/a	n/a	n/a	n/a
cheddar	1	1190	84	33.0	1930	50	2	11	64	n/a	n/a	n/a	n/a
Cheeseburger	1	280	13	6.0	560	27	1	7	15	n/a	n/a	n/a	n/a
bacon	1	320	16	7.0	710	27	1	7	17	n/a	n/a	n/a	n/a
bacon double	1	420	24	10.0	740	27	1	7	25				
double	1	390	21	9.0	590	27	1	7	23	n/a	n/a	n/a	n/a
extra long	1	630	37	14.0	1050	45	2	9	29	n/a	n/a	n/a	n/a
Hamburger	1	240	10	3.5	380	26	1	6	13	n/a	n/a	n/a	n/a
double	1	350	18	7.0	410	26	1	6	21	n/a	n/a	n/a	n/a
King													
single quarter pound	1	580	29	13.0	1310	49	2	10	32	n/a	n/a	n/a	n/a
double quarter pound	1	900	54	25.0	1740	50	2	11	56	n/a	n/a	n/a	n/a
Stacker King													
single	1	700	42	16.0	1360	48	1	10	35	n/a	n/a	n/a	n/a
double	1	1050	68	28.0	1870	49	1	11	61	n/a	n/a	n/a	n/a
Chicken & More													
Big Fish sandwich	1	510	28	4.5	1180	51	2	7	16	n/a	n/a	n/a	n/a
Chicken fries	9 pcs	280	17	2.5	850	20	1	1	13	n/a	n/a	n/a	n/a
Chicken nuggets	10 pcs	430	27	4.5	780	27	2	0	20	n/a	n/a	n/a	n/a
spicy	10 pcs	530	37	7.0	1420	28	4	1	20	n/a	n/a	n/a	n/a

RESTAURANT & FAST FOOD CHAINS

	Amount	Calories	Fat (g)	Saturated Fat (g)	Sodium (mg)	Carbohydrate (g)	Fiber (g)	Sugar (g)	Protein (g)	Vitamin D (mcg)	Calcium (mcg)	Iron (mg)	Potassium
Chicken sandwich	1	660	40	7.0	1170	48	2	5	28	n/a	n/a	n/a	n/a
bacon & cheese crispy	1	800	52	13.0	1650	55	2	8	30	n/a	n/a	n/a	n/a
BBQ bacon crispy	1	790	49	10.0	1630	60	2	13	28	n/a	n/a	n/a	n/a
crispy	1	670	41	7.0	1080	54	2	8	23	n/a	n/a	n/a	n/a
spicy crispy	1	700	42	7.0	1140	57	3	8	25	n/a	n/a	n/a	n/a
Crispy taco	1	170	9	3.0	410	19	2	1	5	n/a	n/a	n/a	n/a
Whopper Sandwiches													
Impossible Whopper	1	630	34	11.0	1080	58	4	12	25	n/a	n/a	n/a	n/a
Whopper	1	660	40	12.0	980	49	2	11	28	n/a	n/a	n/a	n/a
bacon & cheese	1	790	51	17.0	1560	50	2	11	35	n/a	n/a	n/a	n/a
cheese	1	740	46	21.0	50	50	2	11	32	n/a	n/a	n/a	n/a
double	1	900	58	20.0	1050	49	2	11	48	n/a	n/a	n/a	n/a
double cheese	1	980	64	24.0	1410	50	2	11	52	n/a	n/a	n/a	n/a
triple	1	1130	75	28.0	1120	49	2	11	67	n/a	n/a	n/a	n/a
triple cheese	1	1220	82	32.0	1470	50	2	11	71	n/a	n/a	n/a	n/a
Salads & Dressing													
Club salad w/ crispy chicken	1	540	33	10.0	1380	31	3	5	25	n/a	n/a	n/a	n/a
Garden chicken salad w/ crispy chicken	1	440	25	7.0	930	31	3	4	25	n/a	n/a	n/a	n/a
Garden side salad	1	60	4	2.5	95	3	1	2	4	n/a	n/a	n/a	n/a
Buttery garlic croutons	1 pkt	60	3	0.0	180	9	0	1	1	n/a	n/a	n/a	n/a
Ken's dressing													
golden Italian	1 pkt	160	17	2.5	380	4	0	3	0	n/a	n/a	n/a	n/a
lite balsamic vinaigrette	1 pkt	120	8	1.0	220	14	0	11	0	n/a	n/a	n/a	n/a
ranch	1 pkt	260	28	4.0	240	2	0	2	1	n/a	n/a	n/a	n/a
Sides													
French fries, unsalted	medium	380	16	2.0	360	58	6	1	4	n/a	n/a	n/a	n/a
Onion rings	medium	410	21	3.5	1080	53	4	5	4	n/a	n/a	n/a	n/a
Desserts													
Chocolate chip cookie	1	160	8	4.0	125	24	1	15	2	n/a	n/a	n/a	n/a
Oreo cookie cheesecake	1 order	350	18	8.0	310	41	1	25	6	n/a	n/a	n/a	n/a
Pies													
Hershey's sundae	1 order	310	19	12.0	220	32	1	22	3	n/a	n/a	n/a	n/a
Twix	1 order	370	20	13.0	330	45	1	30	4	n/a	n/a	n/a	n/a
Soft serve													
cone	1	190	5	3.0	150	32	0	24	5	n/a	n/a	n/a	n/a
cup	1	170	5	3.0	150	28	0	24	5	n/a	n/a	n/a	n/a
Sundaes													
caramel	1	240	5	3.5	210	42	0	33	5	n/a	n/a	n/a	n/a
Hershey's chocolate	1	260	5	3.0	160	49	1	43	5	n/a	n/a	n/a	n/a

RESTAURANT & FAST FOOD CHAINS

Chick-fil-A

	Amount	Calories	Fat (g)	Saturated Fat (g)	Sodium (mg)	Carbohydrate (g)	Fiber (g)	Sugar (g)	Protein (g)	Vitamin D (mcg)	Calcium (mg)	Iron (mg)	Potassium (mg)
Breakfast													
Bacon, egg & cheese													
biscuit	1	420	23	11.0	1290	38	2	4	15	n/a	n/a	n/a	n/a
muffin	1	310	14	6.0	810	29	1	2	16	n/a	n/a	n/a	n/a
Buttered biscuit	1	290	15	6.0	760	37	2	4	4	n/a	n/a	n/a	n/a
Chicken biscuit	1	460	23	8.0	1510	45	2	6	19	n/a	n/a	n/a	n/a
Chik-n-Minis	4 pcs	360	13	4.0	1050	41	2	8	19	n/a	n/a	n/a	n/a
Egg white grill	1	290	8	3.5	980	30	1	2	26	n/a	n/a	n/a	n/a
English muffin	1	140	2	0.0	220	29	0	1	5	n/a	n/a	n/a	n/a
Greek yogurt parfait													
cookie crumbles	1	240	8	3.5	85	33	1	26	12	n/a	n/a	n/a	n/a
granola	1	270	9	3.5	80	36	1	26	12	n/a	n/a	n/a	n/a
Hash brown scramble													
bowl	1	470	30	9.0	1340	19	2	2	29	n/a	n/a	n/a	n/a
burrito	1	700	40	12.0	1750	51	3	2	34	n/a	n/a	n/a	n/a
Hash browns	1 order	270	18	2.5	440	23	3	0	3	n/a	n/a	n/a	n/a
Sausage, egg & cheese													
biscuit	1	610	42	18.0	1510	38	2	4	22	n/a	n/a	n/a	n/a
muffin	1	500	33	12.0	1030	30	1	2	23	n/a	n/a	n/a	n/a
Entrées													
Chick-n-Strips	3 pcs	310	14	2.5	870	16	0	2	29	n/a	n/a	n/a	n/a
Chicken sandwich	1	440	17	4.0	1400	41	1	6	29	n/a	n/a	n/a	n/a
deluxe w/ American cheese	1	500	22	7.0	1640	44	2	7	32	n/a	n/a	n/a	n/a
grilled	1	320	6	1.0	680	41	4	9	28	n/a	n/a	n/a	n/a
spicy	1	460	19	4.0	1670	45	2	6	28	n/a	n/a	n/a	n/a
spicy deluxe w/ pepper Jack cheese	1	550	25	8.0	1810	47	3	7	33	n/a	n/a	n/a	n/a
Cool Wrap	1	350	13	4.0	900	29	13	2	42	n/a	n/a	n/a	n/a
Grilled chicken club sandwich	520	22	8.0	1115	44	4	11	37	n/a	n/a	n/a	n/a	
w/ Colby Jack cheese	1												
Nuggets	8 pcs	250	11	2.5	1210	11	0	1	27	n/a	n/a	n/a	n/a
grilled	8 pcs	130	3	0.5	440	1	0	1	25	n/a	n/a	n/a	n/a
Salads (w/ dressing)													
Cobb w/ nuggets	1	850	61	13.0	2220	34	5	9	42	n/a	n/a	n/a	n/a
Lemon kale Caesar w/ grilled nuggets	1	470	24	6.5	1290	22	4	8	43	n/a	n/a	n/a	n/a
Market w/ grilled filet	1	540	31	6.0	1020	41	4	26	28	n/a	n/a	n/a	n/a
Spicy southwest w/ spicy grilled filet	1	690	49	10.0	1570	29	8	8	33	n/a	n/a	n/a	n/a
Sides													
Buddy Fruits applesauce	1 pkt	45	0	0.0	0	12	1	8	0	n/a	n/a	n/a	n/a
Chicken noodle soup	1 cup	255	6	2.0	1970	34	3	2	16	n/a	n/a	n/a	n/a
Fruit cup	medium	60	0	0.0	0	15	2	11	1	n/a	n/a	n/a	n/a
Kale crunch	1	120	9	1.0	140	8	1	3	3	n/a	n/a	n/a	n/a

RESTAURANT & FAST FOOD CHAINS

Chick-fil-A	Amount	Calories	Fat (g)	Saturated Fat (g)	Sodium (mg)	Carbohydrate (g)	Fiber (g)	Sugar (g)	Protein (g)	Vitamin D (mcg)	Calcium (mg)	Iron (mg)	Potassium (mg)
Macaroni & cheese	medium	450	29	16.0	1190	28	3	3	20	n/a	n/a	n/a	n/a
Side salad w/ avocado lime ranch dressing	1	470	42	8.0	690	16	4	5	7	n/a	n/a	n/a	n/a
Waffle potato chips	1 pkt	220	13	3.5	250	25	2	0	3	n/a	n/a	n/a	n/a
Waffle potato fries	medium	420	24	4.0	240	45	5	1	5	n/a	n/a	n/a	n/a
Drinks													
Lemonade	medium	220	0	0.0	10	58	0	55	0	n/a	n/a	n/a	n/a
diet	medium	50	0	0.0	10	14	0	10	0	n/a	n/a	n/a	n/a
Treats													
Chocolate chunk cookie	1	370	17	9.0	230	49	3	26	5	n/a	n/a	n/a	n/a
Chocolate fudge brownie	1	380	21	2.0	150	48	2	36	4	n/a	n/a	n/a	n/a
Frosted coffee	1	250	6	4.0	120	43	0	39	6	n/a	n/a	n/a	n/a
Frosted lemonade	1	330	6	4.0	120	65	0	63	6	n/a	n/a	n/a	n/a
Icedream cone	1	180	4	2.5	90	32	0	25	4	n/a	n/a	n/a	n/a
Milkshakes													
chocolate	1	590	22	14.0	350	90	0	87	12	n/a	n/a	n/a	n/a
cookies & cream	1	630	25	1.0	410	90	0	84	13	n/a	n/a	n/a	n/a
strawberry	1	570	19	12.0	380	93	0	87	11	n/a	n/a	n/a	n/a
vanilla	1	580	23	15.0	380	82	0	80	13	n/a	n/a	n/a	n/a
Chili's													
Appetizers													
Awesome Blossom Petals	1 order	760	50	8.0	1650	70	5	10	9	n/a	n/a	n/a	n/a
Bone-in wings													
Buffalo	1 order	890	65	11.0	2800	4	1	2	73	n/a	n/a	n/a	n/a
honey chipotle	1 order	1060	54	9.0	2460	74	1	53	73	n/a	n/a	n/a	n/a
house BBQ	1 order	860	55	10.0	2240	19	1	16	74	n/a	n/a	n/a	n/a
mango habanero	1 order	900	54	9.0	2630	30	2	25	74	n/a	n/a	n/a	n/a
Boneless wings													
Buffalo	1 order	1060	71	12.0	3840	58	4	2	49	n/a	n/a	n/a	n/a
honey chipotle	1 order	1200	57	10.0	2990	126	4	53	48	n/a	n/a	n/a	n/a
house BBQ	1 order	1100	60	10.0	3610	89	5	30	50	n/a	n/a	n/a	n/a
mango habanero	1 order	1060	58	10.0	3210	84	5	25	50	n/a	n/a	n/a	n/a
Chips w/ salsa	1 order	910	45	7.0	1920	113	8	5	13	n/a	n/a	n/a	n/a
add fresh guacamole	1 order	230	21	3.0	430	14	10	2	3	n/a	n/a	n/a	n/a
add house-made ranch	1 order	450	47	8.0	810	6	0	4	3	n/a	n/a	n/a	n/a
add skillet queso	1 order	420	31	14.0	1810	13	2	10	21	n/a	n/a	n/a	n/a
add white spinach queso	1 order	520	42	21.0	1190	14	4	5	24	n/a	n/a	n/a	n/a
Chips w/ guacamole & salsa	1 order	1140	66	10.0	2350	128	18	7	16	n/a	n/a	n/a	n/a
Classic nachos	1 order	1010	67	34.0	2360	55	6	8	48	n/a	n/a	n/a	n/a
beef	1 order	1390	87	40.0	3810	55	6	8	99	n/a	n/a	n/a	n/a
chicken	1 order	1170	70	35.0	3400	57	6	9	79	n/a	n/a	n/a	n/a

RESTAURANT & FAST FOOD CHAINS

Chili's

	Amount	Calories	Fat (g)	Saturated Fat (g)	Sodium (mg)	Carbohydrate (g)	Fiber (g)	Sugar (g)	Protein (g)	Vitamin D (mcg)	Calcium (mg)	Iron (mg)	Potassium (mg)
Crispy cheddar bites	1 order	990	77	32.0	2530	33	3	5	42	n/a	n/a	n/a	n/a
Fried pickles	1 order	610	45	8.0	3610	45	4	2	7	n/a	n/a	n/a	n/a
Loaded boneless wings	1 order	1370	92	27.0	3230	64	4	6	72	n/a	n/a	n/a	n/a
Skillet queso	1 order	1330	77	22.0	3730	126	10	15	34	n/a	n/a	n/a	n/a
Southwestern egg rolls	1 order	800	41	10.0	2180	82	8	9	28	n/a	n/a	n/a	n/a
Texas cheese fries	1 order	1650	110	45.0	3650	99	8	3	68	n/a	n/a	n/a	n/a
w/ chili	1 order	2110	138	56.0	5080	112	9	6	94	n/a	n/a	n/a	n/a
White spinach queso	1 order	1430	87	28.0	3110	127	12	10	37	n/a	n/a	n/a	n/a
Baby Back Ribs (w/o sides)													
Dry rub half rack	1	780	54	20.0	2960	23	2	19	50	n/a	n/a	n/a	n/a
Honey chipotle BBQ half rack	1	760	53	20.0	900	23	0	17	49	n/a	n/a	n/a	n/a
House BBQ half rack	1	720	53	20.0	1090	11	1	9	49	n/a	n/a	n/a	n/a
Original BBQ half rack	1	710	53	20.0	960	10	0	9	49	n/a	n/a	n/a	n/a
Big Mouth Burgers (w/o fries)													
Alex's Santa Fe	1	930	62	25.0	1120	45	5	11	51	n/a	n/a	n/a	n/a
Big Mouth Bites	4 pcs	1210	72	26.0	2680	77	5	20	65	n/a	n/a	n/a	n/a
The Boss	1	1530	107	43.0	3120	49	4	16	92	n/a	n/a	n/a	n/a
Chili's Chili	1	1010	65	28.0	1510	49	3	11	56	n/a	n/a	n/a	n/a
Just Bacon	1	1030	71	28.0	1330	43	3	11	55	n/a	n/a	n/a	n/a
Mushroom Swiss	1	1010	70	27.0	1040	45	5	12	52	n/a	n/a	n/a	n/a
Oldtimer w/ cheese	1	860	55	24.0	1200	42	4	10	51	n/a	n/a	n/a	n/a
Queso	1	940	62	26.0	1140	47	3	11	51	n/a	n/a	n/a	n/a
Southern Smokehouse	1	1260	83	31.0	2360	68	4	25	62	n/a	n/a	n/a	n/a
Additions													
applewood smoked bacon	1 order	70	6	2.0	210	0	0	0	5	n/a	n/a	n/a	n/a
avocado slices	1 order	80	7	1.0	0	4	3	0	1	n/a	n/a	n/a	n/a
The Original Chili	1 order	150	9	3.5	480	4	0	1	0	n/a	n/a	n/a	n/a
patty, black bean	1	200	8	1.0	540	22	8	2	17	n/a	n/a	n/a	n/a
patty, classic beef	1	510	39	17.0	350	0	0	0	38	n/a	n/a	n/a	n/a
sautéed mushrooms	1 order	60	4.5	1.5	150	3	1	1	1	n/a	n/a	n/a	n/a
Chicken Crispers													
Crispy	1 order	1380	72	12.0	3070	130	12	13	55	n/a	n/a	n/a	n/a
add BBQ	1 order	70	0	0.0	590	16	0	14	1	n/a	n/a	n/a	n/a
add BBQ house	1 order	80	1	0.0	790	16	1	14	1	n/a	n/a	n/a	n/a
add honey mustard	1 order	200	18	3.0	330	10	0	10	1	n/a	n/a	n/a	n/a
add ranch	1 order	170	18	3.0	300	2	0	2	1	n/a	n/a	n/a	n/a
Honey chipotle	1 order	1830	90	15.0	4380	203	13	66	56	n/a	n/a	n/a	n/a
w/ waffles	1 order	2590	126	42.0	5180	303	14	128	63	n/a	n/a	n/a	n/a
Mango habanero	1 order	1670	90	15.0	4550	159	13	37	56	n/a	n/a	n/a	n/a
Original tempura w/ honey mustard	1 order	1320	67	11.0	3060	120	12	23	61	n/a	n/a	n/a	n/a

Chili's

	Amount	Calories	Fat (g)	Saturated Fat (g)	Sodium (mg)	Carbohydrate (g)	Fiber (g)	Sugar (g)	Protein (g)	Vitamin D (mcg)	Calcium (mg)	Iron (mg)	Potassium (mg)
Chicken & Seafood													
Ancho salmon	1 order	620	30	5.0	1860	42	5	5	48	n/a	n/a	n/a	n/a
Cajun pasta													
grilled chicken	1 order	1180	53	23.0	3470	110	8	5	66	n/a	n/a	n/a	n/a
grilled shrimp	1 order	1090	51	22.0	3580	109	7	5	47	n/a	n/a	n/a	n/a
Fresh Mex bowl													
chipotle chicken	1 order	1000	49	11.0	2520	80	7	7	61	n/a	n/a	n/a	n/a
chipotle shrimp	1 order	860	46	11.0	2870	79	7	7	33	n/a	n/a	n/a	n/a
Mango-chili chicken	1 order	510	20	3.5	1570	50	7	12	36	n/a	n/a	n/a	n/a
Margarita grilled chicken	1 order	650	17	3.0	2340	68	7	9	55	n/a	n/a	n/a	n/a
Fajitas													
Fillings (w/o toppings/tortillas)													
black bean & veggie	1 order	670	38	7.0	2370	66	19	20	28	n/a	n/a	n/a	n/a
carnitas	1 order	680	48	14.0	2490	26	3	14	36	n/a	n/a	n/a	n/a
grilled chicken	1 order	510	20	4.5	2200	22	3	10	63	n/a	n/a	n/a	n/a
grilled steak	1 order	580	30	9.0	2230	25	3	11	57	n/a	n/a	n/a	n/a
mushroom Jack chicken	1 order	670	40	15.0	2550	28	5	12	53	n/a	n/a	n/a	n/a
shrimp	1 order	320	16	3.5	2670	21	3	10	25	n/a	n/a	n/a	n/a
Toppings	1 order	230	17	10.0	850	7	1	4	12	n/a	n/a	n/a	n/a
guacamole	1 order	50	5	0.5	95	3	2	0	1	n/a	n/a	n/a	n/a
grilled carnitas	1 order	240	18	6.0	650	1	0	1	17	n/a	n/a	n/a	n/a
grilled chicken	1 order	160	4	1.0	570	1	0	0	30	n/a	n/a	n/a	n/a
grilled steak	1 order	200	9	3.0	590	2	0	1	27	n/a	n/a	n/a	n/a
peppers & onions	1 order	190	12	2.5	1050	20	3	9	3	n/a	n/a	n/a	n/a
seared shrimp	1 order	60	2	0.0	810	1	0	0	11	n/a	n/a	n/a	n/a
side beans	1 order	120	1	0.0	710	20	6	2	7	n/a	n/a	n/a	n/a
side rice	1 order	160	5	1.0	480	27	1	1	3	n/a	n/a	n/a	n/a
tortillas, corn	4	250	5	0.5	0	51	5	1	5	n/a	n/a	n/a	n/a
tortillas, flour	4	360	10	4.5	430	58	4	4	9	n/a	n/a	n/a	n/a
white queso & pico de gallo	1 order	150	12	6.0	440	5	1	3	6	n/a	n/a	n/a	n/a
Sandwiches (w/o fries)													
Bacon avocado chicken	1	1160	61	15.0	2390	75	9	15	83	n/a	n/a	n/a	n/a
Buffalo chicken ranch	1	960	51	10.0	4260	81	6	12	46	n/a	n/a	n/a	n/a
California turkey club	1	1030	59	16.0	2220	78	9	17	48	n/a	n/a	n/a	n/a
Chicky Chicky Bleu	1	1260	77	17.0	3510	90	0	16	56	n/a	n/a	n/a	n/a
Smokehouse Combos													
Brisket quesadilla	1 order	860	68	21.0	1540	38	2	7	24	n/a	n/a	n/a	n/a
Cheesy bacon BBQ chicken	1 order	370	18	7.0	1450	13	1	10	40	n/a	n/a	n/a	n/a
Crispers													
crispy w/o sauce	1 order	470	29	5.0	1230	25	3	1	27	n/a	n/a	n/a	n/a
honey chipotle w/ ranch	1 order	780	47	8.0	2030	62	3	28	28	n/a	n/a	n/a	n/a

RESTAURANT & FAST FOOD CHAINS

	Amount	Calories	Fat (g)	Saturated Fat (g)	Sodium (mg)	Carbohydrate (g)	Fiber (g)	Sugar (g)	Protein (g)	Vitamin D (mcg)	Calcium (mg)	Iron (mg)	Potassium (mg)
mango-habanero chipotle w/ ranch	1 order	700	47	8.0	2120	40	3	14	28	n/a	n/a	n/a	n/a
original w/ honey mustard	1 order	510	34	6.0	1350	23	3	10	31	n/a	n/a	n/a	n/a
Jalapeño-cheddar smoked sausage	1 order	380	31	13.0	1340	4	1	0	21	n/a	n/a	n/a	n/a
Ribs													
dry rub	1 order	780	54	20.0	2960	23	2	19	50	n/a	n/a	n/a	n/a
honey-chipotle BBQ	1 order	760	53	20.0	900	23	0	17	49	n/a	n/a	n/a	n/a
house BBQ	1 order	720	53	20.0	1090	11	1	9	49	n/a	n/a	n/a	n/a
original BBQ	1 order	710	53	20.0	960	10	0	9	49	n/a	n/a	n/a	n/a
Smoked brisket	1 order	290	22	8.0	710	5	0	5	16	n/a	n/a	n/a	n/a
Steaks (w/o sides)													
Classic ribeye	1 order	630	40	17.0	1450	0	0	0	67	n/a	n/a	n/a	n/a
Classic sirloin	6 oz	260	13	4.5	640	1	0	0	34	n/a	n/a	n/a	n/a
	10 oz	390	19	7.0	960	2	0	1	55	n/a	n/a	n/a	n/a
Country-fried steak w/ gravy	1 order	600	36	8.0	1390	29	3	3	39	n/a	n/a	n/a	n/a
add seared shrimp	1 order	60	2	0.0	810	1	0	0	11	n/a	n/a	n/a	n/a
Tacos & Quesadillas													
Quesadillas													
bacon ranch chicken	1 order	1570	117	36.0	3600	71	5	10	62	n/a	n/a	n/a	n/a
bacon ranch steak	1 order	1720	128	39.0	3890	70	4	10	76	n/a	n/a	n/a	n/a
brisket	1 order	1600	122	40.0	2860	77	0	16	49	n/a	n/a	n/a	n/a
Tacos													
ranchero chicken	1 order	1020	44	13.0	3050	100	13	9	56	n/a	n/a	n/a	n/a
spicy shrimp	1 order	1000	43	11.0	3190	111	15	18	38	n/a	n/a	n/a	n/a
Salads & Dressing													
Salads													
Boneless Buffalo chicken	1	1020	64	14.0	4780	60	7	7	52	n/a	n/a	n/a	n/a
Caesar	1	310	27	5.0	510	14	2	2	5	n/a	n/a	n/a	n/a
Caribbean	1	530	24	3.5	310	80	8	67	5	n/a	n/a	n/a	n/a
w/ grilled chicken	1	710	28	4.5	1010	86	8	71	34	n/a	n/a	n/a	n/a
w/ shrimp	1	600	26	4.0	1120	81	8	67	16	n/a	n/a	n/a	n/a
Grilled chicken	1	430	23	5.0	970	22	5	11	37	n/a	n/a	n/a	n/a
House	1	140	6	2.5	270	15	2	4	6	n/a	n/a	n/a	n/a
Quesadilla explosion	1	1340	87	24.0	2140	82	9	17	58	n/a	n/a	n/a	n/a
Sante Fe chicken	1	630	44	7.0	1460	27	7	8	36	n/a	n/a	n/a	n/a
w/ crispers	1	940	69	12.0	1990	50	10	8	33	n/a	n/a	n/a	n/a
Southwestern chicken Caesar	1	630	44	10.0	1100	21	5	4	39	n/a	n/a	n/a	n/a
Southwestern shrimp Caesar	1	530	42	9.0	1340	21	5	4	21	n/a	n/a	n/a	n/a
Dressing													
ancho chili ranch	2 oz	220	22	4.0	470	4	0	2	2	n/a	n/a	n/a	n/a
avocado ranch	2 oz	190	19	3.0	330	4	1	2	1	n/a	n/a	n/a	n/a
blue cheese	2 oz	330	35	6.0	350	2	0	1	1	n/a	n/a	n/a	n/a
Caesar	2 oz	290	31	5.0	330	3	0	1	2	n/a	n/a	n/a	n/a

RESTAURANT & FAST FOOD CHAINS

	Amount	Calories	Fat (g)	Saturated Fat (g)	Sodium (mg)	Carbohydrate (g)	Fiber (g)	Sugar (g)	Protein (g)	Vitamin D (mcg)	Calcium (mg)	Iron (mg)	Potassium
Chili's													
citrus balsamic vinaigrette	2 oz	330	33	5.0	310	7	0	6	0	n/a	n/a	n/a	n/a
honey lime	2 oz	270	23	3.5	270	16	0	15	1	n/a	n/a	n/a	n/a
honey lime vinaigrette	2 oz	180	17	2.0	300	7	0	6	0	n/a	n/a	n/a	n/a
honey mustard	2 oz	270	24	4.0	440	14	0	13	1	n/a	n/a	n/a	n/a
ranch	2 oz	230	23	4.0	410	3	0	2	2	n/a	n/a	n/a	n/a
Santa Fe	2 oz	280	30	4.5	710	3	0	2	1	n/a	n/a	n/a	n/a
Thousand Island	2 oz	270	26	4.0	490	9	0	8	1	n/a	n/a	n/a	n/a
Sides													
Asparagus	1 order	35	1	0.0	135	5	3	2	3	n/a	n/a	n/a	n/a
Black beans	1 order	120	10	1.0	710	20	6	2	7	n/a	n/a	n/a	n/a
Chili-garlic toast	1 order	140	7	1.5	380	17	1	1	3	n/a	n/a	n/a	n/a
Coleslaw	1 order	250	19	3.5	270	14	2	11	2	n/a	n/a	n/a	n/a
Garlic dill pickles	1 order	5	0	0.0	220	0	0	0	0	n/a	n/a	n/a	n/a
Homestyle fries	1 order	420	17	2.5	660	60	5	0	6	n/a	n/a	n/a	n/a
Loaded mashed potatoes	1 order	350	20	6.0	820	33	3	3	10	n/a	n/a	n/a	n/a
Mexican rice	1 order	160	5	1.0	480	27	1	1	3	n/a	n/a	n/a	n/a
Roasted street corn	1 order	390	27	5.0	330	31	3	12	6	n/a	n/a	n/a	n/a
Steamed broccoli	1 order	40	0	0.0	250	8	4	2	3	n/a	n/a	n/a	n/a
Sweet corn on the cob	1 order	180	6	1.0	360	29	3	11	4	n/a	n/a	n/a	n/a
Soups & Chili													
Chicken enchilada	1 order	400	25	8.0	1480	24	3	3	20	n/a	n/a	n/a	n/a
Clam chowder	1 order	330	23	13.0	690	21	1	5	11	n/a	n/a	n/a	n/a
Loaded baked potato	1 order	430	29	18.0	1270	25	2	7	16	n/a	n/a	n/a	n/a
The Original Chili	1 order	750	46	18.0	2050	28	2	5	38	n/a	n/a	n/a	n/a
Southwest chicken	1 order	250	11	2.0	1390	28	3	4	10	n/a	n/a	n/a	n/a
Desserts													
Cheesecake	1 order	720	43	23.0	430	73	1	60	11	n/a	n/a	n/a	n/a
Molten chocolate cake	1 order	1170	59	30.0	1030	155	5	109	12	n/a	n/a	n/a	n/a
mini	1 order	570	25	13.0	530	82	3	56	7	n/a	n/a	n/a	n/a
Skillet chocolate chip cookie	1	1180	50	24.0	890	176	4	104	15	n/a	n/a	n/a	n/a
Chipotle													
Meals													
Bases													
taco	1	200	9	1.0	0	29	3	0		n/a	221	1	n/a
flour tortilla													
burrito	1	320	9	0.5	600	50	3	0	8	n/a	0	1	n/a
taco	1	250	8	0.5	480	40	2	0	7	n/a	0	1	n/a
Supergreens lettuce blend	1 order	15	0	0.0	15	3	2	1	1	n/a	26	1	n/a
Toppings													
barbacoa	1 order	170	7	2.5	530	2	1	0	24	n/a	26	3	n/a
beans, black	1 order	130	2	0.0	210	22	7	2	8	n/a	52	2	n/a

RESTAURANT & FAST FOOD CHAINS

Chipotle	Amount	Calories	Fat (g)	Saturated Fat (g)	Sodium (mg)	Carbohydrate (g)	Fiber (g)	Sugar (g)	Protein (g)	Vitamin D (mcg)	Calcium (mg)	Iron (mg)	Potassium (mg)
beans, pinto	1 order	130	2	0.0	210	21	8	1	8	n/a	52	3	n/a
carnitas	1 order	210	12	7.0	450	0	0	0	23	n/a	26	1	n/a
chicken	1 order	180	7	3.0	310	0	0	0	32	n/a	39	1	n/a
cilantro-lime rice													
brown	1 order	210	6	1.0	190	36	5	0	4	n/a	13	1	n/a
cauliflower	1 order	40	1	0.0	210	7	3	2	3	n/a	26	1	n/a
white	1 order	210	4	0.5	350	40	1	0	4	n/a	13	1	n/a
fajita vegetables	1 order	20	0	0.0	150	5	1	2	1	n/a	26	1	n/a
fresh tomato salsa	1 order	25	0	0.0	550	4	1	1	0	n/a	13	1	n/a
guacamole	1 order	230	22	3.5	370	8	6	1	2	n/a	26	1	n/a
Monterey Jack cheese	1 order	110	8	5.0	190	1	0	0	6	n/a	260	0	n/a
quesadilla	1 order	330	24	15.0	570	3	0	0	18	n/a	780	0	n/a
queso blanco	1 order	120	9	6.0	250	4	0	1	5	n/a	130	0	n/a
romaine lettuce	1 order	5	0	0.0	0	1	1	0	0	n/a	0	1	n/a
salsa													
roasted chili-corn	1 order	80	2	0.0	330	16	3	4	3	n/a	0	1	n/a
tomatillo green-chili	1 order	15	0	0.0	260	4	0	2	0	n/a	39	1	n/a
tomatillo red-chili	1 order	30	0	0.0	500	4	1	0	0	n/a	0	1	n/a
Sofritas	1 order	150	10	1.5	560	9	3	5	11	n/a	221	3	n/a
sour cream	1 order	110	9	7.0	30	2	0	2	2	n/a	78	0	n/a
steak	1 order	150	6	2.5	330	1	1	0	21	n/a	26	3	n/a
Lifestyle Bowls													
High protein bowl	1	820	27	11.0	1895	70	11	3	72	n/a	416	8	n/a
Keto bowl, chicken	1	590	38	11.5	1580	20	10	3	43	n/a	351	4	n/a
Keto salad bowl, chicken	1	560	37	11.5	1435	16	9	3	41	n/a	364	5	n/a
Keto salad bowl, steak	1	535	36	11.0	1405	17	10	2	30	n/a	338	6	n/a
Paleo salad bowl	1	460	29	6.5	1105	20	9	6	36	n/a	156	6	n/a
Vegan bowl	1	430	14	1.5	1860	59	18	14	22	n/a	312	8	n/a
Vegetarian bowl	1	460	25	3.5	1505	49	20	9	15	n/a	169	6	n/a
Whole30 bowl	1	500	30	6.5	1990	23	11	5	37	n/a	117	5	n/a
Whole30 salad bowl, carnitas	1	500	34	10.5	1535	20	10	5	27	n/a	117	5	n/a
Whole30 salad bowl, chicken	1	470	29	6.5	1395	20	10	5	36	n/a	130	5	n/a
Sides													
Chips	regular	540	25	3.5	390	73	7	1	7	n/a	520	3	n/a
w/ guacamole	1 order	770	47	7.0	760	81	13	2	9	n/a	546	5	n/a
w/ fresh tomato salsa	1 order	570	25	3.5	940	74	8	2	7	n/a	533	4	n/a
w/ queso	1 order	780	43	16.0	880	80	7	3	17	n/a	780	3	n/a
w/ roasted chili-corn salsa	1 order	620	27	3.5	720	89	10	5	10	n/a	520	4	n/a
w/ tomatillo green-chili salsa	1 order	560	25	3.5	650	77	7	3	7	n/a	559	4	n/a
w/ tomatillo red-chili salsa	1 order	570	25	3.5	890	77	8	1	7	n/a	520	4	n/a
Guacamole	large	460	44	7.0	740	16	12	2	4	n/a	52	3	n/a
Queso blanco	side	240	18	12.0	490	7	0	2	10	n/a	260	0	n/a

RESTAURANT & FAST FOOD CHAINS

Country Style

	Amount	Calories	Fat (g)	Saturated Fat (g)	Sodium (mg)	Carbohydrate (g)	Fiber (g)	Sugar (g)	Protein (g)	Vitamin D (mcg)	Calcium (mg)	Iron (mg)	Potas
Bagels													
Cheddar & herb	1	250	4	1.5	440	45	2	5	8	n/a	4	30	n/a
Cinnamon raisin	1	230	1	0.0	380	48	2	8	8	n/a	2	30	n/a
Everything	1	240	5	0.5	960	43	3	5	8	n/a	6	20	n/a
Jalapeño & cheddar	1	210	4	1.5	590	37	2	4	8	n/a	4	25	n/a
Plain	1	230	3	0.0	410	46	2	5	8	n/a	2	30	n/a
Sesame	1	260	6	0.5	390	44	3	5	8	n/a	6	35	n/a
Whole wheat & honey	1	220	1	0.0	390	45	5	5	8	n/a	2	35	n/a
Baked Goods													
Brownie	1	390	23	8.0	120	42	3	31	5	n/a	2	15	n/a
Cookies													
chocolate chunk	1	250	12	6.0	200	34	1	21	3	n/a	2	10	n/a
double chocolate chip	1	260	12	7.0	210	34	1	23	3	n/a	2	15	n/a
oatmeal raisin	1	240	10	6.0	200	34	2	19	3	n/a	2	8	n/a
peanut butter	1	260	14	5.0	250	30	1	18	4	n/a	2	15	n/a
white chocolate macadamia nut	1	260	13	6.0	190	33	1	2	3	n/a	4	6	n/a
Croissants													
butter	1	260	15	10.0	350	26	2	2	5	n/a	2	15	n/a
cheese	1	320	20	13.0	450	26	2	2	8	n/a	10	15	n/a
Fruit danish	1	280	13	4.0	250	37	1	13	5	n/a	2	8	n/a
Muffins													
apple oatmeal	1	460	18	1.5	310	68	4	33	4	n/a	2	20	n/a
banana nut	1	440	18	2.0	340	65	1	36	1	n/a	2	15	n/a
blueberry	1	390	16	1.5	560	59	1	27	1	n/a	6	10	n/a
carrot	1	400	17	1.5	300	59	3	30	3	n/a	6	15	n/a
chocolate chip	1	400	18	4.0	570	69	1	38	1	n/a	6	15	n/a
corn	1	480	21	2.0	300	68	3	29	3	n/a	6	25	n/a
fruit & fiber	1	330	8	0.5	290	59	8	30	8	n/a	2	20	n/a
lemon cranberry	1	390	16	1.5	430	56	1	25	1	n/a	6	10	n/a
morning glory	1	390	16	1.5	290	60	4	34	4	n/a	2	10	n/a
Pecan tart	1	370	19	4.0	180	45	1	25	4	n/a	4	20	n/a
Tea biscuits	1	210	6	1.5	650	31	1	5	5	n/a	4	10	n/a
cheese	1	220	8	3.0	640	28	1	5	7	n/a	10	10	n/a
Breakfast Sandwiches													
B.L.T.													
English muffin	1	250	12	5.0	520	28	2	4	8	n/a	4	10	n/a
plain bagel	1	370	13	5.0	810	50	3	4	12	n/a	6	25	n/a
Breakfast club													
English muffin	1	230	8	2.5	660	26	1	2	13	n/a	4	10	n/a
plain bagel	1	340	9	3.0	950	49	2	3	17	n/a	8	25	n/a
Classic													
English muffin	1	300	12	5.0	940	27	1	3	19	n/a	15	15	n/a
plain bagel	1	510	14	6.0	1430	68	2	4	27	n/a	20	35	n/a

RESTAURANT & FAST FOOD CHAINS

Country Style	Amount	Calories	Fat (g)	Saturated Fat (g)	Sodium (mg)	Carbohydrate (g)	Fiber (g)	Sugar (g)	Protein (g)	Vitamin D (mcg)	Calcium (mg)	Iron (mg)	Potassium (mg)
Garden omelet													
English muffin	1	370	15	7.0	730	31	1	4	20	n/a	25	15	n/a
plain bagel	1	460	17	8.0	950	53	2	4	23	n/a	25	30	n/a
Sausage & egg													
English muffin	1	500	36	15.0	860	27	1	3	18	n/a	15	15	n/a
plain bagel	1	620	37	15.0	1140	49	2	3	23	n/a	20	30	n/a
Sunriser													
English muffin	1	270	12	5.0	620	27	1	2	13	n/a	15	10	n/a
plain bagel	1	33	18	9.0	670	28	2	4	15	n/a	15	15	n/a
Western													
English muffin	1	400	19	9.0	960	31	1	4	24	n/a	25	15	n/a
plain bagel	1	510	21	9.0	1250	53	2	4	28	n/a	30	30	n/a
Donuts													
Apple & spice	1	290	12	5.0	360	41	1	17	5	n/a	2	10	n/a
Apple fritter	1	300	12	5.0	350	42	1	19	5	n/a	2	10	n/a
Boston cream	1	280	11	5.0	340	40	1	15	5	n/a	2	10	n/a
Cinnamon ring	1	370	17	7.0	490	52	5	9	8	n/a	20	50	n/a
Cinnamon twist	1	370	17	7.0	490	52	5	9	8	n/a	20	50	n/a
Coconut													
toasted	1	260	15	8.0	270	30	1	14	3	n/a	2	10	n/a
white	1	270	16	9.0	270	28	2	14	4	n/a	2	10	n/a
Cream delite	1	290	18	11.0	320	28	1	2	5	n/a	2	15	n/a
Cruller													
chocolate walnut	1	330	20	6.0	310	33	2	14	7	n/a	4	15	n/a
French	1	160	11	5.0	100	15	0	5	1	n/a	0	0	n/a
orange	1	340	18	9.0	380	39	1	17	4	n/a	2	10	n/a
walnut	1	340	21	7.0	300	32	1	14	7	n/a	2	15	n/a
Double chocolate	1	250	10	5.0	270	35	1	18	3	n/a	2	15	n/a
Dutchie	1	260	11	5.0	320	37	1	11	5	n/a	2	10	n/a
Éclair	1	420	22	13.0	450	49	1	14	6	n/a	2	15	n/a
Glazed													
chocolate	1	220	10	5.0	270	28	1	13	3	n/a	2	10	n/a
honey	1	210	10	4.0	280	26	1	7	4	n/a	2	10	n/a
plain	1	220	11	5.0	270	27	1	13	3	n/a	2	8	n/a
sour cream	1	310	19	9.0	250	31	·1	15	3	n/a	2	10	n/a
Hawaiian	1	240	14	5.0	290	33	1	13	4	n/a	2	10	n/a
Lemon	1	290	11	5.0	350	42	1	19	5	n/a	2	10	n/a
Marble	1	250	11	5.0	270	34	1	19	3	n/a	2	10	n/a
Plain	1	200	11	5.0	260	21	1	8	3	n/a	2	8	n/a
Raised													
chocolate	1	230	10	4.5	280	33	1	13	4	n/a	2	10	n/a
maple	1	230	10	4.0	280	33	1	13	4	n/a	2	10	n/a
Sour cream	1	290	19	9.0	250	25	1	10	3	n/a	2	10	n/a
Strawberry	1	290	11	5.0	330	42	1	19	5	n/a	2	10	n/a
Sugar twist	1	260	12	3.5	290	32	1	8	5	n/a	0	10	n/a

RESTAURANT & FAST FOOD CHAINS

Sandwiches	Amount	Calories	Fat (g)	Saturated Fat (g)	Sodium (mg)	Carbohydrate (g)	Fiber (g)	Sugar (g)	Protein (g)	Vitamin D (mcg)	Calcium (mg)	Iron (mg)	Potassium (mg)
Albacore tuna salad													
white sliced bread	1	210	18	0.5	690	40	2	7	23	n/a	2	25	n/a
whole wheat sliced bread	1	210	18	0.5	680	40	5	3	24	n/a	2	15	n/a
Clubhouse													
baguette	1	950	39	11.0	2640	98	8	5	49	n/a	20	50	n/a
white ciabatta	1	610	22	6.0	1640	69	5	3	31	n/a	10	35	n/a
whole wheat ciabatta	1	610	22	6.0	1640	69	5	3	31	n/a	10	35	n/a
Egg salad													
white sliced bread	1	320	11	2.0	530	41	3	6	16	n/a	6	30	n/a
whole wheat sliced bread	1	320	11	2.0	520	40	5	3	17	n/a	6	25	n/a
Grilled chicken													
baguette	1	1000	40	10.0	2140	97	8	4	60	n/a	20	45	n/a
white ciabatta	1	620	21	5.0	1350	69	5	3	32	n/a	10	35	n/a
whole wheat ciabatta	1	620	21	5.0	1350	69	5	3	32	n/a	10	35	n/a
Roast beef & cheddar													
baguette	1	840	27	9.0	2450	98	8	4	50	n/a	20	60	n/a
white ciabatta	1	560	16	4.5	1600	69	6	2	31	n/a	10	35	n/a
whole wheat ciabatta	1	560	16	4.5	1600	69	6	2	31	n/a	10	35	n/a
Smoked turkey													
white sliced bread	1	205	14	3.5	1010	41	2	7	17	n/a	15	25	n/a
whole wheat sliced bread	1	205	14	3.5	1000	41	5	4	18	n/a	15	15	n/a
Spicy Buffalo chicken													
baguette	1	1110	45	11.0	3260	125	9	5	47	n/a	20	45	n/a
white ciabatta	1	750	27	6.0	2350	90	6	2	33	n/a	10	30	n/a
whole wheat ciabatta	1	750	27	6.0	2350	90	6	2	33	n/a	10	30	n/a
Wraps													
Chicken Caesar													
white	1	230	15	4.0	1090	30	2	2	31	n/a	2	15	n/a
whole wheat	1	230	16	4.0	1130	31	4	2	32	n/a	4	15	n/a
Chicken feta													
white	1	255	24	7.0	1320	33	2	2	30	n/a	15	15	n/a
whole wheat	1	255	25	7.0	1360	34	4	2	21	n/a	15	15	n/a
Garden													
white	1	430	21	9.0	900	33	4	2	21	n/a	25	20	n/a
whole wheat	1	450	22	9.0	900	32	4	2	21	n/a	25	20	n/a
Roast beef & cheddar													
white	1	220	18	8.0	1180	32	2	1	23	n/a	25	20	n/a
whole wheat	1	220	19	6.0	1220	33	4	1	24	n/a	25	20	n/a
Western													
white	1	460	24	9.0	1340	34	4	2	27	n/a	25	20	n/a
whole wheat	1	480	25	9.0	1340	33	4	2	27	n/a	25	20	n/a

RESTAURANT & FAST FOOD CHAINS

	Amount	Calories	Fat (g)	Saturated Fat (g)	Sodium (mg)	Carbohydrate (g)	Fiber (g)	Sugar (g)	Protein (g)	Vitamin D (mcg)	Calcium (mg)	Iron (mg)	Potassium (mg)
Salads													
Chicken Caesar	1	460	31	7.0	1310	12	3	3	36	n/a	25	10	n/a
Chicken Greek	1	450	34	7.0	1020	13	3	5	22	n/a	10	10	n/a
Cobb	1	550	40	11.0	1120	11	3	6	36	n/a	20	20	n/a
Soups & Chili													
Beef chili	1	160	6	2.0	870	18	4	4	10	n/a	88	20	n/a
Broccoli & cheese	1	170	10	6.0	870	16	1	0	1	n/a	10	20	n/a
Chicken noodle	1	110	3	0.5	810	17	1	0	4	n/a	2	20	n/a
Cream of mushroom	1	150	9	5.0	890	14	1	0	3	n/a	8	4	n/a
Creamy tomato & roasted red pepper	1	120	3	1.0	860	20	2	0	4	n/a	10	6	n/a
Harvest vegetable	1	60	1	0.0	720	10	1	0	1	n/a	2	4	n/a
Italian style wedding	1	140	4	1.0	980	21	1	0	4	n/a	0	8	n/a
Minestrone	1	100	0	0.0	790	21	3	0	4	n/a	0	0	n/a
Red Thai curry chicken w/ rice	1	170	8	5.0	890	22	1	0	4	n/a	2	15	n/a
Smoked turkey w/ wild rice	1	80	1	0.0	640	14	1	0	3	n/a	2	8	n/a
Vegetable beef & barley	1	90	1	0.5	790	18	3	0	3	n/a	2	6	n/a
Extras													
Becel	1 pkg	70	8	1.0	70	0	0	0	0	n/a	0	0	n/a
Cream cheese	1 pkg	90	9	6.0	110	1	0	1	3	n/a	2	0	n/a
cheddar	1 pkg	110	9	6.0	190	1	0	0	7	n/a	20	0	n/a
herb & garlic	1 pkg	60	5	2.5	110	3	0	2	2	n/a	4	0	n/a
light	1 pkg	60	2	3.0	120	2	0	2	2	n/a	4	0	n/a
Peanut butter	1 pkg	110	9	2.0	85	4	1	2	5	n/a	0	2	n/a
Strawberry jam	1 pkg	60	0	0.0	4	14	0	12	0	n/a	0	0	n/a
Breadstick	1	190	1	0.0	310	37	2	1	7	n/a	0	20	n/a
Hash brown	1	130	8	2.0	250	14	3	0	0	n/a	0	2	n/a
Drinks													
Cappuccino													
iced	medium	240	3	0.0	230	38	0	26	1	n/a	10	2	n/a
iced mocha	medium	320	4	0.0	240	50	0	36	1	n/a	10	2	n/a
Coffee													
decaf	medium	0	0	0.0	1	0	0	0	0	n/a	0	0	n/a
iced	medium	150	6	6.0	135	24	0	19	1	n/a	6	0	n/a
original blend/dark roast	medium	0	0	0.0	1	0	0	0	0	n/a	0	0	n/a
French vanilla	medium	170	5	5.0	5	30	0	21	1	n/a	4	0	n/a
Hot chocolate	medium	170	3	1.0	280	32	1	32	1	n/a	15	2	n/a
Iced tea	medium	150	0	0.0	10	36	0	36	0	n/a	4	0	n/a
Lemonade	medium	150	0	0.0	20	36	0	36	0	n/a	4	0	n/a
Smoothie													
mango	medium	320	0	0.0	10	81	0	76	0	n/a	0	0	n/a
piña colada	medium	390	8	7.0	60	81	1	76	1	n/a	0	0	n/a
strawberry	medium	350	0	0.0	0	90	0	87	0	n/a	4	0	n/a
strawberry banana	medium	320	0	0.0	0	81	1	78	1	n/a	4	4	n/a

	Amount	Calories	Fat (g)	Saturated Fat (g)	Sodium (mg)	Carbohydrate (g)	Fiber (g)	Sugar (g)	Protein (g)	Vitamin D (mcg)	Calcium (mg)	Iron (mg)	Potas*
Burgers & Sandwiches													
Burger, ⅓ pound double w/ cheese	1	560	31	13.0	1040	36	1	8	36	n/a	n/a	n/a	n/a
Cheeseburger	1	400	18	8.0	910	36	1	8	22	n/a	n/a	n/a	n/a
Chicken sandwich													
crispy	1	550	28	4.5	980	49	3	5	25	n/a	n/a	n/a	n/a
grilled	1	390	15	2.5	970	34	1	5	29	n/a	n/a	n/a	n/a
Grillburger													
¼ pound bacon cheese	1	630	36	13.0	1220	44	2	12	33	n/a	n/a	n/a	n/a
¼ pound cheese	1	540	29	11.0	960	43	2	12	26	n/a	n/a	n/a	n/a
½ pound cheese	1	800	49	20.0	1030	44	2	12	46	n/a	n/a	n/a	n/a
½ pound flame thrower	1	980	70	25.0	1380	40	2	12	46	n/a	n/a	n/a	n/a
Chicken													
Chicken strip basket	4 pcs	1020	48	8.0	2120	111	6	3	35	n/a	n/a	n/a	n/a
	6 pcs	1300	61	11.0	2750	139	8	5	48	n/a	n/a	n/a	n/a
honey BBQ glazed	4 pcs	1140	48	8.0	2640	142	7	32	35	n/a	n/a	n/a	n/a
	6 pcs	1480	61	11.0	3570	186	9	48	49	n/a	n/a	n/a	n/a
Rotisserie-style chicken bites	6 pcs	610	27	5.0	1300	57	3	1	35	n/a	n/a	n/a	n/a
Hot Dogs													
Bacon cheese	1	420	26	11.0	1140	27	1	3	19	n/a	n/a	n/a	n/a
Cheese	1	360	22	8.0	970	27	1	4	14	n/a	n/a	n/a	n/a
Chili	1	360	22	8.0	970	27	1	4	14	n/a	n/a	n/a	n/a
Snacks & Sides													
Cheese curds	regular	500	34	19.0	990	26	0	1	24	n/a	n/a	n/a	n/a
Fries	regular	280	31	2.0	590	36	3	0	5	n/a	n/a	n/a	n/a
Onion rings	regular	360	16	2.5	840	48	2	3	6	n/a	n/a	n/a	n/a
Pretzel sticks w/ zesty queso	1 order	330	9	3.0	2060	52	2	7	9	n/a	n/a	n/a	n/a
Salads													
Rotisserie-style chicken bites salad bowl	1	320	15	6.0	870	10	3	5	37	n/a	n/a	n/a	n/a
Side salad	1	25	0	0.0	15	5	2	3	1	n/a	n/a	n/a	n/a
Dressing, Sauces & Dips													
Dipping sauce													
BBQ	1 cup	90	0	0.0	430	21	1	16	1	n/a	n/a	n/a	n/a
country gravy	1 cup	70	5	1.5	360	6	0	1	0	n/a	n/a	n/a	n/a
honey mustard	1 cup	240	20	3.0	450	15	0	14	1	n/a	n/a	n/a	n/a
house made Hidden Valley Ranch	1 cup	220	22	4.0	370	3	0	2	1	n/a	n/a	n/a	n/a
wild Buffalo	1 cup	90	10	1.0	1000	1	0	0	0	n/a	n/a	n/a	n/a
zesty queso	1 cup	110	10	3.0	570	3	0	1	2	n/a	n/a	n/a	n/a
Marzetti Dressing													
balsamic vinaigrette	1 order	130	12	2.0	470	4	0	4	0	n/a	n/a	n/a	n/a
blue cheese	1 order	200	21	4.0	430	2	0	1	1	n/a	n/a	n/a	n/a
creamy Caesar	1 order	180	18	3.0	400	2	0	1	1	n/a	n/a	n/a	n/a

RESTAURANT & FAST FOOD CHAINS

Dairy Queen

	Amount	Calories	Fat (g)	Saturated Fat (g)	Sodium (mg)	Carbohydrate (g)	Fiber (g)	Sugar (g)	Protein (g)	Vitamin D (mcg)	Calcium (mg)	Iron (mg)	Potassium (mg)
Dijon honey mustard	1 order	180	16	2.5	230	7	0	7	0	n/a	n/a	n/a	n/a
fat-free California French style	1 order	40	0	0.0	270	10	0	8	0	n/a	n/a	n/a	n/a
honey French	1 order	190	15	2.5	300	13	0	12	0	n/a	n/a	n/a	n/a
light Italian	1 order	15	1	0.0	730	2	0	2	0	n/a	n/a	n/a	n/a
light ranch	1 order	60	3	0.0	220	9	1	3	1	n/a	n/a	n/a	n/a
Thousand Island	1 order	210	21	3.0	310	6	0	6	0	n/a	n/a	n/a	n/a
Blizzards													
Brownie batter	mini	400	17	9.0	170	56	2	45	8	n/a	n/a	n/a	n/a
	medium	1050	48	24.0	460	145	6	114	20	n/a	n/a	n/a	n/a
Butterfinger	mini	350	12	7.0	150	52	1	41	9	n/a	n/a	n/a	n/a
	medium	730	26	15.0	330	107	2	81	18	n/a	n/a	n/a	n/a
Choco brownie extreme	mini	400	17	10.0	180	56	2	45	9	n/a	n/a	n/a	n/a
	medium	810	36	21.0	370	111	4	87	16	n/a	n/a	n/a	n/a
Chocolate chip cookie dough	mini	420	16	9.0	220	61	1	46	8	n/a	n/a	n/a	n/a
	medium	1030	41	24.0	570	151	2	111	17	n/a	n/a	n/a	n/a
Heath	mini	370	15	9.0	180	53	0	46	8	n/a	n/a	n/a	n/a
	medium	860	37	23.0	440	119	1	106	16	n/a	n/a	n/a	n/a
M&M's	mini	370	12	8.0	125	58	1	50	8	n/a	n/a	n/a	n/a
	medium	800	27	17.0	250	124	1	107	16	n/a	n/a	n/a	n/a
Oreo	mini	380	14	7.0	180	56	0	44	8	n/a	n/a	n/a	n/a
	medium	790	31	15.0	400	117	1	88	14	n/a	n/a	n/a	n/a
Reese's	mini	360	14	7.0	170	50	1	43	9	n/a	n/a	n/a	n/a
	medium	750	31	16.0	380	102	2	88	19	n/a	n/a	n/a	n/a
Rocky road trip	mini	500	19	8.0	230	73	2	57	11	n/a	n/a	n/a	n/a
	medium	1180	52	21.0	590	160	7	122	27	n/a	n/a	n/a	n/a
Royal New York cheesecake	mini	450	18	8.0	220	65	1	53	8	n/a	n/a	n/a	n/a
	medium	1040	46	21.0	530	140	2	112	19	n/a	n/a	n/a	n/a
Snicker's	mini	350	21	7.0	150	53	0	45	8	n/a	n/a	n/a	n/a
	medium	800	28	15.0	340	120	1	102	19	n/a	n/a	n/a	n/a
Cakes													
Blizzard cake													
Oreo	⅛ cake	560	25	17.5	251	77	1	59	9	n/a	n/a	n/a	n/a
choco brownie extreme	⅛ cake	575	26	19.5	244	77	2	59	9	n/a	n/a	n/a	n/a
chocolate chip cookie dough	⅛ cake	601	27	19.5	284	83	2	62	9	n/a	n/a	n/a	n/a
Reese's	⅛ cake	556	25	18.5	253	74	2	60	10	n/a	n/a	n/a	n/a
TreatZZa pizza													
choco brownie	⅛ pizza	190	10	6.0	95	26	1	18	3	n/a	n/a	n/a	n/a
Heath	⅛ pizza	190	9	6.0	90	26	1	19	2	n/a	n/a	n/a	n/a
M&M's	⅛ pizza	200	9	7.0	85	28	1	20	3	n/a	n/a	n/a	n/a
Reese's peanut butter cup	⅛ pizza	200	10	6.0	110	24	1	17	3	n/a	n/a	n/a	n/a
Cones													
Chocolate	medium	340	10	6.0	130	52	0	35	8	n/a	n/a	n/a	n/a

RESTAURANT & FAST FOOD CHAINS

	Amount	Calories	Fat (g)	Saturated Fat (g)	Sodium (mg)	Carbohydrate (g)	Fiber (g)	Sugar (g)	Protein (g)	Vitamin D (mcg)	Calcium (mg)	Iron (mg)	Pota...
Dipped													
butterscotch	medium	460	21	17.0	150	59	0	45	8	n/a	n/a	n/a	n/a
cherry	medium	460	22	18.0	140	58	0	44	8	n/a	n/a	n/a	n/a
chocolate	medium	460	22	17.0	140	58	1	43	9	n/a	n/a	n/a	n/a
Vanilla	medium	320	10	6.0	130	50	0	36	8	n/a	n/a	n/a	n/a
Frozen Drinks													
Misty Freeze	medium	450	12	8.0	160	77	0	68	10	n/a	n/a	n/a	n/a
Misty Slush	medium	260	0	0.0	40	65	0	64	0	n/a	n/a	n/a	n/a
Moolatté													
caramel	medium	620	18	13.0	240	103	0	87	10	n/a	n/a	n/a	n/a
mocha	medium	620	23	14.0	240	94	2	82	11	n/a	n/a	n/a	n/a
vanilla	medium	560	17	12.0	190	93	0	84	9	n/a	n/a	n/a	n/a
Shakes													
banana	medium	590	22	16.0	240	83	1	68	16	n/a	n/a	n/a	n/a
caramel	medium	750	25	17.0	330	115	0	93	17	n/a	n/a	n/a	n/a
chocolate	medium	710	23	16.0	290	110	1	96	16	n/a	n/a	n/a	n/a
hot fudge	medium	750	30	23.0	330	105	1	85	17	n/a	n/a	n/a	n/a
peanut butter	medium	930	53	20.0	590	91	3	69	22	n/a	n/a	n/a	n/a
strawberry	medium	630	23	16.0	260	92	1	80	16	n/a	n/a	n/a	n/a
vanilla	medium	660	23	16.0	260	97	0	85	16	n/a	n/a	n/a	n/a
add Make It a Malt	medium	80	1	0.5	80	18	1	12	1	n/a	n/a	n/a	n/a
Smoothies													
Orange Julius	medium	260	0	0.0	45	65	0	62	1	n/a	n/a	n/a	n/a
mango pineapple	medium	340	0	0.0	125	80	1	72	4	n/a	n/a	n/a	n/a
strawberry banana	medium	360	0	0.0	135	85	3	73	5	n/a	n/a	n/a	n/a
Strawberry Banana Julius	medium	460	7	7.0	105	99	3	86	2	n/a	n/a	n/a	n/a
tripleberry	medium	380	0	0.0	125	90	2	83	5	n/a	n/a	n/a	n/a
Sundaes													
Caramel	medium	430	11	7.0	190	73	0	58	9	n/a	n/a	n/a	n/a
Chocolate	medium	400	10	6.0	160	70	1	60	8	n/a	n/a	n/a	n/a
Hot fudge	medium	430	15	11.0	190	66	1	52	9	n/a	n/a	n/a	n/a
Peanut butter	medium	560	32	10.0	380	56	2	40	13	n/a	n/a	n/a	n/a
Pineapple	medium	330	10	6.0	120	54	1	47	8	n/a	n/a	n/a	n/a
Strawberry	medium	340	10	6.0	135	56	1	49	8	n/a	n/a	n/a	n/a
Add DQ sprinkles	1 order	35	2	1.0	0	6	0	3	0	n/a	n/a	n/a	n/a
Treats													
Banana split	1	520	14	9.0	150	94	4	74	9	n/a	n/a	n/a	n/a
Brownie and Oreo Cupfection	1	720	23	9.0	330	122	2	96	10	n/a	n/a	n/a	n/a
Peanut Buster parfait	1	710	31	18.0	340	95	3	68	17	n/a	n/a	n/a	n/a
Triple chocolate brownie dessert	1	540	25	9.0	260	74	3	57	8	n/a	n/a	n/a	n/a

RESTAURANT & FAST FOOD CHAINS

Denny's

	Amount	Calories	Fat (g)	Saturated Fat (g)	Sodium (mg)	Carbohydrate (g)	Fiber (g)	Sugar (g)	Protein (g)	Vitamin D (mcg)	Calcium (mg)	Iron (mg)	Potassium (mg)
Breakfast													
Benny													
classic w/ hash browns	1 order	710	37	11.0	2180	61	2	2	33	n/a	n/a	n/a	n/a
prime rib w/ hash browns	1 order	1020	65	20.0	2990	56	1	3	50	n/a	n/a	n/a	n/a
southwestern w/ hash browns	1 order	950	60	20.0	2100	65	3	5	36	n/a	n/a	n/a	n/a
Country-fried steak & eggs w/ gravy & hash browns	1 order	570	33	11.0	1450	51	2	2	16	n/a	n/a	n/a	n/a
Moons Over My Hammy w/ hash browns	1 order	960	56	19.0	2650	65	2	4	44	n/a	n/a	n/a	n/a
Skillet													
Sante Fe Sizzlin'	1 order	720	55	18.0	1750	33	3	4	26	n/a	n/a	n/a	n/a
Supreme	1 order	580	45	14.0	1260	30	4	5	15	n/a	n/a	n/a	n/a
T-bone steak w/ hash browns	1 order	670	38	14.0	1790	24	1	1	53	n/a	n/a	n/a	n/a
The Grand Slamwich w/ hash browns	1 order	1320	81	27.0	3410	95	3	4	52	n/a	n/a	n/a	n/a
Crepes													
Berry vanilla													
à la carte	1	270	12	4.5	210	36	2	22	4	n/a	n/a	n/a	n/a
breakfast	1	440	20	6.0	670	60	3	23	5	n/a	n/a	n/a	n/a
Omelets													
Build Your Own													
American cheese	1 slice	80	7	4.0	390	1	0	1	4	n/a	n/a	n/a	n/a
bacon	2 slices	100	8	3.0	350	1	0	1	7	n/a	n/a	n/a	n/a
carmelized onions	1 order	70	7	1.0	210	2	1	1	0	n/a	n/a	n/a	n/a
cheddar cheese	1 order	80	6	3.5	120	0	0	0	5	n/a	n/a	n/a	n/a
chorizo sausage	1 order	330	27	10.0	830	4	0	0	17	n/a	n/a	n/a	n/a
fire-roasted bell peppers & onions	1 order	70	6	1.0	110	4	1	2	0	n/a	n/a	n/a	n/a
fresh avocado	1 order	90	8	1.0	0	5	4	0	1	n/a	n/a	n/a	n/a
fresh spinach	1 order	5	0	0.0	10	0	0	0	0	n/a	n/a	n/a	n/a
ham	1 order	100	4	1.5	1020	3	0	0	14	n/a	n/a	n/a	n/a
jalapeños	1 order	5	0	0.0	440	1	0	1	0	n/a	n/a	n/a	n/a
omelet, egg white, plain	1	110	2	0.0	340	1	0	1	20	n/a	n/a	n/a	n/a
omelet, plain	1	340	26	7.0	540	2	0	0	21	n/a	n/a	n/a	n/a
pepper Jack queso	1 order	100	7	3.0	360	5	0	2	3	n/a	n/a	n/a	n/a
pico de gallo	1 order	15	0	0.0	75	3	1	2	1	n/a	n/a	n/a	n/a
sausage	1 order	180	17	5.0	330	0	0	0	6	n/a	n/a	n/a	n/a
sautéed mushrooms	1 order	50	6	1.0	55	1	0	0	1	n/a	n/a	n/a	n/a
Swiss cheese	1 slice	80	6	4.0	45	0	0	0	6	n/a	n/a	n/a	n/a
tomatoes	1 order	10	0	0.0	0	2	1	1	0	n/a	n/a	n/a	n/a
turkey bacon	2 slices	70	4	1.0	330	1	0	1	7	n/a	n/a	n/a	n/a
Loaded veggie	1 order	500	38	12.0	680	9	2	4	29	n/a	n/a	n/a	n/a

RESTAURANT & FAST FOOD CHAINS

Denny's

	Amount	Calories	Fat (g)	Saturated Fat (g)	Sodium (mg)	Carbohydrate (g)	Fiber (g)	Sugar (g)	Protein (g)	Vitamin D (mcg)	Calcium (mg)	Iron (mg)	Potassium (mg)
Mile High Denver	1 order	660	48	18.0	2430	11	1	3	44	n/a	n/a	n/a	n/a
Ultimate	1 order	720	59	19.0	1250	9	1	4	37	n/a	n/a	n/a	n/a
Pancakes													
Caramel & banana cream	2	930	24	15.0	1590	166	6	81	15	n/a	n/a	n/a	n/a
Choconana	2	870	27	15.0	1360	152	9	75	14	n/a	n/a	n/a	n/a
Cinnamon roll													
w/ cream cheese icing	2	1030	25	11.0	1660	188	4	127	10	n/a	n/a	n/a	n/a
w/ salted caramel	2	1010	24	10.0	1750	188	4	123	11	n/a	n/a	n/a	n/a
Double berry banana	2	540	10	4.0	1360	103	8	36	12	n/a	n/a	n/a	n/a
Hearty 9-grain	2	410	11	4.0	880	68	5	21	10	n/a	n/a	n/a	n/a
Slams													
All-American Slam w/ hash browns	1 order	930	69	25.0	1940	28	2	2	44	n/a	n/a	n/a	n/a
FitSlam	1 order	450	12	2.5	860	59	5	22	27	n/a	n/a	n/a	n/a
French Toast Slam	1 order	790	52	16.0	1570	54	3	12	30	n/a	n/a	n/a	n/a
Grand Slam Slugger	1 order	710	34	11.0	2100	79	3	21	22	n/a	n/a	n/a	n/a
Lumberjack Slam w/ hash browns	1 order	980	45	14.0	3570	107	4	22	38	n/a	n/a	n/a	n/a
Original Grand Slam	1 order	700	34	11.0	2100	79	3	21	22	n/a	n/a	n/a	n/a
Super Slam	1 order	880	41	13.0	2550	103	4	22	23	n/a	n/a	n/a	n/a
Breakfast Sides													
Bacon strips	4	210	16	6.0	700	2	0	1	14	n/a	n/a	n/a	n/a
Buttermilk biscuits	2	470	26	13.0	1320	54	2	4	8	n/a	n/a	n/a	n/a
Cheddar cheese hash browns	1 order	250	14	6.0	580	24	1	1	6	n/a	n/a	n/a	n/a
Eggs													
boiled	1	60	4	1.5	60	0	0	0	6	n/a	n/a	n/a	n/a
fried/basted	1	90	8	2.0	100	0	0	0	6	n/a	n/a	n/a	n/a
scrambled	1	110	9	2.5	180	1	0	0	7	n/a	n/a	n/a	n/a
white	1	40	0	0.0	115	0	0	0	7	n/a	n/a	n/a	n/a
English muffins													
w/ margarine	1	190	6	1.0	270	29	1	1	5	n/a	n/a	n/a	n/a
gluten-free	1	210	6	0.5	540	36	1	7	4	n/a	n/a	n/a	n/a
w/o margarine	1	140	1	0.0	220	29	1	1	5	n/a	n/a	n/a	n/a
gluten-free	1	180	2	0.0	500	36	1	7	4	n/a	n/a	n/a	n/a
Grilled ham slice	1	100	4	1.5	1020	3	0	0	14	n/a	n/a	n/a	n/a
Hash browns	1 order	180	8	1.5	460	24	1	1	1	n/a	n/a	n/a	n/a
everything	1 order	310	17	7.0	790	32	2	3	7	n/a	n/a	n/a	n/a
Red-skinned potatoes	1 order	200	10	2.0	670	24	3	1	3	n/a	n/a	n/a	n/a
Sausage links	4	310	29	9.0	700	3	2	1	10	n/a	n/a	n/a	n/a
Seasonal fruit	1 order	110	0	0.0	5	27	3	19	1	n/a	n/a	n/a	n/a
Toast													
sourdough w/ margarine	2	280	12	2.5	460	37	1	2	6	n/a	n/a	n/a	n/a
sourdough w/o margarine	2	210	3	1.0	380	37	1	2	6	n/a	n/a	n/a	n/a
wheat w/ margarine	2	230	11	1.5	400	29	2	2	6	n/a	n/a	n/a	n/a
wheat w/o margarine	2	150	2	0.0	310	29	2	2	6	n/a	n/a	n/a	n/a

RESTAURANT & FAST FOOD CHAINS

Denny's	Amount	Calories	Fat (g)	Saturated Fat (g)	Sodium (mg)	Carbohydrate (g)	Fiber (g)	Sugar (g)	Protein (g)	Vitamin D (mcg)	Calcium (mg)	Iron (mg)	Potassium (mg)
white w/ margarine	2	240	10	2.0	400	31	0	2	5	n/a	n/a	n/a	n/a
white w/o margarine	2	160	2	0.0	320	31	0	2	5	n/a	n/a	n/a	n/a
Tortillas, flour	3	260	8	3.5	660	40	5	3	7	n/a	n/a	n/a	n/a
Turkey bacon strips	4	140	8	2.0	660	2	0	15	2	n/a	n/a	n/a	n/a
Appetizers													
Bacon cheddar tots w/ sour cream	10	500	32	13.0	1900	39	0	1	15	n/a	n/a	n/a	n/a
Beer-battered onion rings	1 order	800	54	9.0	1430	71	6	11	9	n/a	n/a	n/a	n/a
Boneless chicken wings													
w/ BBQ sauce	8	770	36	5.0	3020	80	5	37	35	n/a	n/a	n/a	n/a
w/ Buffalo sauce	8	770	52	8.0	3750	42	5	1	34	n/a	n/a	n/a	n/a
w/ Nashville hot sauce	8	720	42	8.0	3300	52	6	8	35	n/a	n/a	n/a	n/a
Burgers													
America's Dinner single	1	820	50	20.0	1640	51	2	12	41	n/a	n/a	n/a	n/a
America's Dinner double	1	1250	83	36.0	2520	52	2	13	74	n/a	n/a	n/a	n/a
Bacon avocado cheeseburger	1	1080	72	25.0	1650	57	8	12	51	n/a	n/a	n/a	n/a
Bourbon bacon burger	1	910	51	21.0	1700	64	4	22	50	n/a	n/a	n/a	n/a
Build Your Own													
bacon strips	2 slices	100	8	3.0	350	1	0	1	7	n/a	n/a	n/a	n/a
brioche bun	1	250	5	2.0	380	45	2	9	8	n/a	n/a	n/a	n/a
carmelized onions	1 order	70	7	1.0	210	2	1	1	0	n/a	n/a	n/a	n/a
cheese													
American	1 slice	80	7	4.0	390	1	0	1	4	n/a	n/a	n/a	n/a
cheddar	1 slice	80	6	3.5	120	0	0	0	5	n/a	n/a	n/a	n/a
Swiss	1 slice	80	6	4.0	45	0	0	0	6	n/a	n/a	n/a	n/a
chicken breast													
fried	1	410	26	5.0	1280	18	2	0	27	n/a	n/a	n/a	n/a
grilled seasoned	1	200	9	2.5	820	1	0	0	29	n/a	n/a	n/a	n/a
fresh avocado	1 order	90	8	1.0	0	5	4	0	1	n/a	n/a	n/a	n/a
jalapeños	1 order	5	0	0.0	440	1	0	1	0	n/a	n/a	n/a	n/a
lettuce	1 order	5	0	0.0	5	1	0	0	0	n/a	n/a	n/a	n/a
mayonnaise	1 order	100	11	2.0	75	0	0	0	0	n/a	n/a	n/a	n/a
patty													
100% beef	1	360	26	12.0	480	0	0	0	29	n/a	n/a	n/a	n/a
Beyond Burger	1	320	25	7.0	860	6	2	0	20	n/a	n/a	n/a	n/a
pickles	4 slices	0	0	0.0	180	0	0	0	0	n/a	n/a	n/a	n/a
red onions	3 rings	5	0	0.0	0	2	0	1	0	n/a	n/a	n/a	n/a
sauce													
All-American	1 order	120	12	2.0	230	2	0	1	0	n/a	n/a	n/a	n/a
BBQ	1 order	70	0	0.0	310	20	0	19	0	n/a	n/a	n/a	n/a
bourbon	1 order	110	0	0.0	270	26	0	24	0	n/a	n/a	n/a	n/a
sautéed mushrooms	1 order	50	6	1.0	55	1	0	0	1	n/a	n/a	n/a	n/a
tomato	2 slices	5	0	0.0	0	2	0	1	0	n/a	n/a	n/a	n/a
Double cheeseburger	1	980	56	25.0	1540	50	3	11	66	n/a	n/a	n/a	n/a
Slamburger	1	870	49	21.0	1830	59	2	10	48	n/a	n/a	n/a	n/a

RESTAURANT & FAST FOOD CHAINS

Denny's

Denny's

	Amount	Calories	Fat (g)	Saturated Fat (g)	Sodium (mg)	Carbohydrate (g)	Fiber (g)	Sugar (g)	Protein (g)	Vitamin D (mcg)	Calcium (mg)	Iron (mg)	Potassium
Dinners													
Brooklyn spaghetti & meatballs	1 order	1080	51	17.0	2460	111	8	17	40	n/a	n/a	n/a	n/a
Chicken Addiction bowl	1 order	870	39	12.0	2200	84	9	8	47	n/a	n/a	n/a	n/a
Country-fried steak	1 order	960	56	21.0	2240	78	3	4	35	n/a	n/a	n/a	n/a
Fried fish platter	1 order	1010	68	11.0	1680	65	1	6	33	n/a	n/a	n/a	n/a
Mama D's pot roast bowl	1 order	760	32	11.0	3040	65	5	11	54	n/a	n/a	n/a	n/a
Plate Lickin' Chicken fried chicken	1 order	1070	62	14.0	3230	68	6	3	60	n/a	n/a	n/a	n/a
Premium chicken tenders	1 order	860	47	7.0	2860	63	3	2	51	n/a	n/a	n/a	n/a
Sirloin steak	1 order	530	25	7.0	1420	27	1	2	49	n/a	n/a	n/a	n/a
Sizzlin' Skillet, bourbon chicken	1 order	840	35	7.0	2920	69	7	36	65	n/a	n/a	n/a	n/a
Sizzlin' Skillet, Crazy Spicy	1 order	990	66	23.0	3500	43	5	9	59	n/a	n/a	n/a	n/a
T-bone steak	1 order	680	38	14.0	1690	26	1	2	57	n/a	n/a	n/a	n/a
Wild salmon	1 order	540	31	8.0	1130	27	1	2	37	n/a	n/a	n/a	n/a
Melts & Handhelds													
Melts													
All-American patty	1	1100	70	25.0	2030	69	3	7	49	n/a	n/a	n/a	n/a
The Big Dipper	1	1140	69	22.0	220	63	2	11	65	n/a	n/a	n/a	n/a
Nashville hot chicken	1	1260	81	25.0	3080	84	6	19	50	n/a	n/a	n/a	n/a
Sandwiches													
Cali club	1	890	55	14.0	2070	59	10	12	44	n/a	n/a	n/a	n/a
Chick 'n BBQ	1	740	28	6.0	2400	91	5	33	42	n/a	n/a	n/a	n/a
Chick 'n Buffalo	1	740	28	6.0	2400	91	5	33	42	n/a	n/a	n/a	n/a
Chick 'n honey	1	770	40	13.0	2020	70	4	21	34	n/a	n/a	n/a	n/a
The Super Bird	1	680	35	14.0	1830	44	2	5	46	n/a	n/a	n/a	n/a
Salads													
Cobb	1 order	480	34	12.0	610	23	7	6	22	n/a	n/a	n/a	n/a
House	1 order	190	9	4.5	340	19	3	6	9	n/a	n/a	n/a	n/a
Toppings													
fresh avocado	1 order	90	8	1.0	0	5	4	0	1	n/a	n/a	n/a	n/a
grilled chicken	1 order	200	9	2.5	820	1	0	0	25	n/a	n/a	n/a	n/a
premium chicken tenders	3	410	24	3.0	1500	23	2	0	27	n/a	n/a	n/a	n/a
prime rib	1 order	140	8	2.0	430	2	0	0	14	n/a	n/a	n/a	n/a
wild Alaskan salmon	1 order	350	23	6.0	780	2	0	1	32	n/a	n/a	n/a	n/a
Dinner Sides													
Broccoli	1 order	35	0	0.0	180	6	3	1	3	n/a	n/a	n/a	n/a
Build Your Own Sampler													
…eer-battered onion rings	1 order	400	27	4.5	710	35	3	5	4	n/a	n/a	n/a	n/a
…eless Buffalo wings	4	460	34	5.0	2550	22	3	0	17	n/a	n/a	n/a	n/a
…& queso	1 order	570	34	9.0	620	57	4	3	10	n/a	n/a	n/a	n/a
…lla sticks	4	570	11	6.0	1230	30	1	2	16	n/a	n/a	n/a	n/a
…hicken tenders	2	270	16	2.0	1000	15	1	0	18	n/a	n/a	n/a	n/a

95

RESTAURANT & FAST FOOD CHAINS

	Amount	Calories	Fat (g)	Saturated Fat (g)	Sodium (mg)	Carbohydrate (g)	Fiber (g)	Sugar (g)	Protein (g)	Vitamin D (mcg)	Calcium (mg)	Iron (mg)	Potassium (mg)
Denny's													
fries, seasoned	1 order	490	26	5.0	1100	57	8	1	7	n/a	n/a	n/a	n/a
fries, wavy-cut	1 order	400	22	4.0	470	46	4	0	4	n/a	n/a	n/a	n/a
Cinnamon Sugar Pancake Puppies	6	530	18	6.0	780	87	1	53	4	n/a	n/a	n/a	n/a
Fresh sauteed zucchini & squash	1 order	70	6	1.0	220	3	1	2	1	n/a	n/a	n/a	n/a
Loaded bacon cheddar tots	10	730	50	22.0	2550	45	0	3	27	n/a	n/a	n/a	n/a
add seasoned taco meat	1 order	200	14	5.0	1060	7	1	3	10	n/a	n/a	n/a	n/a
Mozzarella cheese sticks	8	560	22	13.0	2460	60	2	4	32	n/a	n/a	n/a	n/a
Garlic toast	2 pcs	190	7	2.0	360	25	1	2	6	n/a	n/a	n/a	n/a
Red-skinned mashed potatoes	1 order	140	6	4.0	530	18	0	3	3	n/a	n/a	n/a	n/a
Sweet petite corn	1 order	210	13	2.5	280	20	5	9	4	n/a	n/a	n/a	n/a
Wavy-cut fries	1 order	400	22	4.0	470	46	4	0	4	n/a	n/a	n/a	n/a
Whole grain rice	1 order	240	2.5	0.5	360	48	5	2	6	n/a	n/a	n/a	n/a
Zesty nachos	1 order	870	55	19.0	1820	69	6	9	25	n/a	n/a	n/a	n/a
Soups													
Chicken noodle	cup	260	10	4.0	2580	28	2	4	14	n/a	n/a	n/a	n/a
	bowl	390	15	6.0	3880	43	2	5	21	n/a	n/a	n/a	n/a
Loaded baked potato	cup	340	23	11.0	1180	22	1	5	10	n/a	n/a	n/a	n/a
	bowl	440	29	15.0	1650	32	2	5	12	n/a	n/a	n/a	n/a
Vegetable beef	cup	200	11	2.0	2280	27	2	3	11	n/a	n/a	n/a	n/a
	bowl	310	16	3.0	3420	40	3	4	16	n/a	n/a	n/a	n/a
Desserts													
Caramel apple pie crisp	1 order	830	27	15.0	690	142	4	100	7	n/a	n/a	n/a	n/a
New York–style cheesecake	1 order	490	32	19.0	370	42	1	29	9	n/a	n/a	n/a	n/a
Signature Skookie	1 order	820	40	25.0	460	108	0	73	10	n/a	n/a	n/a	n/a
Domino's													
Pizza*													
Buffalo chicken	1 slice	350	16	8.0	840	33	1	2	15	n/a	n/a	n/a	n/a
Cali chicken bacon ranch	1 slice	410	23	8.0	890	33	1	3	16	n/a	n/a	n/a	n/a
Cheese	1 slice	130	10	6.0	400	3	0	0	8	n/a	n/a	n/a	n/a
Chicken taco	1 slice	350	16	8.0	780	35	1	4	16	n/a	n/a	n/a	n/a
Cheeseburger	1 slice	380	19	8.0	880	35	1	4	15	n/a	n/a	n/a	n/a
Deluxe	1 slice	310	13	5.0	640	35	2	4	12	n/a	n/a	n/a	n/a
ExtravaganZZa	1 slice	390	19	8.0	940	36	2	4	16	n/a	n/a	n/a	n/a
Honolulu Hawaiian	1 slice	330	14	7.0	770	35	2	5	14	n/a	n/a	n/a	n/a
MeatZZa	1 slice	370	18	8.0	890	34	1	3	16	n/a	n/a	n/a	n/a
Memphis BBQ chicken	1 slice	350	14	7.0	670	39	1	7	15	n/a	n/a	n/a	n/a
Philly cheesesteak	1 slice	310	13	7.0	720	33	1	3	13	n/a	n/a	n/a	n/a
Pacific veggie	1 slice	310	13	6.0	640	35	2	3	12	n/a	n/a	n/a	n/a
Spinach & feta	1 slice	320	15	8.0	610	33	1	2	13	n/a	n/a	n/a	n/'
Ultimate pepperoni	1 slice	370	18	8.0	860	34	2	3	15	n/a	n/a	n/a	n
Wisconsin 6 cheese	1 slice	340	15	8.0	660	35	2	3	15	n/a	n/a	n/a	

* Based on a 12-in medium pizza (8 slices).

Domino's

	Amount	Calories	Fat (g)	Saturated Fat (g)	Sodium (mg)	Carbohydrate (g)	Fiber (g)	Sugar (g)	Protein (g)	Vitamin D (mcg)	Calcium (mg)	Iron (mg)	Potassium
Chicken													
Boneless chicken	3 pcs	170	7	1.5	660	18	0	1	9	n/a	n/a	n/a	n/a
Specialty chicken													
classic hot Buffalo	4 pcs	190	11	3.5	1040	14	0	1	9	n/a	n/a	n/a	n/a
crispy bacon & tomato	4 pcs	260	18	5.0	810	14	0	1	11	n/a	n/a	n/a	n/a
spicy jalapeño pineapple	4 pcs	190	11	3.5	1040	14	0	1	9	n/a	n/a	n/a	n/a
sweet BBQ bacon	4 pcs	220	10	4.0	790	20	0	7	11	n/a	n/a	n/a	n/a
Wings	4 pcs	250	20	5.0	720	8	0	0	14	n/a	n/a	n/a	n/a
garlic Parmesan	4 pcs	390	34	8.0	960	10	0	1	15	n/a	n/a	n/a	n/a
honey BBQ	4 pcs	310	20	5.0	940	22	0	13	15	n/a	n/a	n/a	n/a
hot Buffalo	4 pcs	260	20	5.0	1520	9	0	0	15	n/a	n/a	n/a	n/a
sweet mango habanero	4 pcs	310	20	5.0	790	21	0	10	15	n/a	n/a	n/a	n/a
Pasta													
Chicken Alfredo	1 order	600	29	17.0	1110	60	2	5	25	n/a	n/a	n/a	n/a
Chicken carbonara	1 order	690	34	19.0	1370	63	2	6	30	n/a	n/a	n/a	n/a
Italian sausage marinara	1 order	700	36	15.0	1650	68	3	13	27	n/a	n/a	n/a	n/a
Pasta primavera	1 order	530	26	16.0	880	62	3	6	15	n/a	n/a	n/a	n/a
Sandwiches													
Buffalo chicken	½	420	21	8.0	1300	37	1	2	20	n/a	n/a	n/a	n/a
Chicken bacon ranch	½	440	22	8.0	1260	35	1	2	22	n/a	n/a	n/a	n/a
Chicken habanero	½	400	16	8.0	1120	42	1	7	22	n/a	n/a	n/a	n/a
Chicken parm	½	380	15	7.0	1080	36	2	2	24	n/a	n/a	n/a	n/a
Italian	½	410	20	9.0	1470	35	2	2	21	n/a	n/a	n/a	n/a
Mediterranean veggie	½	350	15	8.0	1210	38	2	4	16	n/a	n/a	n/a	n/a
Philly cheesesteak	½	360	15	8.0	1320	37	2	3	19	n/a	n/a	n/a	n/a
Bread													
Bread twists													
garlic	2 pcs	230	11	4.5	220	27	1	1	5	n/a	n/a	n/a	n/a
Parmesan	2 pcs	230	11	4.5	240	27	1	1	5	n/a	n/a	n/a	n/a
Parmesan bread bites	4 pcs	220	10	4.5	220	27	1	1	5	n/a	n/a	n/a	n/a
Stuffed cheesy bread	1 pc	150	7	3.0	250	16	0	1	6	n/a	n/a	n/a	n/a
w/ bacon & jalapeño	1 pc	170	8	3.5	350	16	1	1	7	n/a	n/a	n/a	n/a
w/ spinach & feta	1 pc	160	7	3.5	270	16	1	1	6	n/a	n/a	n/a	n/a
Salads													
ken Caesar	1 order	220	8	3.0	570	14	2	3	18	n/a	n/a	n/a	n/a
garden	1 order	80	4	2.0	120	8	1	2	3	n/a	n/a	n/a	n/a
va crunch cake	1	360	19	10.0	160	46	0	29	4	n/a	n/a	n/a	n/a
d twists	2 pcs	250	12	4.5	170	31	1	6	5	n/a	n/a	n/a	n/a
brownie	1	200	10	3.5	125	26	1	19	2	n/a	n/a	n/a	n/a

Dunkin'

	Amount	Calories	Fat (g)	Saturated Fat (g)	Sodium (mg)	Carbohydrate (g)	Fiber (g)	Sugar (g)	Protein (g)	Vitamin D (mcg)	Calcium (mg)	Iron (mg)	Potassium (mg)
Americano													
Hot	medium	10	0	0.0	30	2	0	0	0	0	15	0	142
Iced	medium	10	0	0.0	30	2	0	0	0	0	18	0	116
Cappuccino, Hot & Iced													
Caramel swirl													
w/ skim milk	medium	230	0	0.0	150	49	0	47	8	2	314	0	615
w/ whole milk	medium	280	6	3.5	150	48	0	47	8	2	296	0	570
French vanilla swirl													
w/ skim milk	medium	230	0	0.0	140	48	0	46	8	2	299	0	587
w/ whole milk	medium	280	6	3.5	140	48	0	45	8	2	282	0	542
Hazelnut swirl													
w/ skim milk	medium	230	0	0.0	150	49	0	46	8	2	299	0	587
w/ whole milk	medium	280	6	3.5	150	48	0	45	8	2	282	0	543
Mocha swirl													
w/ skim milk	medium	220	1	0.5	115	48	2	43	7	2	244	1	618
w/ whole milk	medium	270	7	4.0	120	48	2	43	7	2	227	1	573
Regular													
w/ skim milk	medium	70	0	0.0	95	10	0	9	6	2	236	0	354
w/ skim milk & sugar	medium	170	0	0.0	95	36	0	35	6	2	236	0	355
w/ whole milk	medium	120	6	3.5	100	10	0	9	6	2	219	0	310
w/ whole milk & sugar	medium	220	6	3.5	100	36	0	35	6	2	219	0	310
Coffee, Cold Brew													
Regular													
	medium	5	0	0.0	15	0	0	0	0	0	21	0	275
w/ cream	medium	90	9	4.5	45	1	0	1	2	0	55	0	247
w/ cream & sugar	medium	190	9	4.5	45	27	0	27	2	0	55	0	247
Coffee, Hot & Iced													
Caramel swirl													
black	medium	170	0	0.0	65	39	0	38	3	0	92	0	459
w/ cream	medium	260	9	4.5	95	40	0	40	4	0	132	0	500
French vanilla swirl													
black	medium	170	0	0.0	60	38	0	37	2	0	77	0	432
w/ cream	medium	250	9	4.5	90	40	0	38	4	0	118	0	473
Hazelnut swirl													
black	medium	170	0	0.0	60	38	0	37	2	0	77	0	432
w/ cream	medium	250	9	4.5	90	40	0	38	4	0	118	0	473
Mocha swirl													
black	medium	160	0.5	0.0	35	38	2	34	2	0	23	1	462
w/ cream	medium	240	9	5.0	65	39	2	35	3	0	63	1	503
Regular													
black	medium	5	0	0.0	15	0	0	0	1	0	15	0	206
black w/ sugar	medium	110	0	0.0	15	26	0	26	1	0	15	0	206
w/ almond milk	medium	25	1	0.0	50	4	0	3	1	1	130	0	221

RESTAURANT & FAST FOOD CHAINS

Dunkin'

	Amount	Calories	Fat (g)	Saturated Fat (g)	Sodium (mg)	Carbohydrate (g)	Fiber (g)	Sugar (g)	Protein (g)	Vitamin D (mcg)	Calcium (mg)	Iron (mg)	Potassium (mg)
w/ cream	medium	90	9	4.5	45	1	0	1	2	0	55	0	257
w/ cream & sugar	medium	190	9	4.5	45	27	0	27	2	0	55	0	247
w/ skim milk	medium	20	0	0.0	35	2	0	2	2	1	70	0	257
w/ skim milk & sugar	medium	120	0	0.0	35	28	0	28	2	1	70	0	257
w/ whole milk	medium	30	2	1.0	35	2	0	2	2	1	66	0	246
w/ whole milk & sugar	medium	130	2	1.0	35	28	0	28	2	1	66	0	246
Coolattas													
Blue raspberry	medium	350	0	0.0	45	84	0	83	0	0	18	0	7
Strawberry	medium	350	0	0.0	15	86	1	83	0	0	24	0	93
Vanilla bean	medium	590	5	2.5	240	129	0	125	7	2	284	0	342
Espresso													
Single shot	1	5	0	0.0	5	1	0	0	0	0	1	0	46
w/ sugar	1	60	0	0.0	5	15	0	14	0	0	1	0	46
Frozen Chocolate													
Caramel swirl	medium	700	14	10.0	290	135	1	126	9	2	302	0	639
Hazelnut swirl	medium	700	14	10.0	280	135	1	124	9	2	287	0	612
French vanilla swirl	medium	700	14	10.0	280	135	1	124	9	2	287	0	612
Regular	medium	690	15	10.0	250	134	3	121	7	2	214	2	643
Frozen Coffee													
Caramel swirl													
w/ cream	medium	860	31	17.0	220	139	0	132	8	2	267	2	1730
w/ skim milk	medium	650	5	3.0	180	142	0	135	9	2	312	2	1760
w/ whole milk	medium	680	9	6.0	180	141	0	134	8	2	299	2	1727
French vanilla swirl													
w/ cream	medium	860	31	17.0	220	138	0	130	8	2	253	2	1703
w/ skim milk	medium	640	5	3.0	180	141	0	133	9	2	297	2	1733
w/ whole milk	medium	680	9	6.0	180	141	0	132	8	2	284	2	1699
Hazelnut swirl													
w/ cream	medium	860	31	17.0	220	138	0	130	8	2	253	2	1703
w/ skim milk	medium	640	5	3.0	180	141	0	133	9	2	297	2	1733
w/ whole milk	medium	680	9	6.0	180	141	0	132	8	2	284	2	1699
Mocha swirl													
w/ cream	medium	850	31	17.0	190	137	2	125	7	2	180	3	1734
w/ skim milk	medium	630	5	3.5	100	99	2	90	5	1	155	2	1206
w/ whole milk	medium	670	10	6.0	150	140	2	129	7	2	211	3	1730
Regular													
w/ cream	medium	590	26	14.0	150	85	0	81	5	1	153	2	1381
w/ skim milk	medium	370	0	0.0	115	88	0	84	6	2	198	2	1411
w/ whole milk	medium	410	5	2.5	115	88	0	84	5	2	185	2	1377
Hot Chocolate													
Dunkaccino	medium	350	15	12.0	340	52	1	38	3	0	67	0	408
Mint	medium	300	10	9.0	260	52	2	42	2	0	23	0	173

RESTAURANT & FAST FOOD CHAINS

Dunkin'	Amount	Calories	Fat (g)	Saturated Fat (g)	Sodium (mg)	Carbohydrate (g)	Fiber (g)	Sugar (g)	Protein (g)	Vitamin D (mcg)	Calcium (mg)	Iron (mg)	Potassium (mg)
Oreo	medium	350	8	6.0	380	66	2	53	4	0	103	3	457
Regular	medium	330	10	9.0	320	59	2	46	3	0	50	0	220
Lattes, Hot & Iced													
Caramel swirl													
w/ skim milk	medium	260	0	0.0	190	53	0	52	11	3	426	0	758
w/ whole milk	medium	340	9	5.0	190	53	0	52	11	4	400	0	690
Chai													
w/ skim milk	medium	220	0	0.0	150	44	2	41	10	3	338	0	488
w/ whole milk	medium	290	9	5.0	150	43	2	40	9	4	312	0	421
French vanilla swirl													
w/ skim milk	medium	260	0	0.0	180	53	0	50	11	3	411	0	730
w/ whole milk	medium	320	9	5.0	180	52	0	50	11	4	385	0	663
Matcha													
w/ skim milk	medium	180	0	0.0	115	34	1	32	11	6	336	0	430
w/ whole milk	medium	250	9	5.0	120	33	1	32	10	6	362	0	310
Mocha swirl													
w/ skim milk	medium	250	1	0.5	160	52	2	48	10	3	356	1	761
w/ whole milk	medium	330	10	6.0	160	52	2	47	10	4	330	1	694
Regular													
w/ almond milk	medium	100	3	0.0	190	17	1	15	1	3	563	1	276
w/ skim milk	medium	100	0	0.0	135	15	0	14	9	3	348	0	498
w/ skim milk & sugar	medium	200	0	0.0	135	41	0	40	9	3	348	0	498
w/ whole milk	medium	170	9	5.0	135	14	0	13	9	4	322	0	430
w/ whole milk & sugar	medium	270	9	5.0	135	40	0	39	9	4	323	0	431
Signature caramel craze													
w/ skim milk	medium	340	5	3.0	190	61	0	57	12	3	442	0	792
w/ whole milk	medium	410	14	8.0	190	61	0	57	11	4	416	0	725
Signature cocoa mocha													
w/ skim milk	medium	330	6	3.5	160	61	2	53	11	3	373	2	798
w/ whole milk	medium	400	14	9.0	170	60	2	52	10	4	347	2	731
Macchiatos, Hot & Iced													
Caramel swirl													
w/ skim milk	medium	240	0	0.0	150	49	0	47	8	2	314	0	661
w/ whole milk	medium	290	6	3.5	150	49	0	47	8	2	297	0	616
French vanilla													
w/ skim milk	medium	230	0	0.0	150	49	0	46	8	2	300	0	633
w/ whole milk	medium	280	6	3.5	150	49	0	45	8	2	283	0	588
Hazelnut swirl													
w/ skim milk	medium	230	0	0.0	150	49	0	46	8	2	300	0	633
w/ whole milk	medium	280	6	0.5	150	49	0	45	8	2	283	0	589
Mocha swirl													
w/ skim milk	medium	230	1	0.5	125	49	2	43	7	2	245	2	664
w/ whole milk	medium	280	7	4.0	125	48	2	43	7	2	228	2	619

RESTAURANT & FAST FOOD CHAINS

Dunkin'

	Amount	Calories	Fat (g)	Saturated Fat (g)	Sodium (mg)	Carbohydrate (g)	Fiber (g)	Sugar (g)	Protein (g)	Vitamin D (mcg)	Calcium (mg)	Iron (mg)	Potassium (mg)
Regular													
w/ skim milk	medium	70	0	0.0	100	11	0	9	6	2	237	0	400
w/ skim milk & sugar	medium	170	0	0.0	100	37	0	35	6	2	237	0	401
w/ whole milk	medium	120	6	3.5	105	10	0	9	6	2	220	0	356
w/ whole milk & sugar	medium	220	6	3.5	105	37	0	35	6	2	220	0	356
Iced Tea													
Blueberry													
sweetened	medium	110	0	0.0	20	29	0	25	0	0	6	0	149
unsweetened	medium	15	0	0.0	20	4	0	0	0	0	6	0	149
Raspberry													
sweetened	medium	110	0	0.0	20	29	0	25	0	0	6	0	149
unsweetened	medium	15	0	0.0	20	4	0	0	0	0	6	0	149
Green													
sweetened	medium	100	0	0.0	10	25	0	25	1	0	6	0	36
unsweetened	medium	5	0	0.0	10	0	0	0	1	0	6	0	36
Regular													
sweetened	medium	100	0	0.0	20	26	0	25	0	0	6	0	159
unsweetened	medium	15	0	0.0	20	3	0	0	0	0	6	0	148
Sweet tea	medium	230	0	0.0	20	60	0	58	0	0	7	0	154
blueberry	medium	250	0	0.0	20	64	0	60	0	0	7	0	167
raspberry	medium	250	0	0.0	20	65	0	60	0	0	7	0	167
Bagels													
Cinnamon raisin	1	320	1	0.0	510	67	4	13	11	0	38	3	160
Everything	1	340	3	0.5	630	67	5	8	12	0	57	4	182
Multigrain	1	380	8	1.0	550	63	8	8	15	0	52	5	297
Plain	1	300	1	0.0	620	64	4	7	11	0	20	4	126
Sesame seed	1	350	5	1.0	630	64	5	7	12	0	24	4	152
White cheddar twist	1	390	8	4.5	760	64	4	7	16	0	171	4	142
Cream Cheese													
Classic plain	1 pkt	120	12	8.0	200	3	0	3	2	0	36	0	0
Garden veggie	1 pkt	100	10	6.0	200	2	0	1	2	0	33	0	0
Strawberry	1 pkt	130	10	6.0	100	9	0	8	2	0	32	0	0
Donuts													
Apple crumb	1	290	11	4.5	310	44	1	21	5	1	12	2	73
Apple fritter	1	510	28	12.0	470	57	2	24	6	0	26	1	110
Bavarian kreme	1	240	11	4.0	310	31	1	11	4	1	12	2	59
Boston kreme	1	270	11	4.5	320	39	1	18	5	1	13	2	80
Chocolate frosted	1	260	11	4.5	290	34	1	13	4	0	13	2	75
Coffee roll	1	390	19	8.0	440	48	2	17	7	0	27	3	92
Double chocolate	1	370	22	10.0	440	40	1	19	4	0	35	2	185
Éclair	1	370	16	6.0	470	50	2	23	6	2	18	3	106
French cruller	1	230	14	7.0	135	21	0	10	3	0	12	0	17

RESTAURANT & FAST FOOD CHAINS

Dunkin'

	Amount	Calories	Fat (g)	Saturated Fat (g)	Sodium (mg)	Carbohydrate (g)	Fiber (g)	Sugar (g)	Protein (g)	Vitamin D (mcg)	Calcium (mg)	Iron (mg)	Potassium (mg)
Glazed	1	240	11	4.5	270	33	1	13	4	0	12	2	56
blueberry	1	350	18	7.0	380	44	1	21	4	0	20	1	68
chocolate	1	360	22	10.0	420	39	1	18	4	0	34	2	167
Jelly	1	250	10	4.0	290	36	1	13	4	1	13	2	58
Old fashioned	1	310	19	9.0	320	30	1	10	4	0	24	2	64
Powdered	1	330	20	9.0	320	34	1	14	4	0	24	2	64
Strawberry frosted w/ sprinkles	1	270	12	5.0	280	37	1	16	4	0	12	2	59
Vanilla crème	1	300	15	6.0	290	37	1	18	4	1	12	2	61
Vanilla frosted w/ sprinkles	1	270	11	4.5	280	37	1	16	4	0	12	2	60
Munchkins													
Glazed	1	60	3	1.5	60	7	0	3	1	0	2	0	11
blueberry	1	70	4	2.0	65	8	0	4	1	0	4	0	12
chocolate	1	60	4	1.5	80	8	0	4	1	0	6	0	31
old fashioned	1	70	4	1.5	70	8	0	4	1	0	4	0	12
Jelly	1	60	3	1.5	65	8	0	3	1	0	3	0	11
Powdered	1	60	4	1.5	70	6	0	2	1	0	4	0	12
Muffins													
Blueberry	1	460	15	3.0	390	77	1	44	6	0	21	2	93
Chocolate chip	1	550	21	6.0	400	85	2	49	7	0	29	3	175
Coffee cake	1	290	24	8.0	370	88	2	51	7	0	36	3	101
Corn	1	460	16	3.0	670	73	1	30	7	0	17	2	85
Sandwiches													
Bacon, egg & cheese													
bagel	1	520	18	6.0	1200	67	4	8	23	1	137	5	280
croissant	1	560	36	14.0	820	41	1	6	18	4	126	3	210
English muffin	1	400	19	7.0	840	39	1	4	18	2	126	3	209
Wake-Up Wrap	1	220	13	5.0	590	15	0	1	10	1	134	1	112
Beyond Sausage													
English muffin	1	510	26	10.0	820	40	2	3	26	2	245	5	244
Wake-Up Wrap	1	280	18	7.0	500	15	1	1	14	1	224	2	119
Egg & cheese													
bagel	1	460	13	5.0	1010	66	4	8	19	1	135	4	222
croissant	1	500	31	13.0	640	40	1	6	15	4	125	3	153
English muffin	1	340	15	5.0	650	38	1	4	14	2	124	3	151
Wake-Up Wrap	1	180	10	4.0	470	14	0	1	7	1	132	1	74
Ham, egg & cheese													
bagel	1	500	15	5.0	1330	68	4	9	24	1	136	5	293
croissant	1	540	33	13.0	960	41	1	7	9	4	126	3	223
English muffin	1	370	15	5.0	910	39	1	4	19	2	126	3	349
Wake-Up Wrap	1	190	11	4.0	600	15	0	1	9	1	133	1	172

RESTAURANT & FAST FOOD CHAINS

Dunkin'	Amount	Calories	Fat (g)	Saturated Fat (g)	Sodium (mg)	Carbohydrate (g)	Fiber (g)	Sugar (g)	Protein (g)	Vitamin D (mcg)	Calcium (mg)	Iron (mg)	Potassium
Sausage, egg & cheese													
bagel	1	680	34	12.0	1500	68	5	8	26	2	162	5	330
croissant	1	720	52	20.0	1120	42	2	6	21	5	152	4	261
English muffin	1	560	35	12.0	1140	40	2	4	21	2	151	3	260
Wake-Up Wrap	1	290	21	8.0	710	15	1	1	10	1	146	2	128
Turkey sausage													
English muffin	1	460	22	7.0	1120	39	1	4	26	2	137	4	270
Wake-Up Wrap	1	240	15	6.0	680	15	0	1	11	1	135	2	122
Veggie egg white													
multigrain thin	1	290	13	5.0	550	27	5	4	17	0	193	2	246
Wake-Up Wrap	1	190	10	4.5	390	15	1	1	9	0	187	1	93
w/ Beyond Sausage	1	250	15	6.0	530	15	1	1	14	0	217	2	140
Power Breakfast Sandwich	1	420	23	8.0	980	28	5	5	25	0	344	2	199
Grilled cheese	1	480	20	11.0	1120	54	3	1	21	0	407	4	167
w/ ham	1	510	21	11.0	1390	55	3	1	25	0	408	4	365
Hardee's													
Biscuits													
Bacon, egg & cheese	1	620	40	6.0	1520	44	2	4	20	n/a	n/a	n/a	n/a
Beyond Sausage	1	480	26	13.0	1140	44	3	4	16	n/a	n/a	n/a	n/a
w/ egg	1	600	35	17.0	1440	47	3	4	25	n/a	n/a	n/a	n/a
Biscuit 'n' gravy	1	600	38	14.0	1580	54	2	5	10	n/a	n/a	n/a	n/a
Chicken fillet	1	660	43	13.0	1440	50	2	4	19	n/a	n/a	n/a	n/a
Country fried steak	1	650	44	15.0	1350	49	2	4	14	n/a	n/a	n/a	n/a
Country ham	1	510	32	12.0	1780	42	2	4	16	n/a	n/a	n/a	n/a
Frisco breakfast sandwich	1	430	19	8.0	1280	42	2	5	24	n/a	n/a	n/a	n/a
Loaded omelet	1	630	41	16.0	1480	46	2	4	19	n/a	n/a	n/a	n/a
Monster	1	890	63	25.0	2480	45	2	6	35	n/a	n/a	n/a	n/a
Pork chop 'n' gravy	1	550	34	12.0	1230	48	2	4	13	n/a	n/a	n/a	n/a
Sausage	1	630	45	17.0	1320	42	2	4	13	n/a	n/a	n/a	n/a
w/ egg	1	700	50	18.0	1400	44	2	4	19	n/a	n/a	n/a	n/a
Smoked sausage, egg & cheese	1	700	48	22.0	1920	45	2	6	23	n/a	n/a	n/a	n/a
Southwest omelet	1	660	45	18.0	1170	42	2	4	20	n/a	n/a	n/a	n/a
Breakfast Burritos													
Beyond Sausage	1	730	41	16.0	1170	51	0	1	36	n/a	n/a	n/a	n/a
Loaded	1	580	30	12.0	1320	46	3	2	30	n/a	n/a	n/a	n/a
Southwest omelet	1	690	41	16.0	1920	44	3	2	35	n/a	n/a	n/a	n/a
Breakfast Platters & Bowls													
Hardee breakfast platter													
w/ bacon	1	1050	68	21.0	2420	76	12	5	31	n/a	n/a	n/a	n/a
w/ chicken fillet	1	980	58	19.0	2030	63	4	6	29	n/a	n/a	n/a	n/a
w/ country ham	1	990	61	19.0	2600	75	4	6	32	n/a	n/a	n/a	n/a
w/ country steak	1	970	60	20.0	1950	62	4	6	24	n/a	n/a	n/a	n/a

RESTAURANT & FAST FOOD CHAINS

Hardee's	Amount	Calories	Fat (g)	Saturated Fat (g)	Sodium (mg)	Carbohydrate (g)	Fiber (g)	Sugar (g)	Protein (g)	Vitamin D (mcg)	Calcium (mg)	Iron (mg)	Potassium (mg)
w/ pork chop	1	990	56	18.0	2020	66	2	5	33	n/a	n/a	n/a	n/a
w/ sausage	1	1150	79	26.0	2420	76	12	5	30	n/a	n/a	n/a	n/a
w/ smoked sausage	1	1000	26	26.0	2340	56	2	7	25	n/a	n/a	n/a	n/a
Loaded hash round bowl	1	510	36	10.0	1060	30	3	1	16	n/a	n/a	n/a	n/a
Low carb breakfast bowl	1	760	68	21.0	1490	0	0	1	33	n/a	n/a	n/a	n/a
Croissants													
Bacon Sunrise	1	420	26	10.0	770	29	0	4	18	n/a	n/a	n/a	n/a
Ham Sunrise	1	390	23	9.0	860	29	0	4	18	n/a	n/a	n/a	n/a
Sausage Sunrise	1	550	40	15.0	870	30	0	4	18	n/a	n/a	n/a	n/a
Burgers													
The Big Hardee	1	920	58	23.0	1380	55	0	12	47	n/a	n/a	n/a	n/a
Cheeseburger													
small	1	300	14	4.0	790	33	1	8	13	n/a	n/a	n/a	n/a
double	1	530	26	11.0	1470	56	2	11	25	n/a	n/a	n/a	n/a
big	1	540	23	11.0	1240	56	0	13	28	n/a	n/a	n/a	n/a
Western Bacon	1	810	38	14.0	1750	80	0	16	38	n/a	n/a	n/a	n/a
Double Western Bacon	1	1060	57	24.0	2080	81	0	17	58	n/a	n/a	n/a	n/a
Hamburger	1	250	9	3.5	570	32	1	7	11	n/a	n/a	n/a	n/a
Slider													
single	1	210	11	4.0	360	21	1	7	10	n/a	n/a	n/a	n/a
double	1	360	24	10.0	700	22	1	8	19	n/a	n/a	n/a	n/a
Star													
Famous w/ cheese	1	660	37	13.0	1270	55	0	12	28	n/a	n/a	n/a	n/a
Super w/ cheese	1	920	56	23.0	1530	59	3	13	48	n/a	n/a	n/a	n/a
Thickburger	1	820	51	16.0	1440	56	4	14	39	n/a	n/a	n/a	n/a
bacon cheese	1	790	49	15.0	1400	54	3	11	38	n/a	n/a	n/a	n/a
Beyond	1	780	46	13.0	1450	61	5	13	33	n/a	n/a	n/a	n/a
Frisco	1	760	50	17.0	1550	43	3	7	38	n/a	n/a	n/a	n/a
Monster Double	1	1400	97	35.0	2780	53	4	13	86	n/a	n/a	n/a	n/a
mushroom & Swiss	1	620	33	13.0	1310	52	3	10	31	n/a	n/a	n/a	n/a
Hand-Breaded Chicken Tenders													
	3 pcs	260	213	2.5	770	13	2	0	25	n/a	n/a	n/a	n/a
	5 pcs	440	21	4.5	1290	21	3	0	41	n/a	n/a	n/a	n/a
	10 pcs	880	42	9.0	2580	42	6	0	82	n/a	n/a	n/a	n/a
Red Burrito													
Bowls													
beef	1	500	19	8.0	1500	55	6	5	27	n/a	n/a	n/a	n/a
chicken	1	430	11	3.0	1370	55	5	4	27	n/a	n/a	n/a	n/a
Burritos													
bean, rice & cheese	1	540	21	11.0	1360	67	7	4	21	n/a	n/a	n/a	n/a
grilled beef	1	850	35	15.0	1720	90	8	7	41	n/a	n/a	n/a	n/a
grilled chicken	1	630	23	11.0	1650	70	7	4	21	n/a	n/a	n/a	n/a

RESTAURANT & FAST FOOD CHAINS

Hardee's	Amount	Calories	Fat (g)	Saturated Fat (g)	Sodium (mg)	Carbohydrate (g)	Fiber (g)	Sugar (g)	Protein (g)	Vitamin D (mcg)	Calcium (mg)	Iron (mg)	Potass.
Chips & salsa	1 order	310	17	3.5	380	37	5	2	4	n/a	n/a	n/a	n/a
Nachos													
beef super	1 order	560	29	8.0	1390	57	9	5	17	n/a	n/a	n/a	n/a
chicken super	1 order	570	27	8.0	1490	57	9	4	25	n/a	n/a	n/a	n/a
Quesadillas													
cheese	1	550	32	18.0	1110	40	2	1	25	n/a	n/a	n/a	n/a
chicken	1	640	34	19.0	1410	43	2	1	39	n/a	n/a	n/a	n/a
Taco salads													
beef	1	920	56	17.0	1920	72	8	5	35	n/a	n/a	n/a	n/a
chicken	1	940	49	14.0	2060	73	7	4	49	n/a	n/a	n/a	n/a
Tacos													
beef, hard shell	1	170	12	5.0	320	13	2	1	11	n/a	n/a	n/a	n/a
beef, soft shell	1	210	11	5.0	560	17	1	0	11	n/a	n/a	n/a	n/a
chicken, hard shell	1	210	9	4.0	320	14	1	0	16	n/a	n/a	n/a	n/a
chicken, soft shell	1	200	8	4.0	650	17	0	0	16	n/a	n/a	n/a	n/a
Toppings													
beans	1 order	140	2	0.0	590	24	8	1	8	n/a	n/a	n/a	n/a
rice	1 order	200	3	0.0	660	40	1	1	4	n/a	n/a	n/a	n/a
sour cream	1 order	50	4	2.0	40	3	0	3	2	n/a	n/a	n/a	n/a
Sandwiches													
Big chicken fillet	1	590	29	6.0	1060	61	7	9	21	n/a	n/a	n/a	n/a
Big hot ham 'n' cheese	1	530	20	8.0	2190	51	2	10	34	n/a	n/a	n/a	n/a
Big roast beef	1	500	22	7.0	1350	49	3	9	30	n/a	n/a	n/a	n/a
Charbroiled chicken club	1	650	29	7.0	1870	53	0	5	43	n/a	n/a	n/a	n/a
Jumbo chili dog	1	390	26	9.0	1300	23	1	5	15	n/a	n/a	n/a	n/a
Monster roast beef	1	870	33	13.0	3150	52	2	10	54	n/a	n/a	n/a	n/a
Sides													
French fries, crispy curls	medium	420	21	5.0	1050	53	4	0	5	n/a	n/a	n/a	n/a
French fries, natural cut	medium	420	21	3.5	850	55	5	0	5	n/a	n/a	n/a	n/a
Hash rounds	medium	370	22	4.5	460	33	4	1	3	n/a	n/a	n/a	n/a
Onion rings	1 order	670	35	6.0	750	77	0	7	10	n/a	n/a	n/a	n/a
Ice Cream Shakes													
Chocolate	1	690	36	24.0	300	84	1	59	12	n/a	n/a	n/a	n/a
Strawberry	1	690	35	24.0	250	83	0	64	12	n/a	n/a	n/a	n/a
Vanilla	1	700	35	24.0	240	86	0	65	12	n/a	n/a	n/a	n/a
Desserts													
Apple turnover	1	270	13	3.5	260	35	1	11	3	n/a	n/a	n/a	n/a
Chocolate chip cookie	1	200	10	5.0	180	26	0	15	2	n/a	n/a	n/a	n/a

RESTAURANT & FAST FOOD CHAINS

IHOP

	Amount	Calories	Fat (g)	Saturated Fat (g)	Sodium (mg)	Carbohydrate (g)	Fiber (g)	Sugar (g)	Protein (g)	Vitamin D (mcg)	Calcium (mg)	Iron (mg)	Potassium (mg)
Appetizers													
Appetizer sampler w/ marinara	1 order	1410	72	18.0	3760	132	9	12	60	n/a	n/a	n/a	n/a
Mozza sticks w/ marinara	1 order	620	30	12.0	2070	58	4	8	28	n/a	n/a	n/a	n/a
Blintzes													
Cheese													
w/ blueberry compote	1	920	54	27.0	1210	77	3	39	27	n/a	n/a	n/a	n/a
w/ glazed strawberries	1	900	53	27.0	1190	72	4	34	27	n/a	n/a	n/a	n/a
w/ strawberry preserves	1	1090	54	27.0	1190	118	12	78	27	n/a	n/a	n/a	n/a
Crepes (w/o syrup)													
Strawberries & cream	1	700	29	10.0	880	97	5	45	17	n/a	n/a	n/a	n/a
Swedish	1	590	28	9.0	830	71	3	26	16	n/a	n/a	n/a	n/a
French Toast & Waffles (w/o syrup)													
Chicken & waffles	1 order	1050	52	21.0	1980	101	5	17	45	n/a	n/a	n/a	n/a
Gluten-friendly waffles	1 order	410	13	6.0	850	66	2	12	8	n/a	n/a	n/a	n/a
Original French toast	1 order	740	36	14.0	830	84	4	28	20	n/a	n/a	n/a	n/a
Strawberry banana French toast	1 order	840	31	11.0	790	121	7	55	21	n/a	n/a	n/a	n/a
Omelets (w/o cheese)													
Bacon temptation	1 (3 egg)	1190	90	35.0	2940	20	0	6	72	n/a	n/a	n/a	n/a
Big steak	1 (3 egg)	1030	69	24.0	1790	39	5	7	66	n/a	n/a	n/a	n/a
Chicken fajita	1 (3 egg)	900	57	23.0	1860	23	3	7	74	n/a	n/a	n/a	n/a
Colorado	1 (3 egg)	1250	98	35.0	2700	19	2	6	74	n/a	n/a	n/a	n/a
Egg white	1 (3 egg)	100	3	0.0	290	0	0	0	18	n/a	n/a	n/a	n/a
Plain	1 (3 egg)	400	28	8.0	440	8	0	0	28	n/a	n/a	n/a	n/a
Spicy poblano	1 (3 egg)	1010	75	32.0	1850	30	5	7	56	n/a	n/a	n/a	n/a
Spinach & mushroom	1 (3 egg)	910	71	28.0	1870	23	3	6	47	n/a	n/a	n/a	n/a
Toppings													
American cheese	1 order	100	8	5.0	490	2	0	1	5	n/a	n/a	n/a	n/a
avocado	1 order	80	7	1.0	0	4	3	0	1	n/a	n/a	n/a	n/a
diced bacon	1 order	80	6	2.0	350	0	0	0	6	n/a	n/a	n/a	n/a
diced ham	1 order	35	1	0.0	310	1	0	0	5	n/a	n/a	n/a	n/a
fire roasted poblano salsa	1 order	20	0	0.0	180	4	0	2	0	n/a	n/a	n/a	n/a
pepper Jack cheese	1 order	160	13	8.0	270	1	0	0	10	n/a	n/a	n/a	n/a
pork sausage link	1 order	200	20	7.0	330	0	0	0	5	n/a	n/a	n/a	n/a
sautéed green peppers & onions	1 order	70	7	1.5	45	2	0	0	0	n/a	n/a	n/a	n/a
sautéed mushrooms	1 order	70	7	1.5	45	2	0	1	2	n/a	n/a	n/a	n/a
sautéed spinach	1 order	80	7	1.5	85	2	1	0	2	n/a	n/a	n/a	n/a
sharp white cheddar cheese	1 order	170	14	8.0	270	1	0	0	10	n/a	n/a	n/a	n/a
shredded cheddar cheese	1 order	230	18	10.0	360	2	0	0	13	n/a	n/a	n/a	n/a
shredded cheese blend	1 order	220	17	10.0	340	2	0	0	13	n/a	n/a	n/a	n/a
sour cream	1 order	60	6	3.5	15	1	0	0	0	n/a	n/a	n/a	n/a
Swiss cheese	1 order	110	9	5.0	50	0	0	0	8	n/a	n/a	n/a	n/a
tomato	1 order	10	0	0.0	0	2	0	2	0	n/a	n/a	n/a	n/a

RESTAURANT & FAST FOOD CHAINS

	Amount	Calories	Fat (g)	Saturated Fat (g)	Sodium (mg)	Carbohydrate (g)	Fiber (g)	Sugar (g)	Protein (g)	Vitamin D (mcg)	Calcium (mg)	Iron (mg)	Potassium
Pancakes (w/o syrup)													
Buttermilk	3	450	18	7.0	1560	59	3	11	13	n/a	n/a	n/a	n/a
Chocolate chip	4	760	25	11.0	2000	122	9	48	21	n/a	n/a	n/a	n/a
w/ buttermilk	4	750	25	10.0	2000	118	7	48	19	n/a	n/a	n/a	n/a
Cinn-a-Stack	4	880	29	11.0	2160	138	6	67	17	n/a	n/a	n/a	n/a
Cupcake	4	810	23	12.0	2030	134	4	59	17	n/a	n/a	n/a	n/a
Double blueberry	4	620	15	4.5	2010	105	6	36	17	n/a	n/a	n/a	n/a
Gluten-friendly	4	540	15	6.0	1140	90	2	11	11	n/a	n/a	n/a	n/a
Harvest grain 'n' nut	4	800	42	10.0	1730	83	6	20	21	n/a	n/a	n/a	n/a
Mexican tres leches	4	700	26	11.0	2080	99	5	32	19	n/a	n/a	n/a	n/a
New York cheesecake	4	890	34	14.0	2220	126	6	49	22	n/a	n/a	n/a	n/a
Strawberry banana	4	680	15	4.5	2000	120	8	41	19	n/a	n/a	n/a	n/a
Syrup													
Blueberry/strawberry	¼ cup	105	0	0.0	6	27	0	19	0	n/a	n/a	n/a	n/a
Maple/butter pecan	¼ cup	110	0	0.0	11	27	0	19	0	n/a	n/a	n/a	n/a
Burritos & Bowls													
Classic													
bowl w/ bacon	1	870	65	22.0	1700	30	3	3	42	n/a	n/a	n/a	n/a
bowl w/ sausage	1	910	73	25.0	1340	30	3	3	35	n/a	n/a	n/a	n/a
burrito w/ bacon	1	1150	73	25.0	2380	74	4	5	48	n/a	n/a	n/a	n/a
burrito w/ sausage	1	1190	80	28.0	2010	74	4	4	42	n/a	n/a	n/a	n/a
Country													
bowl w/ country gravy	1	1020	76	26.0	1930	38	3	4	45	n/a	n/a	n/a	n/a
bowl w/ sausage gravy	1	1050	79	28.0	2070	39	3	5	46	n/a	n/a	n/a	n/a
burrito w/ country gravy	1	1290	84	29.0	2610	83	5	6	52	n/a	n/a	n/a	n/a
burrito w/ sausage gravy	1	1330	87	30.0	2740	84	5	6	53	n/a	n/a	n/a	n/a
New Mexico chicken													
bowl	1	940	46	31.0	2880	85	13	7	47	n/a	n/a	n/a	n/a
burrito	1	1220	54	34.0	3550	129	14	9	54	n/a	n/a	n/a	n/a
Southwest chicken													
bowl	1	1100	79	39.0	2500	42	8	8	57	n/a	n/a	n/a	n/a
burrito	1	1380	87	41.0	3180	87	9	9	63	n/a	n/a	n/a	n/a
Spicy poblano fajita													
bowl	1	1050	75	25.0	2000	42	7	6	55	n/a	n/a	n/a	n/a
burrito	1	1330	83	28.0	2680	86	9	7	62	n/a	n/a	n/a	n/a
Spicy shredded beef													
bowl	1	900	42	17.0	2370	84	12	5	45	n/a	n/a	n/a	n/a
burrito	1	1180	50	20.0	3050	129	14	6	52	n/a	n/a	n/a	n/a
Entrées													
Boneless Buffalo chicken strips & fries	1 order	930	44	8.0	5220	84	7	0	47	n/a	n/a	n/a	n/a

RESTAURANT & FAST FOOD CHAINS

IHOP

	Amount	Calories	Fat (g)	Saturated Fat (g)	Sodium (mg)	Carbohydrate (g)	Fiber (g)	Sugar (g)	Protein (g)	Vitamin D (mcg)	Calcium (mg)	Iron (mg)	Potassium (mg)
Buttermilk crispy chicken													
w/ fries	1 order	890	43	8.0	2600	81	7	0	47	n/a	n/a	n/a	n/a
w/ mashed potatoes, country gravy & corn	1 order	1050	53	14.0	2490	97	10	10	51	n/a	n/a	n/a	n/a
w/ mashed potatoes, sausage gravy & corn	1 order	1120	59	17.0	2270	99	10	10	53	n/a	n/a	n/a	n/a
Cheesy chicken bacon ranch													
w/ crispy chicken	1 order	1540	101	30.0	3790	83	6	6	74	n/a	n/a	n/a	n/a
w/ grilled chicken	1 order	1300	80	27.0	4710	49	6	7	95	n/a	n/a	n/a	n/a
Grilled tilapia w/ broccoli & rice	1 order	430	11	2.0	1790	39	6	2	44	n/a	n/a	n/a	n/a
Pot roast w/ mashed potatoes & corn	1 order	790	44	15.0	2750	65	8	12	40	n/a	n/a	n/a	n/a
Roasted turkey breast w/ mashed potatoes & broccoli	1 order	710	26	6.0	1600	73	6	35	51	n/a	n/a	n/a	n/a
Sirloin steak tips w/ mashed potatoes & corn	1 order	860	46	13.0	2100	70	10	27	47	n/a	n/a	n/a	n/a
T-bone steak w/ mashed potatoes & broccoli	10 oz	560	24	7.0	1290	35	6	3	56	n/a	n/a	n/a	n/a
	12 oz	650	32	11.0	1690	35	6	3	61	n/a	n/a	n/a	n/a
Sandwiches													
B.L.T.A.	1	1170	84	23.0	1960	74	10	7	32	n/a	n/a	n/a	n/a
Ham & egg melt	1	960	51	23.0	2760	68	3	7	57	n/a	n/a	n/a	n/a
Philly Cheese Steak Stacker	1	820	46	17.0	2250	58	3	9	46	n/a	n/a	n/a	n/a
Spicy Buffalo chicken	1	630	31	8.0	2800	58	3	8	29	n/a	n/a	n/a	n/a
Turkey cheddar club	1	1190	76	25.0	2100	66	4	6	59	n/a	n/a	n/a	n/a
Ultimate Steakburgers													
Big Brunch	1	990	64	23.0	2200	58	4	10	46	n/a	n/a	n/a	n/a
w/ crispy chicken	1	960	54	16.0	2180	76	4	9	44	n/a	n/a	n/a	n/a
w/ grilled chicken	1	843	43	14.0	2650	59	4	10	54	n/a	n/a	n/a	n/a
Classic	1	670	42	17.0	1780	42	3	11	33	n/a	n/a	n/a	n/a
w/ bacon	1	770	49	20.0	2090	42	3	11	38	n/a	n/a	n/a	n/a
w/ crispy chicken	1	640	32	10.0	1760	59	3	10	30	n/a	n/a	n/a	n/a
w/ bacon	1	740	39	13.0	2080	60	3	11	36	n/a	n/a	n/a	n/a
w/ grilled chicken	1	520	21	8.0	2220	42	3	11	41	n/a	n/a	n/a	n/a
w/ bacon	1	620	29	11.0	2540	43	3	11	47	n/a	n/a	n/a	n/a
Cowboy BBQ	1	950	54	21.0	2560	76	4	22	41	n/a	n/a	n/a	n/a
w/ crispy chicken	1	920	43	13.0	2550	93	4	22	39	n/a	n/a	n/a	n/a
w/ grilled chicken	1	790	33	12.0	3010	76	4	23	50	n/a	n/a	n/a	n/a
Jalapeño Kick	1	1000	74	25.0	1890	42	3	10	41	n/a	n/a	n/a	n/a
w/ crispy chicken	1	970	64	18.0	1880	60	4	10	39	n/a	n/a	n/a	n/a
w/ grilled chicken	1	850	53	16.0	2340	43	4	10	50	n/a	n/a	n/a	n/a
Mega Monster cheeseburger	1	1060	72	31.0	2650	43	3	11	60	n/a	n/a	n/a	n/a

IHOP

	Amount	Calories	Fat (g)	Saturated Fat (g)	Sodium (mg)	Carbohydrate (g)	Fiber (g)	Sugar (g)	Protein (g)	Vitamin D (mcg)	Calcium (mg)	Iron (mg)	Potas.
Salads													
Chicken & veggie	1	600	35	5.0	1790	38	9	24	38	n/a	n/a	n/a	n/a
w/ crispy chicken	1	790	49	7.0	1530	60	10	24	32	n/a	n/a	n/a	n/a
House w/o dressing	1	30	0	0.0	20	7	2	4	2	n/a	n/a	n/a	n/a
Sides													
Broccoli florets	1 order	25	0	0.0	25	4	2	1	3	n/a	n/a	n/a	n/a
Buttered corn	1 order	180	10	6.0	70	20	5	8	4	n/a	n/a	n/a	n/a
Buttered English muffin	1	180	5	3.0	240	28	1	0	5	n/a	n/a	n/a	n/a
Crispy breakfast potatoes	1 order	280	13	2.5	1050	37	5	0	5	n/a	n/a	n/a	n/a
Crispy potato pancakes	1 order	370	24	4.0	660	35	4	1	4	n/a	n/a	n/a	n/a
French fries	1 order	50	0	0.0	5	14	1	12	0	n/a	n/a	n/a	n/a
Garlic bread	1 order	140	8	1.5	240	15	0	0	2	n/a	n/a	n/a	n/a
Grilled buttermilk biscuit	1	450	25	15.0	1190	50	1	2	6	n/a	n/a	n/a	n/a
Grits	1 order	120	0	0.0	85	27	1	0	3	n/a	n/a	n/a	n/a
Ham slice	1	120	3	1.0	1290	4	0	2	20	n/a	n/a	n/a	n/a
Hash browns	1 order	210	14	2.5	230	19	2	0	2	n/a	n/a	n/a	n/a
Oatmeal	1 order	210	4	1.5	110	41	4	20	6	n/a	n/a	n/a	n/a
Onion rings	1 order	530	30	5.0	1060	60	4	7	7	n/a	n/a	n/a	n/a
Red skin mashed potatoes	1 order	240	13	2.5	680	30	3	1	5	n/a	n/a	n/a	n/a
Rice & barley medley	1 order	160	1	0.0	430	33	3	0	3	n/a	n/a	n/a	n/a
Scrapple	1 order	290	18	7.0	960	16	0	0	18	n/a	n/a	n/a	n/a
Seasoned fries	1 order	320	15	3.0	1060	41	4	0	4	n/a	n/a	n/a	n/a
Spam	2 slices	170	14	5.0	550	2	0	1	8	n/a	n/a	n/a	n/a
Tortilla, corn	1	110	2	0.0	50	23	2	0	2	n/a	n/a	n/a	n/a
Tortilla, flour	1	280	8	3.0	670	45	2	2	7	n/a	n/a	n/a	n/a

KFC

	Amount	Calories	Fat (g)	Saturated Fat (g)	Sodium (mg)	Carbohydrate (g)	Fiber (g)	Sugar (g)	Protein (g)	Vitamin D (mcg)	Calcium (mg)	Iron (mg)	Potas.
Chicken Sandwiches													
Chicken Littles	1	300	15	2.5	620	27	1	3	14	n/a	n/a	n/a	n/a
Buffalo	1	310	17	2.5	790	27	1	3	14	n/a	n/a	n/a	n/a
Classic chicken	1	650	35	4.5	1260	49	1	6	34	n/a	n/a	n/a	n/a
Crispy Colonel's	1	470	24	3.5	1170	39	0	4	24	n/a	n/a	n/a	n/a
honey BBQ	1	510	25	3.5	1290	48	0	12	24	n/a	n/a	n/a	n/a
Honey BBQ	1	350	4	0.5	1350	55	2	22	24	n/a	n/a	n/a	n/a
Spicy chicken	1	620	33	4.0	2140	49	1	6	34	n/a	n/a	n/a	n/a
Extra Crispy Chicken													
Breast	1	530	35	6.0	1150	18	0	0	35	n/a	n/a	n/a	n/a
Drumstick	1	170	12	2.0	390	5	0	0	10	n/a	n/a	n/a	n/a
Thigh	1	330	23	4.5	700	9	0	0	22	n/a	n/a	n/a	n/a
Whole wing	1	170	13	2.0	340	5	0	0	10	n/a	n/a	n/a	n/a

	Amount	Calories	Fat (g)	Saturated Fat (g)	Sodium (mg)	Carbohydrate (g)	Fiber (g)	Sugar (g)	Protein (g)	Vitamin D (mcg)	Calcium (mg)	Iron (mg)	Potassium (mg)
Kentucky Fried Wings													
Buffalo	1	100	7	1.5	310	3	0	0	5	n/a	n/a	n/a	n/a
Honey BBQ	1	100	6	1.0	210	8	0	4	5	n/a	n/a	n/a	n/a
Nashville hot	1	130	11	2.0	230	4	0	0	5	n/a	n/a	n/a	n/a
Kentucky Grilled Chicken													
Breast	1	210	7	2.0	710	0	0	0	38	n/a	n/a	n/a	n/a
Drumstick	1	80	4	1.0	220	0	0	0	11	n/a	n/a	n/a	n/a
Thigh	1	150	9	3.0	420	0	0	0	17	n/a	n/a		n/a
Whole wing	1	70	3	1.0	180	0	0	0	9	n/a	n/a	n/a	n/a
Nashville Hot Chicken													
Extra crispy													
breast	1	770	60	10.0	1530	21	1	1	35	n/a	n/a	n/a	n/a
drumstick	1	250	21	3.5	530	6	1	0	11	n/a	n/a	n/a	n/a
thigh	1	500	40	7.0	970	11	1	1	22	n/a	n/a	n/a	n/a
whole wing	1	290	25	4.0	520	6	1	1	10	n/a	n/a	n/a	n/a
Kentucky grilled													
breast	1	260	12	3.0	790	1	0	0	38	n/a	n/a	n/a	n/a
drumstick	1	100	6	1.5	260	0	0	0	11	n/a	n/a	n/a	n/a
thigh	1	180	12	3.5	470	0	0	0	17	n/a	n/a	n/a	n/a
whole wing	1	90	6	1.5	210	10	0	0	9	n/a	n/a	n/a	n/a
Original Recipe Chicken													
Breast	1	390	21	4.0	1190	11	2	0	39	n/a	n/a	n/a	n/a
Drumstick	1	130	8	1.5	430	4	1	0	12	n/a	n/a	n/a	n/a
Thigh	1	280	19	4.5	910	8	1	0	19	n/a	n/a	n/a	n/a
Whole wing	1	130	8	2.0	380	3	0	0	10	n/a	n/a	n/a	n/a
Other Chicken													
Famous Bowl w/ mashed potato & gravy	1 order	740	35	6.0	2350	81	6	2	26	n/a	n/a	n/a	n/a
snack size	1 order	270	14	3.5	850	27	2	1	11	n/a	n/a	n/a	n/a
Pot pie	1	720	41	25.0	1750	60	7	5	26	n/a	n/a	n/a	n/a
Tenders, extra crispy	1	140	7	1.0	320	8	0	0	10	n/a	n/a	n/a	n/a
Tenders, Nashville hot extra crispy	1	220	16	2.5	460	9	0	0	10	n/a	n/a	n/a	n/a
Sides													
BBQ baked beans	1 order	190	1	0.0	650	34	7	15	11	n/a	n/a	n/a	n/a
Biscuit	1	180	8	4.5	520	22	1	1	4	n/a	n/a	n/a	n/a
Coleslaw	1 order	170	12	2.0	180	14	4	10	1	n/a	n/a	n/a	n/a
Corn on the cob	1	70	1	0.0	0	17	2	3	2	n/a	n/a	n/a	n/a
Cornbread muffin	1	210	9	1.5	240	28	0	11	3	n/a	n/a	n/a	n/a
Green beans	1 order	25	0	0.0	300	5	3	1	1	n/a	n/a	n/a	n/a
Macaroni & cheese	1 order	140	6	1.5	590	17	1	2	5	n/a	n/a	n/a	n/a

RESTAURANT & FAST FOOD CHAINS

KFC

	Amount	Calories	Fat (g)	Saturated Fat (g)	Sodium (mg)	Carbohydrate (g)	Fiber (g)	Sugar (g)	Protein (g)	Vitamin D (mcg)	Calcium (mg)	Iron (mg)	Potassium
Mashed potatoes	1 order	110	4	0.5	330	17	1	0	2	n/a	n/a	n/a	n/a
w/ gravy	1 order	130	5	1.0	520	2	1	0	3	n/a	n/a	n/a	n/a
Popcorn nuggets	large	620	39	5.0	1820	39	2	0	27	n/a	n/a	n/a	n/a
Secret recipe fries	1 order	320	15	2.0	1100	41	3	0	5	n/a	n/a	n/a	n/a
Sweet kernel corn	1 order	70	1	0.0	0	16	2	2	2	n/a	n/a	n/a	n/a
Salads & Dressing													
Salads													
Caesar side	1	40	2	1.0	90	2	1	1	3	n/a	n/a	n/a	n/a
house side	1	15	0	0.0	10	3	2	2	1	n/a	n/a	n/a	n/a
potato	1	340	28	4.5	290	19	2	3	2	n/a	n/a	n/a	n/a
Parmesan garlic croutons	1 order	60	3	0.0	135	8	0	0	2	n/a	n/a	n/a	n/a
Dressing													
Heinz buttermilk	1 pkt	160	17	2.0	220	1	0	1	0	n/a	n/a	n/a	n/a
Hidden Valley fat-free ranch	1 pkt	35	0	0.0	410	8	0	2	1	n/a	n/a	n/a	n/a
KFC creamy Parmesan Caesar	1 pkt	260	26	5.0	540	4	0	2	2	n/a	n/a	n/a	n/a
Marzetti light Italian	1 pkt	15	1	0.0	510	2	0	1	0	n/a	n/a	n/a	n/a
Desserts													
Apple turnover	1	230	10	2.5	140	32	0	12	2	n/a	n/a	n/a	n/a
Café Valley chocolate chip cake	1 slice	300	15	3.0	260	39	1	27	4	n/a	n/a	n/a	n/a
mini	1	300	12	2.5	190	49	1	35	3	n/a	n/a	n/a	n/a
Café Valley lemon cake	1 slice	220	10	2.0	170	30	0	20	2	n/a	n/a	n/a	n/a
mini	1	300	13	2.5	230	43	0	31	3	n/a	n/a	n/a	n/a
Chocolate chip cookie	1	120	6	3.0	70	18	1	12	1	n/a	n/a	n/a	n/a
Oreo and créme pie	1 slice	270	13	8.0	210	35	1	24	3	n/a	n/a	n/a	n/a
Reese's peanut butter pie	1 slice	300	17	9.0	270	33	1	22	5	n/a	n/a	n/a	n/a

Little Caesars

	Amount	Calories	Fat (g)	Saturated Fat (g)	Sodium (mg)	Carbohydrate (g)	Fiber (g)	Sugar (g)	Protein (g)	Vitamin D (mcg)	Calcium (mg)	Iron (mg)	Potassium
*Pizza**													
Classic													
cheese	1 slice	240	8	4.0	460	31	2	1	12	n/a	208	1	120
Italian sausage	1 slice	280	11	5.0	560	32	2	2	14	n/a	211	2	125
pepperoni	1 slice	280	11	5.0	580	31	2	2	13	n/a	210	2	120
seasoned beef	1 slice	270	10	5.0	550	32	2	1	14	n/a	210	2	140
DEEP!DEEP! dish specialty													
3 Meat Treat	1 slice	440	22	9.0	900	40	2	2	20	n/a	249	2	150
5 Meat Feast	1 slice	440	21	9.0	1010	40	2	2	21	n/a	249	2	160
Hula Hawaiian	1 slice	340	11	4.5	690	43	2	4	17	n/a	244	2	160
Ultimate Supreme	1 slice	380	16	7.0	780	41	3	3	18	n/a	251	2	180
veggie	1 slice	340	12	5.0	720	42	3	3	15	n/a	251	3	180
ExtraMostBestest													
cheese	1 slice	280	11	6.0	560	32	2	1	15	n/a	300	1	140
thin crust	1 slice	120	7	3.0	210	9	n/a	n/a	6	n/a	143	n/a	60

* Based on a 12-in large pizza (8 slices)

RESTAURANT & FAST FOOD CHAINS

Little Caesars	Amount	Calories	Fat (g)	Saturated Fat (g)	Sodium (mg)	Carbohydrate (g)	Fiber (g)	Sugar (g)	Protein (g)	Vitamin D (mcg)	Calcium (mg)	Iron (mg)	Potassium (mg)
Italian sausage	1 slice	330	16	7.0	700	32	2	2	16	n/a	228	2	125
pepperoni	1 slice	310	14	6.0	700	31	2	2	15	n/a	225	2	125
stuffed crust	1 slice	380	20	9.0	900	32	2	2	18	n/a	339	2	125
thin crust	1 slice	140	8	3.0	280	9	n/a	n/a	6	n/a	105	n/a	55
seasoned beef	1 slice	320	15	7.0	700	31	2	1	16	n/a	226	2	160
Specialty													
3 Meat Treat	1 slice	340	17	7.0	760	31	2	2	16	n/a	214	2	120
5 Meat Feast	1 slice	340	17	7.0	840	31	2	2	17	n/a	213	2	130
Hula Hawaiian	1 slice	270	9	4.0	690	34	2	4	15	n/a	209	2	135
Slices-N-Stix	1 slice	550	26	13.0	1250	49	3	3	30	0	641	3	250
Ultimate Supreme	1 slice	300	13	6.0	670	32	2	2	14	0	214	2	150
veggie	1 slice	280	11	5.0	670	33	2	3	13	0	217	3	160
Add stuffed crust													
DEEP!DEEP! dish	1 slice	66	5	3.0	214	1	n/a	n/a	4	n/a	130	n/a	n/a
round pizza	1 slice	70	6	3.0	201	1	n/a	n/a	4	n/a	114	n/a	n/a
Toppings													
Round pizza	1 slice	240	8	4.0	460	31	2	1	12	n/a	208	1	120
bacon	1 slice	45	5	1.5	130	n/a	n/a	n/a	2	n/a	n/a	n/a	n/a
black olives	1 slice	35	3	1.0	135	1	n/a	n/a	0	n/a	n/a	2	n/a
extra cheese	1 slice	35	3	1.5	85	1	n/a	n/a	3	n/a	78	n/a	15
green peppers	1 slice	0	n/a	n/a	0	1	n/a	n/a	0	n/a	1	n/a	20
Italian sausage	1 slice	50	5	1.5	150	0	n/a	n/a	2	n/a	4	n/a	n/a
jalapeño peppers	1 slice	10	1	n/a	250	1	n/a	n/a	n/a	n/a	n/a	n/a	n/a
mild banana peppers	1 slice	5	n/a	n/a	350	1	n/a	n/a	0	n/a	15	n/a	n/a
mozzarella	1 slice	25	2	1.0	45	0	n/a	n/a	2	n/a	31	n/a	0
mushrooms, canned	1 slice	0	n/a	n/a	70	1	n/a	n/a	0	n/a	2	n/a	20
mushrooms, fresh	1 slice	0	0	n/a	0	1	n/a	n/a	1	0	n/a	n/a	65
onions	1 slice	0	n/a	n/a	0	1	n/a	n/a	0	n/a	2	n/a	15
pepperoni	1 slice	35	3	1.0	125	0	n/a	n/a	1	n/a	1	n/a	n/a
pineapple	1 slice	10	n/a	n/a	n/a	3	n/a	2	n/a	n/a	1	n/a	15
seasoned beef	1 slice	40	4	1.5	135	0	n/a	n/a	2	n/a	2	n/a	25
smoky ham	1 slice	20	1	n/a	230	0	n/a	n/a	3	n/a	n/a	n/a	n/a
DEEP!DEEP! dish pizza	1 slice	310	11	4.5	520	40	2	2	15	n/a	243	2	150
bacon	1 slice	45	5	1.5	130	n/a	n/a	n/a	2	n/a	n/a	n/a	n/a
black olives	1 slice	25	2	1.0	100	0	n/a	n/a	0	n/a	n/a	1	n/a
extra cheese	1 slice	40	4	1.5	115	0	n/a	n/a	2	n/a	3	n/a	n/a
green peppers	1 slice	10	1	n/a	180	0	n/a	n/a	n/a	n/a	n/a	n/a	n/a
Italian sausage	1 slice	35	3	1.5	85	1	n/a	n/a	3	n/a	78	n/a	15
jalapeño peppers	1 slice	25	2	1.0	45	0	n/a	n/a	2	n/a	31	n/a	0
mild banana peppers	1 slice	0	n/a	n/a	0	0	n/a	n/a	0	n/a	n/a	n/a	15
mozzarella	1 slice	0	n/a	n/a	270	1	n/a	n/a	0	n/a	11	n/a	n/a
mushrooms, canned	1 slice	0	n/a	n/a	70	1	n/a	n/a	0	n/a	2	n/a	20
mushrooms, fresh	1 slice	0	0	n/a	0	1	n/a	n/a	1	0	n/a	n/a	65

Little Caesars

	Amount	Calories	Fat (g)	Saturated Fat (g)	Sodium (mg)	Carbohydrate (g)	Fiber (g)	Sugar (g)	Protein (g)	Vitamin D (mcg)	Calcium (mg)	Iron (mg)	Potassium
onions	1 slice	0	n/a	n/a	0	1	n/a	n/a	0	n/a	1	n/a	10
pepperoni	1 slice	35	3	1.0	130	0	n/a	n/a	1	n/a	2	n/a	n/a
pineapple	1 slice	10	n/a	n/a	n/a	3	n/a	2	n/a	n/a	1	n/a	15
seasoned beef	1 slice	30	3	1.0	105	0	n/a	n/a	2	n/a	2	n/a	20
smoky ham	1 slice	15	0	n/a	170	0	n/a	n/a	2	n/a	n/a	n/a	n/a
Wings													
BBQ	1 order	620	35	9.0	2300	32	n/a	24	48	n/a	63	2	n/a
Buffalo	1 order	510	35	9.0	3330	3	n/a	n/a	47	n/a	63	2	n/a
Garlic parmesan	1 order	670	51	13.0	2510	5	n/a	n/a	49	n/a	127	2	n/a
Oven roasted	1 order	510	35	9.0	1740	3	n/a	n/a	47	n/a	63	2	n/a
Sides													
Cheese bread													
Italian	1 pc	130	5	2.0	220	16	n/a	n/a	6	0	97	n/a	40
pepperoni	1 pc	150	7	2.5	280	15	n/a	n/a	7	n/a	99	n/a	40
zesty	1 pc	150	7	2.5	250	16	n/a	n/a	5	0	86	n/a	45
Cookie dough brownie	1	210	11	5.0	75	24	n/a	17	3	n/a	26	1	100
Crazy Bread	1 pc	100	3	0.5	160	16	n/a	n/a	3	n/a	14	n/a	25
stuffed	3 pcs	980	37	13.0	2160	126	6	7	36	n/a	508	8	410
Crazy Sauce	1 cup	30	0	0.0	530	7	2	n/a	1	n/a	33	1	230
Dips													
Buffalo ranch	1 cup	230	23	3.5	580	4	n/a	3	1	n/a	29	n/a	60
Butter garlic flavor	1 cup	370	42	8.0	330	n/a	n/a	n/a	n/a	n/a	12	n/a	0
Cheezy Jalapeño	1 cup	210	21	3.5	460	3	n/a	2	1	n/a	34	n/a	55
Ranch	1 cup	230	23	3.5	480	4	n/a	3	2	n/a	41	n/a	95

McDonald's

	Amount	Calories	Fat (g)	Saturated Fat (g)	Sodium (mg)	Carbohydrate (g)	Fiber (g)	Sugar (g)	Protein (g)	Vitamin D (mcg)	Calcium (mg)	Iron (mg)	Potassium
Biscuits													
2 biscuits & sausage gravy platter	1	890	52	20.0	2510	87	3	6	19	n/a	n/a	n/a	n/a
Bacon	1	340	18	9.0	1030	36	1	3	9	n/a	n/a	n/a	n/a
Bacon & cheese	1	390	22	11.0	1240	38	2	3	11	n/a	n/a	n/a	n/a
Bacon, egg & cheese	1	460	26	13.0	1330	39	2	3	17	n/a	n/a	n/a	n/a
Crispy chicken	1	520	25	9.0	1540	49	1	4	25	n/a	n/a	n/a	n/a
Egg	1	340	17	9.0	910	37	1	2	11	n/a	n/a	n/a	n/a
Egg & cheese	1	390	21	11.0	1110	39	1	3	13	n/a	n/a	n/a	n/a
McChicken	1	420	20	9.0	1090	46	1	2	14	n/a	n/a	n/a	n/a
Sausage	1	460	30	13.0	1090	37	2	2	11	n/a	n/a	n/a	n/a
Sausage & egg	1	530	35	15.0	1190	38	2	3	17	n/a	n/a	n/a	n/a
Steak	1	430	23	12.0	1220	37	2	3	18	n/a	n/a	n/a	n/a
Steak & egg	1	500	28	14.0	1320	39	2	3	24	n/a	n/a	n/a	n/a
McGriddles													
Bacon, egg & cheese	1	430	21	9.0	1320	44	2	15	17	n/a	n/a	n/a	n/a
French toast, bacon, egg & sausage	1	650	37	14.0	1280	50	1	24	31	n/a	n/a	n/a	n/a

RESTAURANT & FAST FOOD CHAINS

McDonald's	Amount	Calories	Fat (g)	Saturated Fat (g)	Sodium (mg)	Carbohydrate (g)	Fiber (g)	Sugar (g)	Protein (g)	Vitamin D (mcg)	Calcium (mg)	Iron (mg)	Potassium (mg)
McChicken	1	380	14	4.5	990	50	2	14	14	n/a	n/a	n/a	n/a
Sausage	1	430	24	9.0	990	41	2	14	11	n/a	n/a	n/a	n/a
Sausage, egg & cheese	1	550	33	13.0	1290	44	2	15	19	n/a	n/a	n/a	n/a
Southern style chicken	1	410	17	4.5	1140	49	2	16	17	n/a	n/a	n/a	n/a
Spam	1	450	23	10.0	1340	44	2	15	17	n/a	n/a	n/a	n/a
Steak, egg & cheese	1	520	26	12.0	1420	45	3	16	27	n/a	n/a	n/a	n/a
Triple breakfast stack	1	860	61	24.0	1990	47	3	16	31	n/a	n/a	n/a	n/a
McMuffins													
Bacon & egg	1	360	19	8.0	770	30	2	3	18	n/a	n/a	n/a	n/a
Egg	1	310	13	6.0	770	30	2	3	17	n/a	n/a	n/a	n/a
McChicken	1	310	12	3.5	550	37	2	2	14	n/a	n/a	n/a	n/a
Sausage	1	400	26	10.0	760	29	2	2	14	n/a	n/a	n/a	n/a
Sausage & egg	1	480	31	12.0	830	30	2	2	20	n/a	n/a	n/a	n/a
Steak & egg	1	450	24	11.0	960	30	3	3	28	n/a	n/a	n/a	n/a
Steak, egg & cheese	1	440	23	11.0	960	31	3	3	28	n/a	n/a	n/a	n/a
Triple breakfast stack	1	790	59	23.0	1530	33	3	3	33	n/a	n/a	n/a	n/a
Burgers & Ribs													
Big Mac	1	550	30	11.0	1010	45	3	9	25	n/a	n/a	n/a	n/a
bacon	1	640	38	13.0	1310	46	3	9	30	n/a	n/a	n/a	n/a
Cheeseburger	1	300	13	6.0	720	32	2	7	15	n/a	n/a	n/a	n/a
bacon	1	370	19	8.0	940	33	2	7	19	n/a	n/a	n/a	n/a
bacon double	1	520	30	13.0	1340	35	2	7	29	n/a	n/a	n/a	n/a
bacon triple	1	610	37	17.0	1500	35	2	7	36	n/a	n/a	n/a	n/a
double	1	450	24	11.0	1120	34	2	7	25	n/a	n/a	n/a	n/a
triple	1	540	31	14.0	1280	34	2	7	32	n/a	n/a	n/a	n/a
Hamburger	1	250	9	3.5	510	31	1	6	12	n/a	n/a	n/a	n/a
double	1	350	16	7.0	710	31	1	6	20	n/a	n/a	n/a	n/a
McDouble	1	400	20	9.0	920	33	2	7	22	n/a	n/a	n/a	n/a
bacon	1	470	26	11.0	1140	33	2	7	26	n/a	n/a	n/a	n/a
deluxe	1	490	31	11.0	810	32	2	6	23	n/a	n/a	n/a	n/a
McRib	1	520	28	9.0	890	46	2	13	24	n/a	n/a	n/a	n/a
Quarter Pounder	1	420	18	8.0	730	40	2	9	25	n/a	n/a	n/a	n/a
w/ cheese	1	520	26	12.0	1140	42	2	10	30	n/a	n/a	n/a	n/a
deluxe	1	630	37	14.0	1210	44	3	11	30	n/a	n/a	n/a	n/a
double	1	740	42	20.0	1360	43	2	10	48	n/a	n/a	n/a	n/a
w/ bacon	1	630	35	15.0	1470	43	3	10	36	n/a	n/a	n/a	n/a
Chicken McNuggets													
	4 pcs	170	10	1.5	330	10	0	0	9	n/a	n/a	n/a	n/a
	6 pcs	250	15	2.5	500	15	1	0	14	n/a	n/a	n/a	n/a
	10 pcs	420	25	4.0	840	25	1	0	23	n/a	n/a	n/a	n/a

McDonald's

	Amount	Calories	Fat (g)	Saturated Fat (g)	Sodium (mg)	Carbohydrate (g)	Fiber (g)	Sugar (g)	Protein (g)	Vitamin D (mcg)	Calcium (mg)	Iron (mg)	Pota
Chicken Sandwiches													
Crispy chicken	1	470	20	5.0	1100	45	1	9	27	n/a	n/a	n/a	n/a
deluxe	1	530	26	4.0	1040	47	2	10	27	n/a	n/a	n/a	n/a
spicy	1	530	26	4.0	1230	47	1	9	27	n/a	n/a	n/a	n/a
spicy deluxe	1	540	26	4.0	1150	48	2	10	27	n/a	n/a	n/a	n/a
McChicken	1	400	21	3.5	560	39	1	5	14	n/a	n/a	n/a	n/a
bacon cheddar	1	520	31	8.0	990	41	2	6	21	n/a	n/a	n/a	n/a
deluxe	1	480	25	6.0	810	47	2	7	18	n/a	n/a	n/a	n/a
double	1	550	29	5.0	830	49	2	5	23	n/a	n/a	n/a	n/a
Fish Sandwiches													
Filet-O-Fish	1	380	18	4.0	580	39	2	5	16	n/a	n/a	n/a	n/a
double	1	530	25	6.0	820	49	2	5	26	n/a	n/a	n/a	n/a
French Fries													
	small	220	10	1.5	180	29	3	0	3	n/a	n/a	n/a	n/a
	medium	320	15	2.0	260	43	4	0	5	n/a	n/a	n/a	n/a
	large	490	23	3.0	400	66	6	0	7	n/a	n/a	n/a	n/a
Bakery													
Apple fritter	1	510	29	12.0	360	58	3	28	5	n/a	n/a	n/a	n/a
Baked apple pie	1	240	10	6.0	105	33	2	14	2	n/a	n/a	n/a	n/a
Blueberry muffin	1	470	22	3.5	360	64	2	36	6	n/a	n/a	n/a	n/a
Chocolate chip cookie	1	170	8	4.0	95	22	1	15	2	n/a	n/a	n/a	n/a
Cinnamon roll	1	560	17	8.0	490	92	8	46	9	n/a	n/a	n/a	n/a
McFlurrys													
M&M's	snack	340	11	5.0	170	53	1	40	8	n/a	n/a	n/a	n/a
	regular	640	21	14.0	200	96	2	83	13	n/a	n/a	n/a	n/a
Oreo	snack	420	14	9.0	130	64	1	55	9	n/a	n/a	n/a	n/a
	regular	510	16	8.0	260	80	1	60	12	n/a	n/a	n/a	n/a
Shakes													
Chocolate	medium	620	16	10.0	300	102	1	81	14	n/a	n/a	n/a	n/a
Strawberry	medium	620	16	11.0	220	102	0	77	14	n/a	n/a	n/a	n/a
Vanilla	medium	610	16	10.0	270	101	0	68	13	n/a	n/a	n/a	n/a
Sundaes & Cones													
Ice cream cones													
twist	1	300	8	5.0	160	49	0	35	8	n/a	n/a	n/a	n/a
vanilla	1	300	8	5.0	120	49	0	36	8	n/a	n/a	n/a	n/a
Sundaes	1	210	6	3.5	85	32	0	27	6	n/a	n/a	n/a	n/a
hot caramel	1	340	7	5.0	160	60	0	42	7	n/a	n/a	n/a	n/a
hot fudge	1	330	10	7.0	180	54	2	45	8	n/a	n/a	n/a	n/a

Olive Garden

	Amount	Calories	Fat (g)	Saturated Fat (g)	Sodium (mg)	Carbohydrate (g)	Fiber (g)	Sugar (g)	Protein (g)	Vitamin D (mcg)	Calcium (mg)	Iron (mg)	Potassium (mg)
Appetizers													
Calamari	1 order	670	42	3.5	1600	48	2	3	24	n/a	n/a	n/a	n/a
w/ marinara	1 order	715	45	3.5	1840	54	2	6	24	n/a	n/a	n/a	n/a
w/ spicy ranch	1 order	920	69	8.0	2300	50	2	3	25	n/a	n/a	n/a	n/a
Classic Shrimp Scampi Fritta	1 order	600	40	12.0	1860	39	1	3	23	n/a	n/a	n/a	n/a
Fried mozzarella	1 order	800	49	17.0	1990	57	4	3	33	n/a	n/a	n/a	n/a
w/ marinara	1 order	845	52	17.0	2230	63	4	3	33	n/a	n/a	n/a	n/a
Italian seafood trio	1 order	1070	65	5.0	3780	81	6	6	39	n/a	n/a	n/a	n/a
w/ marinara	1 order	1115	68	5.0	4020	87	6	9	39	n/a	n/a	n/a	n/a
w/ spicy ranch	1 order	1320	92	9.5	4480	83	6	6	40	n/a	n/a	n/a	n/a
Lasagna Fritta	1 order	1130	76	31.0	1800	75	5	6	39	n/a	n/a	n/a	n/a
Spinach-artichoke dip w/ flatbread crisps	1 order	1100	76	21.0	2170	70	8	7	37	n/a	n/a	n/a	n/a
Stuffed ziti Fritta	1 order	500	26	11.0	1040	40	3	0	27	n/a	n/a	n/a	n/a
w/ Alfredo	1 order	720	48	25.0	1340	43	0	0	31	n/a	n/a	n/a	n/a
w/ marinara	1 order	545	29	11.0	1280	46	0	3	27	n/a	n/a	n/a	n/a
Toasted ravioli	1 order	650	30	6.0	1420	71	6	3	25	n/a	n/a	n/a	n/a
w/ marinara	1 order	695	33	6.0	1660	77	6	6	0	n/a	n/a	n/a	n/a
Entrées													
Asiago tortellini Alfredo w/ grilled chicken	dinner	1980	131	76.0	3720	95	5	9	112	n/a	n/a	n/a	n/a
Chicken Alfredo	dinner	1570	95	56.0	2290	96	5	6	81	n/a	n/a	n/a	n/a
Chicken Marsala	dinner	1080	56	31.0	2690	68	4	8	69	n/a	n/a	n/a	n/a
Chicken parmigiana													
	lunch	660	29	7.0	1740	65	5	12	35	n/a	n/a	n/a	n/a
	dinner	1060	52	14.0	2980	86	7	16	63	n/a	n/a	n/a	n/a
Chicken scampi	dinner	1260	72	28.0	1990	105	4	7	49	n/a	n/a	n/a	n/a
Chicken & shrimp carbonara	dinner	1390	94	50.0	2050	75	3	10	64	n/a	n/a	n/a	n/a
Cheese ravioli													
w/ marinara sauce	lunch	450	22	11.0	1210	40	3	5	24	n/a	n/a	n/a	n/a
	dinner	780	39	20.0	2140	68	5	11	41	n/a	n/a	n/a	n/a
w/ meat sauce	lunch	500	26	14.0	1240	39	2	6	29	n/a	n/a	n/a	n/a
	dinner	860	46	24.0	2190	65	4	11	50	n/a	n/a	n/a	n/a
Eggplant parmigiana													
	lunch	660	32	7.0	1330	74	7	13	21	n/a	n/a	n/a	n/a
	dinner	1060	54	12.0	1990	113	11	23	30	n/a	n/a	n/a	n/a
Fettuccine Alfredo													
	lunch	650	45	27.0	610	47	2	3	15	n/a	n/a	n/a	n/a
	dinner	1310	90	55.0	1210	95	4	5	30	n/a	n/a	n/a	n/a
Five cheese ziti al forno													
	lunch	640	37	19.0	1100	57	4	9	25	n/a	n/a	n/a	n/a
	dinner	1220	71	36.0	2160	103	6	19	45	n/a	n/a	n/a	n/a

RESTAURANT & FAST FOOD CHAINS

Olive Garden

	Amount	Calories	Fat (g)	Saturated Fat (g)	Sodium (mg)	Carbohydrate (g)	Fiber (g)	Sugar (g)	Protein (g)	Vitamin D (mcg)	Calcium (mg)	Iron (mg)	Potassium (mg)
Giant cheese stuffed shells	dinner	1140	68	39.0	2260	91	6	22	44	n/a	n/a	n/a	n/a
Grilled chicken Margherita	dinner	540	27	10.0	1930	14	6	5	65	n/a	n/a	n/a	n/a
Herb-grilled salmon	dinner	460	29	8.0	1110	8	5	3	45	n/a	n/a	n/a	n/a
Lasagna Classico													
	lunch	500	30	16.0	1290	33	3	7	29	n/a	n/a	n/a	n/a
	dinner	940	55	30.0	2260	61	6	11	54	n/a	n/a	n/a	n/a
Seafood Alfredo	dinner	1430	91	55.0	1690	97	4	5	56	n/a	n/a	n/a	n/a
Shrimp Alfredo	dinner	1450	91	55.0	1620	96	4	6	63	n/a	n/a	n/a	n/a
Shrimp scampi													
	lunch	480	19	7.0	850	53	4	5	20	n/a	n/a	n/a	n/a
	dinner	510	20	7.0	960	54	4	5	29	n/a	n/a	n/a	n/a
Spaghetti													
w/ marinara sauce	lunch	310	7	0.0	490	53	3	9	9	n/a	n/a	n/a	n/a
w/ meat sauce	lunch	360	12	3.5	530	51	3	9	14	n/a	n/a	n/a	n/a
w/ meat sauce & meatballs	lunch	680	38	17.0	1230	56	4	9	30	n/a	n/a	n/a	n/a
Steak Alfredo	dinner	930	56	32.0	1680	48	2	3	57	n/a	n/a	n/a	n/a
Tour of Italy	dinner	1550	98	50.0	3150	99	7	12	72	n/a	n/a	n/a	n/a
Gluten-Sensitive													
Grilled chicken parmigiana w/ rotini & marinara	1 order	850	34	13.0	2730	64	7	13	74	n/a	n/a	n/a	n/a
Herb-grilled salmon	1 order	460	29	8.0	1110	8	5	3	45	n/a	n/a	n/a	n/a
Rotini pasta w/ marinara	1 order	560	13	1.0	1220	99	8	13	12	n/a	n/a	n/a	n/a
Rotini pasta w/ meat sauce	1 order	680	22	7.0	1300	96	6	13	23	n/a	n/a	n/a	n/a
Tuscan sirloin	6 oz	310	12	5.0	1340	8	4	3	46	n/a	n/a	n/a	n/a
Breadsticks & Sauces													
Breadstick	1	140	3	0.5	460	25	0	1	4	n/a	n/a	n/a	n/a
Sauces													
Alfredo	regular	440	43	27.0	600	5	0	1	8	n/a	n/a	n/a	n/a
five cheese marinara	regular	220	17	9.0	540	11	1	6	5	n/a	n/a	n/a	n/a
marinara	regular	90	5	0.0	480	11	2	6	1	n/a	n/a	n/a	n/a
Salads													
w/o dressing	1	70	2	0.0	250	11	2	2	2	n/a	n/a	n/a	n/a
w/ signature Italian dressing	1	150	10	1.5	770	13	2	4	3	n/a	n/a	n/a	n/a
w/ signaure low-fat Italian dressing	1	100	4	0.0	660	13	2	4	2	n/a	n/a	n/a	n/a
Soups													
Chicken & gnocchi	1 cup	230	12	4.5	1290	22	1	4	11	n/a	n/a	n/a	n/a
Minestrone	1 cup	110	1	0.0	810	17	4	4	5	n/a	n/a	n/a	n/a
Pasta fagioli	1 cup	150	5	2.0	710	16	3	4	8	n/a	n/a	n/a	n/a
Zuppa Toscana	1 cup	220	15	7.0	790	15	2	2	7	n/a	n/a	n/a	n/a

RESTAURANT & FAST FOOD CHAINS

	Amount	Calories	Fat (g)	Saturated Fat (g)	Sodium (mg)	Carbohydrate (g)	Fiber (g)	Sugar (g)	Protein (g)	Vitamin D (mcg)	Calcium (mg)	Iron (mg)	Potassium (mg)
Desserts													
Black Tie Mousse Cake	1 order	750	50	30.0	290	76	4	59	9	n/a	n/a	n/a	n/a
Chocolate brownie lasagna	1 order	910	52	27.0	580	144	6	103	13	n/a	n/a	n/a	n/a
Dolcini chocolate mousse	1 order	240	18	10.0	125	18	1	12	2	n/a	n/a	n/a	n/a
Dolcini strawberry & white chocolate	1 order	190	11	6.0	100	23	0	18	1	n/a	n/a	n/a	n/a
Pumpkin cheesecake	1 order	790	51	30.0	610	69	4	45	13	n/a	n/a	n/a	n/a
Smoothies													
peach	1	190	0	0.0	10	49	0	47	0	n/a	n/a	n/a	n/a
strawberry banana	1	130	0	0.0	0	34	0	31	0	n/a	n/a	n/a	n/a
Sundae w/ chocolate sauce	1	190	8	5.0	45	28	0	22	2	n/a	n/a	n/a	n/a
Tiramisu	1 order	470	27	17.0	125	54	0	35	6	n/a	n/a	n/a	n/a
Warm Italian donuts	1 order	810	28	3.5	510	119	6	25	20	n/a	n/a	n/a	n/a
w/ chocolate sauce	1 order	1030	31	5.5	620	167	6	67	22	n/a	n/a	n/a	n/a
w/ raspberry sauce	1 order	1020	28	3.5	520	170	6	60	20	n/a	n/a	n/a	n/a

	Amount	Calories	Fat (g)	Saturated Fat (g)	Sodium (mg)	Carbohydrate (g)	Fiber (g)	Sugar (g)	Protein (g)	Vitamin D (mcg)	Calcium (mg)	Iron (mg)	Potassium (mg)
Appetizers													
Chang's chicken lettuce wraps	1 order	710	27	6.0	1830	77	8	38	38	n/a	n/a	n/a	n/a
Chang's vegetarian lettuce wraps	1 order	620	28	4.0	1840	64	8	30	24	n/a	n/a	n/a	n/a
Chili garlic green beans	1 order	530	40	6.0	1580	39	10	23	8	n/a	n/a	n/a	n/a
Dynamite shrimp	1 order	640	48	7.0	790	36	2	6	20	n/a	n/a	n/a	n/a
Edamame	1 order	400	17	2.5	1960	25	12	1	37	n/a	n/a	n/a	n/a
Kung pao brussel sprouts	1 order	720	42	6.0	1260	84	12	53	16	n/a	n/a	n/a	n/a
Spare ribs, BBQ pork	6	810	21	12.0	1060	36	1	32	37	n/a	n/a	n/a	n/a
Spare ribs, Northern style	6	700	21	12.0	1070	11	1	9	37	n/a	n/a	n/a	n/a
Dim Sum													
Crab wontons	6	590	30	13.0	1720	66	1	29	14	n/a	n/a	n/a	n/a
Dumplings													
miso lobster	6	780	61	30.0	1100	38	0	2	18	n/a	n/a	n/a	n/a
pork, pan fried	6	530	29	8.0	1350	43	1	9	19	n/a	n/a	n/a	n/a
pork, steamed	6	460	21	7.0	1350	43	1	7	19	n/a	n/a	n/a	n/a
shrimp, pan fried	6	390	15	3.0	1600	35	1	10	26	n/a	n/a	n/a	n/a
shrimp, steamed	6	310	7	1.0	1600	35	1	10	26	n/a	n/a	n/a	n/a
Egg rolls, pork	2	610	35	7.0	1580	59	3	15	14	n/a	n/a	n/a	n/a
Vegetable spring rolls	2	390	19	3.0	990	53	4	25	4	n/a	n/a	n/a	n/a
Entrées													
Beef w/ broccoli	1 order	670	33	7.0	2110	46	5	33	50	n/a	n/a	n/a	n/a
Buddha's feast	1 order	380	8	1.0	2330	53	9	30	27	n/a	n/a	n/a	n/a
steamed	1 order	260	4	0.0	310	32	9	13	25	n/a	n/a	n/a	n/a
Chang's spicy chicken	1 order	840	33	5.0	1140	77	1	66	61	n/a	n/a	n/a	n/a
steamed	1 order	560	12	3.0	1170	60	2	54	56	n/a	n/a	n/a	n/a
Crispy honey chicken	1 order	1120	60	9.0	750	87	1	38	47	n/a	n/a	n/a	n/a

RESTAURANT & FAST FOOD CHAINS

P.F. Chang's

	Amount	Calories	Fat (g)	Saturated Fat (g)	Sodium (mg)	Carbohydrate (g)	Fiber (g)	Sugar (g)	Protein (g)	Vitamin D (mcg)	Calcium (mg)	Iron (mg)	Potassium (mg)
Crispy honey shrimp	1 order	1020	55	8.0	1170	79	1	38	46	n/a	n/a	n/a	n/a
Ginger chicken w/ broccoli	1 order	480	12	2.0	1370	41	6	26	57	n/a	n/a	n/a	n/a
Korean bulgogi steak	1 order	1370	58	11.0	3740	121	8	44	88	n/a	n/a	n/a	n/a
Kung pao chicken	1 order	960	58	9.0	1430	46	7	27	71	n/a	n/a	n/a	n/a
steamed	1 order	720	39	6.0	1460	30	8	17	67	n/a	n/a	n/a	n/a
Kung pao shrimp	1 order	760	52	6.0	1860	40	15	17	39	n/a	n/a	n/a	n/a
steamed	1 order	570	36	5.0	1880	27	7	18	42	n/a	n/a	n/a	n/a
Miso glazed salmon	1 order	660	37	6.0	1300	30	3	21	49	n/a	n/a	n/a	n/a
Mongolian beef	1 order	770	42	9.0	2300	39	1	32	59	n/a	n/a	n/a	n/a
Oolong Chilean sea bass	1 order	560	35	7.0	2090	30	5	17	34	n/a	n/a	n/a	n/a
Orange chicken	1 order	1160	59	9.0	1780	87	3	55	65	n/a	n/a	n/a	n/a
Pepper steak	1 order	640	36	8.0	2260	29	4	17	51	n/a	n/a	n/a	n/a
steamed	1 order	440	21	6.0	1730	28	4	17	33	n/a	n/a	n/a	n/a
Salt & pepper prawns	1 order	500	22	2.0	2980	37	4	14	32	n/a	n/a	n/a	n/a
Sesame chicken	1 order	920	37	6.0	1740	82	5	61	66	n/a	n/a	n/a	n/a
steamed	1 order	600	14	3.0	1590	58	5	44	62	n/a	n/a	n/a	n/a
Shrimp w/ lobster sauce	1 order	500	27	5.0	2740	22	5	5	38	n/a	n/a	n/a	n/a
steamed	1 order	370	18	4.0	2450	14	3	6	31	n/a	n/a	n/a	n/a
Stir-fried eggplant	1 order	530	34	5.0	2090	57	9	35	4	n/a	n/a	n/a	n/a
Sweet & sour chicken	1 order	860	41	7.0	560	86	3	45	36	n/a	n/a	n/a	n/a

Lunch Rice Bowls (w/o rice)

	Amount	Calories	Fat (g)	Saturated Fat (g)	Sodium (mg)	Carbohydrate (g)	Fiber (g)	Sugar (g)	Protein (g)	Vitamin D (mcg)	Calcium (mg)	Iron (mg)	Potassium (mg)
Beef & broccoli	1 order	370	19	4.5	1380	29	3	22	22	n/a	n/a	n/a	n/a
Chang's spicy chicken	1 order	680	27	4.0	960	127	2	54	54	n/a	n/a	n/a	n/a
Crispy honey chicken	1 order	840	42	7.0	660	71	1	38	35	n/a	n/a	n/a	n/a
Ginger chicken w/ broccoli	1 order	330	9	1.5	1470	31	3	22	32	n/a	n/a	n/a	n/a
Kung pao chicken	1 order	550	33	5.0	960	27	4	17	39	n/a	n/a	n/a	n/a
Kung pao shrimp	1 order	430	30	4.5	1200	24	8	11	21	n/a	n/a	n/a	n/a
Mongolian beef	1 order	490	28	6.0	1440	89	2	20	45	n/a	n/a	n/a	n/a
Sesame chicken	1 order	540	20	3.5	1100	53	4	39	35	n/a	n/a	n/a	n/a
Sweet & sour chicken	1 order	630	30	5.0	420	64	2	35	24	n/a	n/a	n/a	n/a

Noodles & Rice

	Amount	Calories	Fat (g)	Saturated Fat (g)	Sodium (mg)	Carbohydrate (g)	Fiber (g)	Sugar (g)	Protein (g)	Vitamin D (mcg)	Calcium (mg)	Iron (mg)	Potassium (mg)
Fried rice													
beef	1 order	1140	33	8.0	1810	155	5	20	49	n/a	n/a	n/a	n/a
chicken	1 order	1100	26	5.0	1580	159	6	19	52	n/a	n/a	n/a	n/a
pork	1 order	1190	37	9.0	1720	161	5	20	46	n/a	n/a	n/a	n/a
shrimp	1 order	1000	20	4.0	1740	154	5	19	44	n/a	n/a	n/a	n/a
vegetables	1 order	910	16	3.0	1360	164	10	24	25	n/a	n/a	n/a	n/a
combo	1 order	1200	35	8.0	1920	160	6	20	56	n/a	n/a	n/a	n/a
Lo mein													
beef	1 order	980	31	7.0	2630	127	7	20	48	n/a	n/a	n/a	n/a
chicken	1 order	950	24	4.0	2410	130	8	19	51	n/a	n/a	n/a	n/a

RESTAURANT & FAST FOOD CHAINS

P.F. Chang's

	Amount	Calories	Fat (g)	Saturated Fat (g)	Sodium (mg)	Carbohydrate (g)	Fiber (g)	Sugar (g)	Protein (g)	Vitamin D (mcg)	Calcium (mg)	Iron (mg)	Potassium (mg)
pork	1 order	1030	35	8.0	2550	133	7	20	45	n/a	n/a	n/a	n/a
shrimp	1 order	850	18	3.0	2560	126	7	19	43	n/a	n/a	n/a	n/a
vegetable	1 order	760	13	2.0	2190	135	11	24	24	n/a	n/a	n/a	n/a
combo	1 order	1050	33	7.0	2750	132	7	20	55	n/a	n/a	n/a	n/a
Pad thai													
chicken	1 order	1320	39	7.0	2730	190	9	50	53	n/a	n/a	n/a	n/a
shrimp	1 order	1270	37	6.0	3010	190	9	50	46	n/a	n/a	n/a	n/a
combo	1 order	1290	38	7.0	2870	190	9	50	49	n/a	n/a	n/a	n/a
Singapore street noodles	1 order	1180	13	2.0	2670	226	6	22	41	n/a	n/a	n/a	n/a
Ramen													
Spicy miso	1 order	700	22	3.0	4210	106	5	12	20	n/a	n/a	n/a	n/a
Tonkotsu	1 order	790	34	9.0	3520	106	4	15	19	n/a	n/a	n/a	n/a
Toppings													
braised chicken	1 order	120	2.5	0.5	180	2	0	2	22	n/a	n/a	n/a	n/a
braised pork	1 order	210	13	5.0	120	3	0	2	18	n/a	n/a	n/a	n/a
fried egg	1 order	90	7	2.0	60	1	0	1	6	n/a	n/a	n/a	n/a
poached shrimp	1 order	80	1	0.0	260	0	0	0	17	n/a	n/a	n/a	n/a
spicy bomb	1 order	40	1	0.0	820	4	1	1	2	n/a	n/a	n/a	n/a
Sushi													
California roll	1 order	390	16	3.0	1340	53	3	17	10	n/a	n/a	n/a	n/a
Kung pao dragon roll	1 order	510	23	3.0	1550	60	4	18	21	n/a	n/a	n/a	n/a
Shrimp tempura roll	1 order	580	25	4.0	1480	69	4	15	20	n/a	n/a	n/a	n/a
Spicy tuna roll	1 order	300	6	1.0	680	43	2	10	19	n/a	n/a	n/a	n/a
Gluten-Free Appetizers & Soups													
Chicken lettuce wraps	1 order	490	20	3.0	1680	45	5	21	31	n/a	n/a	n/a	n/a
Egg drop soup	cup	40	1	0.0	560	6	0	2	1	n/a	n/a	n/a	n/a
	bowl	270	7	2.0	3760	42	1	14	7	n/a	n/a	n/a	n/a
Gluten-Free Entrées													
Beef w/ broccoli	1 order	680	33	7.0	2280	47	5	34	51	n/a	n/a	n/a	n/a
Chang's spicy chicken	1 order	840	33	5.0	1140	77	1	66	61	n/a	n/a	n/a	n/a
Ginger chicken with broccoli	1 order	490	12	2.5	1640	43	6	28	57	n/a	n/a	n/a	n/a
Mongolian beef	1 order	740	41	9.0	1910	32	1	26	59	n/a	n/a	n/a	n/a
Shrimp w/ lobster sauce	1 order	500	27	5.0	2740	22	5	5	38	n/a	n/a	n/a	n/a
Gluten-Free Lunch Bowls (w/o rice)													
Beef w/ broccoli	1 order	380	19	4.0	1040	31	3	24	22	n/a	n/a	n/a	n/a
Chang's spicy chicken	1 order	460	10	2.0	980	48	1	44	45	n/a	n/a	n/a	n/a
Ginger chicken w/ broccoli	1 order	330	9	1.5	1120	33	3	24	32	n/a	n/a	n/a	n/a
Mongolian beef	1 order	500	27	6.0	1350	23	1	18	39	n/a	n/a	n/a	n/a
Gluten-Free Noodles & Rice													
Brown rice	1 order	250	2	0.0	0	53	4	0	5	n/a	n/a	n/a	n/a

P.F. Chang's

	Amount	Calories	Fat (g)	Saturated Fat (g)	Sodium (mg)	Carbohydrate (g)	Fiber (g)	Sugar (g)	Protein (g)	Vitamin D (mcg)	Calcium (mg)	Iron (mg)	Potass.
Fried rice													
beef	1 order	1140	33	7.0	1730	156	5	20	48	n/a	n/a	n/a	n/a
chicken	1 order	1100	26	5.0	1500	159	6	20	52	n/a	n/a	n/a	n/a
pork	1 order	1190	37	9.0	1650	162	5	21	46	n/a	n/a	n/a	n/a
shrimp	1 order	1000	20	4.0	1660	155	5	20	44	n/a	n/a	n/a	n/a
vegetable	1 order	920	16	3.0	1290	165	9	25	25	n/a	n/a	n/a	n/a
combo	1 order	1200	35	8.0	1850	161	6	20	56	n/a	n/a	n/a	n/a
side	1 order	510	15	3.0	670	77	2	10	13	n/a	n/a	n/a	n/a
Pad thai													
chicken	1 order	1240	34	6.0	2650	188	8	50	48	n/a	n/a	n/a	n/a
shrimp	1 order	1190	32	6.0	2920	187	8	50	41	n/a	n/a	n/a	n/a
combo	1 order	1210	33	6.0	2790	188	8	50	44	n/a	n/a	n/a	n/a
Singapore street noodles	1 order	1180	13	2.0	2670	226	6	22	41	n/a	n/a	n/a	n/a
White rice	1 order	290	0	0.0	0	65	1	1	5	n/a	n/a	n/a	n/a
Salads													
Asian Caesar	1 order	410	30	7.0	880	22	4	3	15	n/a	n/a	n/a	n/a
Mandarin Crunch	1 order	750	46	6.0	1510	75	8	41	14	n/a	n/a	n/a	n/a
Toppings													
chicken	1 order	160	5	1.0	250	4	0	3	22	n/a	n/a	n/a	n/a
salmon	1 order	240	16	3.0	450	0	0	0	22	n/a	n/a	n/a	n/a
Sides													
Brown rice	1 order	190	0	0.0	0	40	3	0	4	n/a	n/a	n/a	n/a
Fried rice	1 order	510	15	3.0	700	77	3	10	13	n/a	n/a	n/a	n/a
White rice	1 order	220	0	0.0	0	49	1	1	4	n/a	n/a	n/a	n/a
Soups													
Egg drop	bowl	270	7	2.0	3760	42	1	14	7	n/a	n/a	n/a	n/a
Wonton	cup	120	3	1.0	570	13	0	2	9	n/a	n/a	n/a	n/a
	bowl	570	17	4.0	2610	53	3	9	49	n/a	n/a	n/a	n/a
Desserts													
Banana spring rolls	1 order	940	35	13.0	480	149	2	47	14	n/a	n/a	n/a	n/a
Bao donuts	1 order	1400	62	30.0	2720	183	2	68	21	n/a	n/a	n/a	n/a
Fire & Ice	1 order	1170	54	33.0	580	148	0	103	18	n/a	n/a	n/a	n/a
The Great Wall of Chocolate	1 order	1700	71	30.0	1410	259	14	190	17	n/a	n/a	n/a	n/a
New York–style cheesecake	1 order	940	61	36.0	660	80	4	64	17	n/a	n/a	n/a	n/a
Vietnamese chocolate lava cake	1 order	820	48	25.0	370	97	5	71	11	n/a	n/a	n/a	n/a

Panda Express

	Amount	Calories	Fat (g)	Saturated Fat (g)	Sodium (mg)	Carbohydrate (g)	Fiber (g)	Sugar (g)	Protein (g)	Vitamin D (mcg)	Calcium (mg)	Iron (mg)	Potass.
Appetizers													
Chicken egg rolls	1	200	10	2.0	340	20	2	2	6	n/a	n/a	n/a	n/a
Chicken pot stickers	3	160	8	5.0	250	20	1	2	6	n/a	n/a	n/a	n/a
Cream cheese rangoons	3	190	8	5.0	180	24	2	1	5	n/a	n/a	n/a	n/a
Vegetable spring rolls	2	190	8	1.5	520	27	2	3	3	n/a	n/a	n/a	n/a

Panda Express

	Amount	Calories	Fat (g)	Saturated Fat (g)	Sodium (mg)	Carbohydrate (g)	Fiber (g)	Sugar (g)	Protein (g)	Vitamin D (mcg)	Calcium (mg)	Iron (mg)	Potassium (mg)
Entrées													
Asian chicken	1 order	340	13	3.5	630	14	3	10	41	n/a	n/a	n/a	n/a
grilled	1 order	300	13	4.0	530	8	0	8	36	n/a	n/a	n/a	n/a
Beijing beef	1 order	470	26	5.0	660	46	1	24	13	n/a	n/a	n/a	n/a
Black pepper Angus steak	1 order	180	7	2.0	750	10	1	6	19	n/a	n/a	n/a	n/a
Black pepper chicken	1 order	280	19	3.5	1130	15	1	7	13	n/a	n/a	n/a	n/a
Broccoli beef	1 order	150	7	1.5	520	13	2	7	9	n/a	n/a	n/a	n/a
Firecracker shrimp	1 order	110	4	0.5	630	7	1	4	11	n/a	n/a	n/a	n/a
Golden treasure shrimp	1 order	360	18	3.0	440	35	2	14	14	n/a	n/a	n/a	n/a
Honey sesame chicken breast	1 order	420	22	4.0	480	40	2	19	16	n/a	n/a	n/a	n/a
Honey walnut shrimp	1 order	360	23	3.5	440	35	2	9	13	n/a	n/a	n/a	n/a
Kung pao chicken	1 order	290	19	3.5	970	14	2	6	16	n/a	n/a	n/a	n/a
Mushroom chicken	1 order	220	14	2.5	840	10	1	5	13	n/a	n/a	n/a	n/a
Orange chicken	1 order	490	23	5.0	820	51	2	19	25	n/a	n/a	n/a	n/a
Potato chicken	1 order	190	10	2.0	680	18	2	4	8	n/a	n/a	n/a	n/a
Shanghai Angus steak	1 order	310	19	4.0	790	17	1	11	19	n/a	n/a	n/a	n/a
Sichuan hot chicken	1 order	400	26	4.5	910	22	2	1	19	n/a	n/a	n/a	n/a
Steamed ginger fish	1 order	220	12	2.5	1990	8	0	6	15	n/a	n/a	n/a	n/a
String bean chicken breast	1 order	190	9	2.0	590	13	4	4	14	n/a	n/a	n/a	n/a
Sweet & sour chicken breast	1 order	300	12	3.0	260	40	1	24	10	n/a	n/a	n/a	n/a
Sweetfire chicken breast	1 order	380	15	3.0	320	47	1	27	13	n/a	n/a	n/a	n/a
Teriyaki chicken	1 order	340	13	3.5	630	14	3	10	41	n/a	n/a	n/a	n/a
grilled	1 order	300	13	4.0	530	8	0	8	36	n/a	n/a	n/a	n/a
Wok-seared steak & shrimp	1 order	240	7	1.5	1090	21	2	10	23	n/a	n/a	n/a	n/a
Sides													
Brown steamed rice	1 order	420	4	1.0	15	86	4	1	9	n/a	n/a	n/a	n/a
Chow fun	1 order	410	9	1.0	1110	73	1	6	9	n/a	n/a	n/a	n/a
Chow mein	1 order	510	20	3.5	860	80	6	9	13	n/a	n/a	n/a	n/a
Eggplant tofu	1 order	340	24	3.5	520	23	3	17	7	n/a	n/a	n/a	n/a
Fried rice	1 order	520	16	3.0	850	85	1	3	11	n/a	n/a	n/a	n/a
Hot & sour soup	cup	120	5	0.5	680	14	1	4	7	n/a	n/a	n/a	n/a
	bowl	170	6	1.0	1260	20	1	6	10	n/a	n/a	n/a	n/a
Super greens	1 order	90	3	0.0	260	10	5	4	6	n/a	n/a	n/a	n/a
White steamed rice	1 order	380	0	0.0	0	87	0	0	7	n/a	n/a	n/a	n/a
Sauces													
Chili	1 order	10	0	0.0	125	2	0	2	0	n/a	n/a	n/a	n/a
Hot mustard	1 order	10	1	0.0	115	0	0	0	0	n/a	n/a	n/a	n/a
Plum	1 order	15	0	0.0	55	3	0	3	0	n/a	n/a	n/a	n/a
Potsticker	1 order	10	0	0.0	290	3	0	2	0	n/a	n/a	n/a	n/a
Soy	1 order	5	0	0.0	375	0	0	0	0	n/a	n/a	n/a	n/a
Sweet & sour	1 order	70	0	0.0	115	21	0	20	0	n/a	n/a	n/a	n/a
Teriyaki	1 order	70	0	0.0	380	16	0	14	0	n/a	n/a	n/a	n/a

RESTAURANT & FAST FOOD CHAINS

Panda Express	Amount	Calories	Fat (g)	Saturated Fat (g)	Sodium (mg)	Carbohydrate (g)	Fiber (g)	Sugar (g)	Protein (g)	Vitamin D (mcg)	Calcium (mg)	Iron (mg)	Potassium
Desserts													
Chocolate chunk cookie	1	160	7	3.0	125	25	1	14	2	n/a	n/a	n/a	n/a
Fortune cookie	1	20	0	0.0	0	5	0	2	0	n/a	n/a	n/a	n/a
Panera Bread													
Breakfast													
Avocado, egg white & spinach	1	360	14	6.0	700	39	5	5	19	n/a	n/a	n/a	n/a
Bacon, egg & cheese													
artisan ciabatta	1	440	20	9.0	890	40	2	1	25	n/a	n/a	n/a	n/a
brioche	1	460	25	12.0	830	33	1	6	24	n/a	n/a	n/a	n/a
Bacon, scrambled egg & cheese													
artisan ciabatta	1	460	21	10.0	900	41	2	1	25	n/a	n/a	n/a	n/a
brioche	1	470	26	14.0	840	33	1	6	25	n/a	n/a	n/a	n/a
Chipotle chicken, scrambled egg & avocado wrap	1	470	27	10.0	750	32	4	4	29	n/a	n/a	n/a	n/a
Egg & cheese													
artisan ciabatta	1	370	14	7.0	620	40	2	1	20	n/a	n/a	n/a	n/a
brioche	1	390	20	10.0	560	32	1	6	20	n/a	n/a	n/a	n/a
Sausage, egg & cheese													
artisan ciabatta	1	520	27	11.0	940	40	2	1	29	n/a	n/a	n/a	n/a
brioche	1	540	32	15.0	870	33	1	6	28	n/a	n/a	n/a	n/a
Sausage, scrambled egg & cheese													
artisan ciabatta	1	540	28	12.0	950	41	2	1	30	n/a	n/a	n/a	n/a
brioche	1	550	33	16.0	880	33	1	6	29	n/a	n/a	n/a	n/a
Scrambled egg & cheese													
artisan ciabatta	1	390	15	8.0	630	40	2	1	21	n/a	n/a	n/a	n/a
brioche	1	400	21	12.0	570	33	1	6	20	n/a	n/a	n/a	n/a
Steel cut oatmeal w/ strawberries & pecans	1	360	15	2.0	150	52	9	17	8	n/a	n/a	n/a	n/a
Souffles													
Four cheese	1	460	28	15.0	840	38	1	9	15	n/a	n/a	n/a	n/a
Spinach & artichoke	1	520	33	18.0	940	39	3	8	19	n/a	n/a	n/a	n/a
Spinach & bacon	1	540	35	18.0	970	38	2	8	20	n/a	n/a	n/a	n/a
Bagels													
Asiago cheese	1	320	5	3.0	530	55	2	4	14	n/a	n/a	n/a	n/a
Blueberry	1	290	1	0.0	390	61	2	10	10	n/a	n/a	n/a	n/a
Chocolate chip	1	320	5	2.5	370	61	2	13	10	n/a	n/a	n/a	n/a
Cinnamon crunch	1	420	7	5.0	380	83	2	32	9	n/a	n/a	n/a	n/a
Cinnamon swirl & raisin	1	310	2	1.0	410	65	3	12	10	n/a	n/a	n/a	n/a
Everything	1	290	2	0.0	560	58	2	4	10	n/a	n/a	n/a	n/a
Plain	1	280	1	0.0	410	57	2	4	10	n/a	n/a	n/a	n/a
Sesame	1	290	3	0.0	410	57	2	4	11	n/a	n/a	n/a	n/a

RESTAURANT & FAST FOOD CHAINS

	Amount	Calories	Fat (g)	Saturated Fat (g)	Sodium (mg)	Carbohydrate (g)	Fiber (g)	Sugar (g)	Protein (g)	Vitamin D (mcg)	Calcium (mg)	Iron (mg)	Potassium (mg)
Bread													
Artisan ciabatta	1 slice	150	2	0.0	280	30	1	0	6	n/a	n/a	n/a	n/a
Asiago cheese focaccia	1 slice	150	3	1.0	320	24	1	0	6	n/a	n/a	n/a	n/a
Black pepper focaccia	1 slice	140	2	0.0	370	26	1	0	5	n/a	n/a	n/a	n/a
Brioche roll	1	210	7	4.0	300	31	1	6	7	n/a	n/a	n/a	n/a
Classic sourdough	1 slice	150	0	0.0	320	31	1	0	6	n/a	n/a	n/a	n/a
Classic white miche	1 slice	160	4	2.0	260	27	1	4	6	n/a	n/a	n/a	n/a
Country rustic sourdough	1 slice	130	0	0.0	260	28	1	0	5	n/a	n/a	n/a	n/a
French baguette	1 slice	150	5	0.0	370	30	1	1	5	n/a	n/a	n/a	n/a
Sourdough bread bowl	1	670	40	4.5	1160	130	4	2	27	n/a	n/a	n/a	n/a
White whole grain	1 slice	130	5	0.5	260	25	3	2	6	n/a	n/a	n/a	n/a
Entrées													
Bowls													
Baja w/ chicken	1	740	35	7.0	1370	80	13	8	31	n/a	n/a	n/a	n/a
Mediterranean w/ chicken	1	690	31	7.0	1400	76	9	6	32	n/a	n/a	n/a	n/a
Teriyaki chicken & broccoli	1	650	21	4.5	1850	78	4	25	43	n/a	n/a	n/a	n/a
Broccoli cheddar mac & cheese	large	770	53	25.0	2250	50	4	11	26	n/a	n/a	n/a	n/a
Flatbread pizza													
chipotle chicken & bacon	1	940	45	17.0	2270	89	3	7	45	n/a	n/a	n/a	n/a
four cheese	1	930	45	26.0	2120	86	2	4	45	n/a	n/a	n/a	n/a
Margherita	1	780	31	17.0	1730	89	3	7	36	n/a	n/a	n/a	n/a
pepperoni	1	950	47	23.0	2410	87	3	5	44	n/a	n/a	n/a	n/a
Macaroni & cheese	large	950	62	35.0	2090	66	2	15	33	n/a	n/a	n/a	n/a
Sandwiches													
Bacon Turkey Bravo	1	870	42	16.0	2240	75	3	9	51	n/a	n/a	n/a	n/a
Chipotle chicken avocado melt	1	930	49	15.0	1980	80	8	5	46	n/a	n/a	n/a	n/a
Classic grilled cheese	1	860	49	31.0	2290	69	2	11	40	n/a	n/a	n/a	n/a
Mediterranean veggie	1	540	12	3.0	1270	88	8	9	21	n/a	n/a	n/a	n/a
Modern caprese	1	890	43	23.0	1910	85	6	12	42	n/a	n/a	n/a	n/a
Napa almond chicken salad	1	550	25	4.0	790	59	4	11	24	n/a	n/a	n/a	n/a
Roasted turkey & avocado BLT	1	850	53	10.0	1530	54	7	5	43	n/a	n/a	n/a	n/a
Smokehouse BBQ chicken	1	770	30	15.0	1690	80	3	18	46	n/a	n/a	n/a	n/a
Toasted Frontega Chicken	1	820	38	12.0	1900	79	4	6	43	n/a	n/a	n/a	n/a
Toasted steak & white cheddar	1	940	45	16.0	1550	85	4	6	48	n/a	n/a	n/a	n/a
Tuna salad	1	740	34	5.0	1670	79	5	5	31	n/a	n/a	n/a	n/a
Turkey	1	520	20	3.5	1350	54	4	4	32	n/a	n/a	n/a	n/a
Salads													
Asian sesame w/ chicken	1	430	23	3.0	720	29	6	7	31	n/a	n/a	n/a	n/a
BBQ chicken salad	1	510	25	4.0	1150	42	10	13	34	n/a	n/a	n/a	n/a
Caesar w/ chicken	1	460	28	7.0	970	21	4	3	34	n/a	n/a	n/a	n/a
Fuji apple w/ chicken	1	580	36	8.0	750	37	6	23	32	n/a	n/a	n/a	n/a

RESTAURANT & FAST FOOD CHAINS

Panera Bread

	Amount	Calories	Fat (g)	Saturated Fat (g)	Sodium (mg)	Carbohydrate (g)	Fiber (g)	Sugar (g)	Protein (g)	Vitamin D (mcg)	Calcium (mg)	Iron (mg)	Potassium
Greek	1	400	35	8.0	1120	14	6	6	9	n/a	n/a	n/a	n/a
Green Goddess Cobb w/ chicken	1	530	30	7.0	940	24	7	10	42	n/a	n/a	n/a	n/a
Strawberry poppy seed w/ chicken	1	360	15	2.0	480	34	8	23	28	n/a	n/a	n/a	n/a
Soups													
Baked potato	bowl	330	21	10.0	1420	33	4	7	9	n/a	n/a	n/a	n/a
Bistro French onion	bowl	310	13	6.0	1660	36	3	15	13	n/a	n/a	n/a	n/a
Broccoli cheddar	bowl	360	21	13.0	1330	30	6	6	14	n/a	n/a	n/a	n/a
Corn chowder	bowl	320	20	12.0	1310	34	3	8	5	n/a	n/a	n/a	n/a
Cream of chicken & wild rice	bowl	260	16	7.0	1390	27	5	4	10	n/a	n/a	n/a	n/a
Creamy tomato	bowl	330	21	11.0	840	34	1	17	5	n/a	n/a	n/a	n/a
Homestyle chicken noodle	bowl	180	5	1.5	2260	153	6	4	40	n/a	n/a	n/a	n/a
Ten vegetable	bowl	100	2	0.0	1090	15	4	6	5	n/a	n/a	n/a	n/a
Turkey chili	bowl	300	10	4.5	690	31	14	8	21	n/a	n/a	n/a	n/a
Smoothies													
Green Passion	16 fl oz	250	2	0.0	45	59	5	50	2	n/a	n/a	n/a	n/a
Mango w/ Greek yogurt	16 fl oz	290	5	3.0	60	51	4	42	13	n/a	n/a	n/a	n/a
Peach & blueberry w/ almond milk	16 fl oz	210	2	0.0	50	49	4	41	2	n/a	n/a	n/a	n/a
Strawberry w/ Greek yogurt	16 fl oz	270	5	2.5	60	44	6	37	12	n/a	n/a	n/a	n/a
Strawberry banana w/ Greek yogurt	16 fl oz	250	3	1.5	35	51	6	35	7	n/a	n/a	n/a	n/a
Superfruit w/ Greek yogurt	16 fl oz	240	5	2.5	50	36	0	28	13	n/a	n/a	n/a	n/a
Pastries & Sweets													
Bear claw	1	500	23	10.0	390	66	2	30	9	n/a	n/a	n/a	n/a
Brownie	1	400	13	8.0	370	68	3	48	6	n/a	n/a	n/a	n/a
Cookies													
candy	1	410	19	11.0	260	59	1	33	5	n/a	n/a	n/a	n/a
Chocolate Chipper	1	390	19	11.0	290	52	2	31	4	n/a	n/a	n/a	n/a
kitchen sink	1	800	44	28.0	760	99	2	56	8	n/a	n/a	n/a	n/a
tulip shortbread	1	420	23	13.0	300	48	1	14	7	n/a	n/a	n/a	n/a
Croissant	1	260	15	11.0	230	27	3	1	6	n/a	n/a	n/a	n/a
chocolate	1	380	22	13.0	240	39	4	11	7	n/a	n/a	n/a	n/a
Muffins													
blueberry	1	460	18	3.0	380	69	1	40	6	n/a	n/a	n/a	n/a
chocolate chip	1	640	28	7.0	410	91	3	55	8	n/a	n/a	n/a	n/a
muffie	1	320	14	3.5	210	46	2	28	4	n/a	n/a	n/a	n/a
cranberry orange	1	480	19	3.0	360	71	2	40	6	n/a	n/a	n/a	n/a
pumpkin	1	570	21	3.5	470	87	3	51	7	n/a	n/a	n/a	n/a
Pecan braid	1	490	28	11.0	280	53	3	23	8	n/a	n/a	n/a	n/a
Scones													
orange	1	540	20	13.0	810	80	2	37	8	n/a	n/a	n/a	n/a
wild blueberry	1	460	19	12.0	900	64	1	26	8	n/a	n/a	n/a	n/a
Vanilla cinnamon roll	1	620	18	8.0	490	109	3	72	8	n/a	n/a	n/a	n/a

RESTAURANT & FAST FOOD CHAINS

Pizza*

	Amount	Calories	Fat (g)	Saturated Fat (g)	Sodium (mg)	Carbohydrate (g)	Fiber (g)	Sugar (g)	Protein (g)	Vitamin D (mcg)	Calcium (mg)	Iron (mg)	Potassium (mg)
Hand-tossed													
cheese	1 slice	220	8	4.0	550	26	1	4	10	n/a	n/a	n/a	n/a
Meat Lover's	1 slice	300	16	7.0	860	26	1	4	14	n/a	n/a	n/a	n/a
pepperoni	1 slice	230	9	4.0	610	25	1	3	10	n/a	n/a	n/a	n/a
Pepperoni Lover's	1 slice	270	13	6.0	770	26	1	4	13	n/a	n/a	n/a	n/a
supreme	1 slice	260	12	5.0	680	26	1	4	12	n/a	n/a	n/a	n/a
Ultimate Cheese Lover's	1 slice	240	11	5.0	590	25	1	3	11	n/a	n/a	n/a	n/a
Veggie Lover's	1 slice	200	6	3.0	530	27	2	4	9	n/a	n/a	n/a	n/a
Pan													
cheese	1 slice	240	10	4.5	530	27	1	2	11	n/a	n/a	n/a	n/a
Meat Lover's	1 slice	330	18	7.0	830	27	1	2	14	n/a	n/a	n/a	n/a
pepperoni	1 slice	250	12	4.5	590	26	1	2	11	n/a	n/a	n/a	n/a
Pepperoni Lover's	1 slice	290	14	6.0	730	27	1	2	13	n/a	n/a	n/a	n/a
supreme	1 slice	290	14	5.0	650	27	2	2	12	n/a	n/a	n/a	n/a
Ultimate Cheese Lover's	1 slice	270	13	5.0	580	26	1	2	12	n/a	n/a	n/a	n/a
Veggie Lover's	1 slice	230	9	3.5	520	27	1	2	10	n/a	n/a	n/a	n/a
Personal pan													
cheese	1 pizza	590	24	10.0	1290	69	3	7	26	n/a	n/a	n/a	n/a
Meat Lover's	1 pizza	830	46	17.0	2110	68	3	7	36	n/a	n/a	n/a	n/a
pepperoni	1 pizza	610	26	10.0	1410	67	3	6	26	n/a	n/a	n/a	n/a
Pepperoni Lover's	1 pizza	720	34	14.0	1760	69	3	7	32	n/a	n/a	n/a	n/a
supreme	1 pizza	720	36	14.0	1680	69	4	7	30	n/a	n/a	n/a	n/a
Ultimate Cheese Lover's	1 pizza	660	30	12.0	1400	68	3	6	29	n/a	n/a	n/a	n/a
Veggie Lover's	1 pizza	550	20	8.0	1190	70	4	8	22	n/a	n/a	n/a	n/a
P'Zone													
meaty	½ order	550	23	10.0	1370	61	2	2	24	n/a	n/a	n/a	n/a
pepperoni	½ order	450	15	7.0	1120	60	2	2	19	n/a	n/a	n/a	n/a
Thin 'N Crispy													
cheese	1 slice	190	8	4.0	550	22	1	4	9	n/a	n/a	n/a	n/a
Meat Lover's	1 slice	280	16	6.0	860	22	1	4	13	n/a	n/a	n/a	n/a
pepperoni	1 slice	200	9	4.0	610	21	1	4	9	n/a	n/a	n/a	n/a
Pepperoni Lover's	1 slice	250	13	6.0	760	22	1	4	12	n/a	n/a	n/a	n/a
supreme	1 slice	240	12	5.0	670	23	1	4	10	n/a	n/a	n/a	n/a
Ultimate Cheese Lover's	1 slice	220	11	5.0	600	21	1	4	10	n/a	n/a	n/a	n/a
Veggie Lover's	1 slice	180	6	3.0	530	23	1	4	8	n/a	n/a	n/a	n/a

Tuscani Pasta

	Amount	Calories	Fat (g)	Saturated Fat (g)	Sodium (mg)	Carbohydrate (g)	Fiber (g)	Sugar (g)	Protein (g)	Vitamin D (mcg)	Calcium (mg)	Iron (mg)	Potassium (mg)
Chicken Alfredo	½ order	580	32	9.0	1250	49	4	4	23	n/a	n/a	n/a	n/a
Meaty marinara	½ order	450	20	8.0	1100	44	5	8	22	n/a	n/a	n/a	n/a

* Based on a 12-in medium pizza (8 slices).

RESTAURANT & FAST FOOD CHAINS

Wings	Amount	Calories	Fat (g)	Saturated Fat (g)	Sodium (mg)	Carbohydrate (g)	Fiber (g)	Sugar (g)	Protein (g)	Vitamin D (mcg)	Calcium (mg)	Iron (mg)	Potassium
Breaded boneless													
Buffalo													
Burnin' Hot	2 pcs	190	8	1.5	1000	18	1	2	10	n/a	n/a	n/a	n/a
medium	2 pcs	190	9	0.0	990	18	1	2	10	n/a	n/a	n/a	n/a
mild	2 pcs	190	9	0.0	1020	18	1	2	10	n/a	n/a	n/a	n/a
garlic Parmesan	2 pcs	260	19	3.5	710	11	1	1	11	n/a	n/a	n/a	n/a
honey BBQ	2 pcs	220	8	1.5	720	27	1	12	10	n/a	n/a	n/a	n/a
lemon pepper dry rub	2 pcs	220	12	2.0	620	18	1	7	10	n/a	n/a	n/a	n/a
naked	2 pcs	150	8	1.5	490	11	1	0	10	n/a	n/a	n/a	n/a
Traditional													
Buffalo													
Burnin' Hot	2 pcs	110	6	1.5	810	8	1	2	8	n/a	n/a	n/a	n/a
medium	2 pcs	110	6	1.5	800	8	1	2	8	n/a	n/a	n/a	n/a
mild	2 pcs	110	6	1.5	830	8	1	2	8	n/a	n/a	n/a	n/a
garlic Parmesan	2 pcs	180	16	3.5	520	1	0	1	8	n/a	n/a	n/a	n/a
honey BBQ	2 pcs	140	5	1.5	530	16	0	12	8	n/a	n/a	n/a	n/a
lemon pepper dry rub	2 pcs	150	10	2.0	430	8	0	7	8	n/a	n/a	n/a	n/a
naked	2 pcs	80	5	1.5	290	0	0	0	7	n/a	n/a	n/a	n/a
Sides													
Breadsticks	1 pc	140	5	1.0	260	19	1	2	5	n/a	n/a	n/a	n/a
Cheese sticks	1 pc	170	6	2.5	390	20	1	2	8	n/a	n/a	n/a	n/a
Fries	1 order	320	18	3.5	530	35	3	0	4	n/a	n/a	n/a	n/a

Breakfast	Amount	Calories	Fat (g)	Saturated Fat (g)	Sodium (mg)	Carbohydrate (g)	Fiber (g)	Sugar (g)	Protein (g)	Vitamin D (mcg)	Calcium (mg)	Iron (mg)	Potassium
Biscuit													
bacon	1	400	25	12.0	780	37	3	2	8	n/a	n/a	n/a	n/a
chicken	1	490	26	14.0	1275	47	1	2	17	n/a	n/a	n/a	n/a
egg	1	510	29	15.0	1155	41	1	2	13	n/a	n/a	n/a	n/a
egg & sausage	1	690	45	22.0	1520	43	1	2	20	n/a	n/a	n/a	n/a
sausage	1	540	36	18.0	1100	41	1	2	13	n/a	n/a	n/a	n/a
Grits	1 order	370	5	0.5	30	80	7	0	5	n/a	n/a	n/a	n/a
Hash rounds	1 order	360	20	9.0	450	41	4	0	3	n/a	n/a	n/a	n/a
Chicken													
Breast	1 pc	380	20	8.0	1230	16	2	0	35	n/a	n/a	n/a	n/a
Leg	1 pc	160	9	4.0	460	5	1	0	14	n/a	n/a	n/a	n/a
Nuggets	9 pcs	338	20	9.0	517	23	2	0	16	n/a	n/a	n/a	n/a
Tenders, spicy/mild	5 pcs	741	34	14.0	3035	48	3	0	63	n/a	n/a	n/a	n/a
Tenders, blackened	5 pcs	283	3	0.0	917	3	0	0	43	n/a	n/a	n/a	n/a
Thigh	1 pc	280	21	8.0	640	7	1	0	14	n/a	n/a	n/a	n/a
Whole wing	1 pc	210	14	4.0	610	8	1	0	13	n/a	n/a	n/a	n/a

Popeyes

	Amount	Calories	Fat (g)	Saturated Fat (g)	Sodium (mg)	Carbohydrate (g)	Fiber (g)	Sugar (g)	Protein (g)	Vitamin D (mcg)	Calcium (mg)	Iron (mg)	Potassium (mg)
Seafood													
Butterfly shrimp	8 pcs	420	25	9.0	1100	34	4	0	16	n/a	n/a	n/a	n/a
Cajun fish filet	3 pcs	380	19	5.0	1650	37	2	4	16	n/a	n/a	n/a	n/a
Catfish filet	2 pcs	460	29	12.0	1140	27	1	0	21	n/a	n/a	n/a	n/a
Popcorn shrimp	¼ lb	390	25	8.0	1391	28	3	0	14	n/a	n/a	n/a	n/a
Chicken Sandwiches													
Classic	1	699	42	14.0	1443	50	2	8	28	n/a	n/a	n/a	n/a
Spicy	1	700	42	14.0	1473	50	2	8	28	n/a	n/a	n/a	n/a
Sides													
Biscuit	1	207	13	6.0	435	20	1	1	3	n/a	n/a	n/a	n/a
Cajun fries	large	804	42	15.0	1761	97	9	1	10	n/a	n/a	n/a	n/a
Cinnamon apple pie	1	236	16	6.0	260	35	1	12	3	n/a	n/a	n/a	n/a
Coleslaw	large	420	30	5.0	570	36	3	27	3	n/a	n/a	n/a	n/a
Homestyle mac & cheese	large	655	28	14.0	2995	70	5	10	24	n/a	n/a	n/a	n/a
Mashed potatoes w/ gravy	large	330	12	6.0	1770	54	3	3	9	n/a	n/a	n/a	n/a
Red beans & rice	large	610	40	13.0	1489	51	15	0	19	n/a	n/a	n/a	n/a

Sonic

	Amount	Calories	Fat (g)	Saturated Fat (g)	Sodium (mg)	Carbohydrate (g)	Fiber (g)	Sugar (g)	Protein (g)	Vitamin D (mcg)	Calcium (mg)	Iron (mg)	Potassium (mg)
Breakfast													
Breakfast burrito													
bacon	1	470	25	11.0	1540	35	1	1	25	n/a	n/a	n/a	n/a
sausage	1	500	30	13.0	1430	35	1	1	23	n/a	n/a	n/a	n/a
ultimate meat & cheese	1	840	58	19.0	2220	47	2	1	30	n/a	n/a	n/a	n/a
Breakfast Toaster													
bacon	1	610	31	10.0	1610	52	2	7	29	n/a	n/a	n/a	n/a
sausage	1	720	43	14.0	1530	52	2	7	29	n/a	n/a	n/a	n/a
Cinnabon Cinnasnacks	5 pcs	630	37	11.0	350	63	4	21	10	n/a	n/a	n/a	n/a
French toast sticks	4 pcs	480	25	4.5	460	54	3	12	8	n/a	n/a	n/a	n/a
SuperSONIC breakfast burrito	1	610	35	14.0	1800	49	3	3	24	n/a	n/a	n/a	n/a
Burgers & Toppings													
Cheeseburger													
	1	720	42	11.0	1400	52	2	12	31	n/a	n/a	n/a	n/a
double	1	1070	71	21.0	2020	54	2	12	53	n/a	n/a	n/a	n/a
bacon double	1	1140	77	23.0	2020	52	5	10	58	n/a	n/a	n/a	n/a
quarter pound double	1	610	39	15.0	1470	34	2	5	28	n/a	n/a	n/a	n/a
Toppings													
American cheese	1 order	70	6	3.0	330	1	0	0	4	n/a	n/a	n/a	n/a
crispy bacon	1 order	80	7	0.5	290	1	0	0	6	n/a	n/a	n/a	n/a
grilled onions	1 order	5	0	0.0	5	1	0	0	0	n/a	n/a	n/a	n/a
hot chili	1 order	60	4	1.5	170	3	1	1	3	n/a	n/a	n/a	n/a
spicy jalapeños	1 order	5	0	0.0	140	1	0	1	0	n/a	n/a	n/a	n/a

Sonic

	Amount	Calories	Fat (g)	Saturated Fat (g)	Sodium (mg)	Carbohydrate (g)	Fiber (g)	Sugar (g)	Protein (g)	Vitamin D (mcg)	Calcium (mg)	Iron (mg)	Potassi
Chicken													
Chicken Slinger	1	350	16	3.5	680	35	3	6	14	n/a	n/a	n/a	n/a
Classic crispy chicken sandwich	1	550	30	6.0	870	48	4	10	21	n/a	n/a	n/a	n/a
Classic grilled chicken sandwich	1	470	22	4.0	1340	39	3	10	30	n/a	n/a	n/a	n/a
Crispy tenders	5 pcs	430	20	2.0	1210	27	3	0	35	n/a	n/a	n/a	n/a
Jumbo popcorn chicken	medium	750	43	8.0	2520	55	6	2	36	n/a	n/a	n/a	n/a
Buffalo	medium	560	35	6.0	2500	37	5	2	24	n/a	n/a	n/a	n/a
honey BBQ	medium	570	28	5.0	2170	53	4	17	24	n/a	n/a	n/a	n/a
Hot Dogs & Sandwiches													
All-American dog	1	410	21	8.0	1120	41	2	12	13	n/a	n/a	n/a	n/a
All beef regular hot dog	1	360	21	8.0	800	31	2	4	12	n/a	n/a	n/a	n/a
Chili cheese coney	1	470	29	12.0	1260	34	2	5	18	n/a	n/a	n/a	n/a
Footlong quarter pound coney	1	790	49	19.0	2300	55	3	9	31	n/a	n/a	n/a	n/a
Grilled cheese sandwich	1	430	19	7.0	1090	51	2	7	14	n/a	n/a	n/a	n/a
Snacks & Sides													
Ched 'R' Peppers	6 pcs	490	48	12.0	2130	56	3	4	13	n/a	n/a	n/a	n/a
Corn dog	1	230	13	4.0	480	23	1	5	6	n/a	n/a	n/a	n/a
Fries	medium	290	13	2.5	300	38	3	0	3	n/a	n/a	n/a	n/a
chili cheese	medium	450	26	10.0	940	42	4	2	12	n/a	n/a	n/a	n/a
Mozzarella sticks	6 pcs	560	29	11.0	1490	61	3	8	23	n/a	n/a	n/a	n/a
Onion rings	medium	580	29	5.0	570.0	74	4	19	8	n/a	n/a	n/a	n/a
Soft pretzel twist	1	250	60	7.0	440	39	2	6	7	n/a	n/a	n/a	n/a
Tots	medium	360	19	3.5	890	43	4	0	3	n/a	n/a	n/a	n/a
chili cheese	medium	530	32	10.0	1540	47	5	2	12	n/a	n/a	n/a	n/a
Limeades													
Cherry	medium	250	0	0.0	50	66	0	65	0	n/a	n/a	n/a	n/a
diet	medium	20	0	0.0	20	3	0	2	0	n/a	n/a	n/a	n/a
Diet lime	medium	10	0	0.0	15	1	0	0	0	n/a	n/a	n/a	n/a
Minute Maid cranberry	medium	240	0	0.0	45	64	0	62	0	n/a	n/a	n/a	n/a
Regular	medium	180	0	0.0	40	47	0	46	0	n/a	n/a	n/a	n/a
Strawberry	medium	220	0	0.0	50	59	1	57	0	n/a	n/a	n/a	n/a
Shakes													
Butterfinger	medium	980	48	28.0	550	118	2	75	18	n/a	n/a	n/a	n/a
Caramel	medium	830	41	28.0	520	97	0	67	12	n/a	n/a	n/a	n/a
Cheesecake	medium	840	43	28.0	680	101	1	68	12	n/a	n/a	n/a	n/a
Chocolate	medium	810	43	29.0	540	95	1	67	12	n/a	n/a	n/a	n/a
Chocolate chip cookie dough	medium	920	45	25.0	450	118	1	73	13	n/a	n/a	n/a	n/a
Fresh banana	medium	850	41	27.0	390	108	3	70	13	n/a	n/a	n/a	n/a
Hot fudge	medium	940	48	33.0	480	113	2	80	13	n/a	n/a	n/a	n/a

RESTAURANT & FAST FOOD CHAINS

Sonic

	Amount	Calories	Fat (g)	Saturated Fat (g)	Sodium (mg)	Carbohydrate (g)	Fiber (g)	Sugar (g)	Protein (g)	Vitamin D (mcg)	Calcium (mg)	Iron (mg)	Potassium (mg)
M&M's	medium	1060	54	34.0	430	127	2	98	15	n/a	n/a	n/a	n/a
Oreo	medium	860	44	24.0	620	103	2	66	13	n/a	n/a	n/a	n/a
Oreo cheesecake	medium	1030	51	30.0	900	131	2	84	13	n/a	n/a	n/a	n/a
Oreo chocolate	medium	1000	51	32.0	760	125	3	84	13	n/a	n/a	n/a	n/a
Oreo peanut butter	medium	1130	67	33.0	740	116	3	75	18	n/a	n/a	n/a	n/a
Peanut butter	medium	940	59	30.0	520	87	2	58	17	n/a	n/a	n/a	n/a
Reese's	medium	990	55	29.0	610	110	2	82	18	n/a	n/a	n/a	n/a
Snickers	medium	890	46	26.0	490	103	1	73	15	n/a	n/a	n/a	n/a
Strawberry	medium	790	41	27.0	400	92	1	66	11	n/a	n/a	n/a	n/a
Strawberry cheesecake	medium	890	43	28.0	680	112	2	78	12	n/a	n/a	n/a	n/a
Vanilla	medium	820	45	30.0	430	89	0	61	13	n/a	n/a	n/a	n/a
Slushes													
Blue coconut	medium	270	0	0.0	45	72	0	72	0	n/a	n/a	n/a	n/a
Blue raspberry	medium	270	0	0.0	45	71	0	71	0	n/a	n/a	n/a	n/a
Cherry	medium	280	0	0.0	45	74	0	74	0	n/a	n/a	n/a	n/a
Grape	medium	290	0	0.0	45	77	1	76	0	n/a	n/a	n/a	n/a
Lemonade	medium	280	0	0.0	40	74	0	72	0	n/a	n/a	n/a	n/a
Limeade	medium	280	0	0.0	40	74	0	72	0	n/a	n/a	n/a	n/a
Strawberry	medium	290	0	0.0	50	78	1	77	0	n/a	n/a	n/a	n/a
Sundaes, Cones & Toppings													
Caramel	1	490	22	15.0	350	61	0	43	7	n/a	n/a	n/a	n/a
Chocolate	1	430	22	15.0	280	51	1	36	7	n/a	n/a	n/a	n/a
Hot fudge	1	520	26	18.0	270	65	1	46	7	n/a	n/a	n/a	n/a
Peanuts	1 order	40	4	0.5	0	2	1	0	2	n/a	n/a	n/a	n/a
Strawberry	1	440	21	14.0	220	55	1	40	7	n/a	n/a	n/a	n/a
Vanilla cone	1	250	12	8.0	140	30	0	17	4	n/a	n/a	n/a	n/a
Whipped topping	1 order	70	3	5.0	0	5	0	5	0	n/a	n/a	n/a	n/a

Starbucks

	Amount	Calories	Fat (g)	Saturated Fat (g)	Sodium (mg)	Carbohydrate (g)	Fiber (g)	Sugar (g)	Protein (g)	Vitamin D (mcg)	Calcium (mg)	Iron (mg)	Potassium (mg)
Cold Coffee													
Cold brew	grande (16 fl oz)	5	0	0.0	15	0	0	0	0	n/a	n/a	n/a	n/a
honey almondmilk	grande (16 fl oz)	50	1	0.0	25	11	0	10	0	n/a	n/a	n/a	n/a
salted caramel	grande (16 fl oz)	230	14	9.0	330	23	0	23	2	n/a	n/a	n/a	n/a
Starbucks Reserve	grande (16 fl oz)	5	0	0.0	15	0	0	0	0	n/a	n/a	n/a	n/a
vanilla sweet cream	grande (16 fl oz)	110	5	3.5	20	14	0	14	1	n/a	n/a	n/a	n/a
w/ milk	grande (16 fl oz)	35	2	1.0	40	3	0	3	2	n/a	n/a	n/a	n/a
Iced caffè americano	grande (16 fl oz)	15	0	0.0	15	2	0	0	1	n/a	n/a	n/a	n/a
Iced caramel macchiato	grande (16 fl oz)	250	7	4.5	150	37	0	34	10	n/a	n/a	n/a	n/a
Iced coffee	grande (16 fl oz)	80	0	0.0	10	20	0	20	0	n/a	n/a	n/a	n/a
w/ milk	grande (16 fl oz)	110	2	1.0	40	23	0	23	2	n/a	n/a	n/a	n/a
Iced espresso	grande (16 fl oz)	10	0	0.0	0	2	0	0	1	n/a	n/a	n/a	n/a
shaken	grande (16 fl oz)	100	2	1.0	0	17	0	14	4	n/a	n/a	n/a	n/a

RESTAURANT & FAST FOOD CHAINS

Starbucks

	Amount	Calories	Fat (g)	Saturated Fat (g)	Sodium (mg)	Carbohydrate (g)	Fiber (g)	Sugar (g)	Protein (g)	Vitamin D (mcg)	Calcium (mg)	Iron (mg)	Potassium
chocolate almondmilk shaken	grande (16 fl oz)	110	3	0.0	80	20	1	16	2	n/a	n/a	n/a	n/a
Iced flat white	grande (16 fl oz)	150	8	4.5	110	13	0	11	8	n/a	n/a	n/a	n/a
honey almondmilk	grande (16 fl oz)	100	3	0.0	70	20	1	17	1	n/a	n/a	n/a	n/a
Iced latte													
caffè	grande (16 fl oz)	130	5	2.5	115	13	0	11	8	n/a	n/a	n/a	n/a
cinnamon dolce	grande (16 fl oz)	300	13	8.0	115	38	0	35	8	n/a	n/a	n/a	n/a
Starbucks Blonde vanilla	grande (16 fl oz)	190	4	2.0	100	30	0	28	7	n/a	n/a	n/a	n/a
Starbucks Reserve	grande (16 fl oz)	210	11	6.0	150	17	0	16	11	n/a	n/a	n/a	n/a
hazelnut bianco	grande (16 fl oz)	280	13	6.0	120	30	1	26	10	n/a	n/a	n/a	n/a
Iced mocha													
caffè	grande (16 fl oz)	350	17	11.0	100	38	4	30	10	n/a	n/a	n/a	n/a
Starbucks Reserve dark chocolate	grande (16 fl oz)	260	10	6.0	115	33	2	28	10	n/a	n/a	n/a	n/a
white chocolate	grande (16 fl oz)	420	20	14.0	200	49	0	48	11	n/a	n/a	n/a	n/a
Cold Drinks													
Blended strawberry lemonade	grande (16 fl oz)	190	0	0.0	200	46	0	45	0	n/a	n/a	n/a	n/a
Dragon drink	grande (16 fl oz)	130	3	2.5	60	26	0	23	1	n/a	n/a	n/a	n/a
Iced guava passionfruit drink	grande (16 fl oz)	190	3	2.5	85	41	0	33	1	n/a	n/a	n/a	n/a
Iced pineapple matcha drink	grande (16 fl oz)	170	5	4.5	115	30	2	27	2	n/a	n/a	n/a	n/a
Pink drink	grande (16 fl oz)	140	3	2.5	65	27	2	24	1	n/a	n/a	n/a	n/a
Refresher													
kiwi starfruit	grande (16 fl oz)	90	0	0.0	15	22	1	18	0	n/a	n/a	n/a	n/a
mango dragonfruit	grande (16 fl oz)	90	0	0.0	15	21	0	19	0	n/a	n/a	n/a	n/a
strawberry açaí	grande (16 fl oz)	90	0	0.0	15	23	1	20	0	n/a	n/a	n/a	n/a
very berry hibiscus	grande (16 fl oz)	70	0	0.0	15	17	1	14	1	n/a	n/a	n/a	n/a
Star drink	grande (16 fl oz)	130	3	2.5	65	26	1	22	1	n/a	n/a	n/a	n/a
Violet drink	grande (16 fl oz)	110	3	2.5	0	22	1	19	0	n/a	n/a	n/a	n/a
Frappucino Blended Beverages													
Caffè vanilla	grande (16 fl oz)	400	14	9.0	230	65	0	64	4	n/a	n/a	n/a	n/a
Caramel	grande (16 fl oz)	380	16	10.0	230	55	0	54	4	n/a	n/a	n/a	n/a
Caramel ribbon crunch	grande (16 fl oz)	470	22	14.0	280	65	0	60	5	n/a	n/a	n/a	n/a
crème	grande (16 fl oz)	420	22	14.0	280	50	0	46	5	n/a	n/a	n/a	n/a
Chai crème	grande (16 fl oz)	340	16	10.0	230	46	0	45	5	n/a	n/a	n/a	n/a
Chocolate cookie crumble crème	grande (16 fl oz)	460	25	16.0	290	52	2	46	7	n/a	n/a	n/a	n/a
Coffee	grande (16 fl oz)	230	3	2.0	230	46	0	45	3	n/a	n/a	n/a	n/a
Double chocolaty chip crème	grande (16 fl oz)	410	20	13.0	270	51	2	47	7	n/a	n/a	n/a	n/a
Espresso	grande (16 fl oz)	210	3	1.5	210	43	0	42	3	n/a	n/a	n/a	n/a
Java chip	grande (16 fl oz)	440	18	12.0	260	65	2	60	6	n/a	n/a	n/a	n/a
Matcha crème	grande (16 fl oz)	420	16	10.0	240	62	1	61	6	n/a	n/a	n/a	n/a

RESTAURANT & FAST FOOD CHAINS

Starbucks

	Amount	Calories	Fat (g)	Saturated Fat (g)	Sodium (mg)	Carbohydrate (g)	Fiber (g)	Sugar (g)	Protein (g)	Vitamin D (mcg)	Calcium (mg)	Iron (mg)	Potassium (mg)
Mocha	grande (16 fl oz)	370	15	10.0	220	54	1	51	5	n/a	n/a	n/a	n/a
Mocha cookie crumble	grande (16 fl oz)	480	24	15.0	270	62	2	55	6	n/a	n/a	n/a	n/a
Strawberry funnel cake crème	grande (16 fl oz)	410	20	12.0	220	53	0	51	4	n/a	n/a	n/a	n/a
	grande (16 fl oz)	380	21	13.0	240	42	0	41	5	n/a	n/a	n/a	n/a
White chocolate mocha	grande (16 fl oz)	420	17	11.0	260	61	0	61	5	n/a	n/a	n/a	n/a
Strawberry crème	grande (16 fl oz)	370	16	10.0	240	51	0	51	5	n/a	n/a	n/a	n/a
Vanilla bean crème	grande (16 fl oz)	380	16	10.0	250	53	0	52	5	n/a	n/a	n/a	n/a
White chocolate crème	grande (16 fl oz)	380	18	12.0	280	49	0	49	6	n/a	n/a	n/a	n/a
Hot Coffee													
Blonde roast	grande (16 fl oz)	5	0	0.0	10	0	0	0	1	n/a	n/a	n/a	n/a
Caffè americano	grande (16 fl oz)	15	0	0.0	10	2	0	0	1	n/a	n/a	n/a	n/a
Caffè latte	grande (16 fl oz)	190	7	4.5	170	19	0	18	13	n/a	n/a	n/a	n/a
Caffè misto	grande (16 fl oz)	110	4	2.0	100	10	0	10	7	n/a	n/a	n/a	n/a
Caffè mocha	grande (16 fl oz)	370	15	10.0	150	43	4	35	14	n/a	n/a	n/a	n/a
Cappuccino	grande (16 fl oz)	140	5	3.0	120	14	0	12	9	n/a	n/a	n/a	n/a
Caramel macchiato	grande (16 fl oz)	250	7	4.5	150	35	0	33	10	n/a	n/a	n/a	n/a
Espresso con panna shot	1.5 fl oz	35	3	1.5	0	2	0	1	1	n/a	n/a	n/a	n/a
Espresso shot	1.5 fl oz	10	0	0.0	0	2	0	0	1	n/a	n/a	n/a	n/a
Espresso macchiato	1.6 fl oz	15	0	0.0	0	2	0	0	1	n/a	n/a	n/a	n/a
Featured Starbucks dark roast coffee	grande (16 fl oz)	5	0	0.0	10	0	0	0	1	n/a	n/a	n/a	n/a
Flat white	grande (16 fl oz)	220	11	7.0	150	18	0	17	12	n/a	n/a	n/a	n/a
honey almondmilk	grande (16 fl oz)	170	5	0.0	135	30	1	24	3	n/a	n/a	n/a	n/a
Latte													
cinnamon dolce	grande (16 fl oz)	340	14	9.0	160	43	0	40	12	n/a	n/a	n/a	n/a
Starbucks Blonde vanilla	grande (16 fl oz)	250	6	3.5	150	37	0	35	12	n/a	n/a	n/a	n/a
Starbucks Reserve	grande (16 fl oz)	230	12	7.0	160	19	0	18	12	n/a	n/a	n/a	n/a
hazelnut bianco	grande (16 fl oz)	380	18	8.0	160	40	1	36	13	n/a	n/a	n/a	n/a
Mocha													
Starbucks Reserve dark chocolate	grande (16 fl oz)	320	14	8.0	150	38	2	33	13	n/a	n/a	n/a	n/a
white chocolate	grande (16 fl oz)	430	18	12.0	240	54	0	53	15	n/a	n/a	n/a	n/a
Pike Place roast	grande (16 fl oz)	5	0	0.0	10	0	0	0	1	n/a	n/a	n/a	n/a
Hot Drinks													
Caramel apple spice	grande (16 fl oz)	380	8	5.0	35	77	0	70	1	n/a	n/a	n/a	n/a
Cinnamon dolce crème	grande (16 fl oz)	360	15	9.0	180	44	0	42	13	n/a	n/a	n/a	n/a
Hot chocolate	grande (16 fl oz)	370	16	10.0	160	43	4	37	14	n/a	n/a	n/a	n/a
white	grande (16 fl oz)	440	19	13.0	260	55	0	55	15	n/a	n/a	n/a	n/a
Steamed apple juice	grande (16 fl oz)	220	0	0.0	20	55	0	50	0	n/a	n/a	n/a	n/a
Steamed milk	grande (16 fl oz)	200	8	4.0	190	19	0	19	13	n/a	n/a	n/a	n/a
Vanilla crème	grande (16 fl oz)	350	14	9.0	180	44	0	43	13	n/a	n/a	n/a	n/a

	Amount	Calories	Fat (g)	Saturated Fat (g)	Sodium (mg)	Carbohydrate (g)	Fiber (g)	Sugar (g)	Protein (g)	Vitamin D (mcg)	Calcium (mg)	Iron (mg)	Potassium (mg)
Hot Tea Lattes													
Chai	grande (16 fl oz)	240	5	2.0	115	45	0	42	8	n/a	n/a	n/a	n/a
London fog	grande (16 fl oz)	180	4	2.5	105	29	0	29	7	n/a	n/a	n/a	n/a
Matcha	grande (16 fl oz)	240	7	4.5	160	34	1	32	12	n/a	n/a	n/a	n/a
Royal English breakfast	grande (16 fl oz)	150	4	2.5	105	21	0	21	7	n/a	n/a	n/a	n/a
Iced Tea													
Black	grande (16 fl oz)	0	0	0.0	10	0	0	0	0	n/a	n/a	n/a	n/a
Green	grande (16 fl oz)	0	0	0.0	10	0	0	0	0	n/a	n/a	n/a	n/a
Guava black	grande (16 fl oz)	70	0	0.0	20	16	0	13	0	n/a	n/a	n/a	n/a
Iced lattes													
chai	grande (16 fl oz)	240	4	2.0	110	44	0	42	7	n/a	n/a	n/a	n/a
London fog	grande (16 fl oz)	140	3	1.5	70	25	0	25	4	n/a	n/a	n/a	n/a
matcha	grande (16 fl oz)	200	5	3.0	120	29	1	28	9	n/a	n/a	n/a	n/a
royal English breakfast	grande (16 fl oz)	140	3	1.5	70	25	0	25	4	n/a	n/a	n/a	n/a
Matcha lemonade	grande (16 fl oz)	120	0	0.0	10	29	1	27	1	n/a	n/a	n/a	n/a
Passion Tango	grande (16 fl oz)	0	0	0.0	10	0	0	0	0	n/a	n/a	n/a	n/a
Peach green	grande (16 fl oz)	60	0	0.0	20	15	0	12	0	n/a	n/a	n/a	n/a
Breakfast													
Berry trio parfait	1	240	3	0.0	125	39	2	25	14	n/a	n/a	n/a	n/a
Oatmeal	1 order	160	3	0.5	125	28	4	0	5	n/a	n/a	n/a	n/a
hearty blueberry	1 order	220	3	0.5	125	43	5	13	5	n/a	n/a	n/a	n/a
Potato, cheddar & chive bake	1	230	14	9.0	460	13	0	4	13	n/a	n/a	n/a	n/a
Sandwiches													
bacon, Gouda & egg	1	360	18	7.0	720	35	1	2	19	n/a	n/a	n/a	n/a
double-smoked bacon, cheddar & egg	1	500	28	13.0	920	42	1	8	22	n/a	n/a	n/a	n/a
Impossible breakfast	1	420	22	8.0	800	36	2	4	21	n/a	n/a	n/a	n/a
roasted ham, Swiss & egg	1	450	21	11.0	880	42	1	8	22	n/a	n/a	n/a	n/a
sausage, cheddar & egg	1	480	29	10.0	890	34	1	2	18	n/a	n/a	n/a	n/a
turkey bacon, cheddar & egg white	1	230	5	2.5	550	28	3	2	17	n/a	n/a	n/a	n/a
Sous vide egg bites													
bacon & Gruyère	2	300	20	12.0	680	9	0	2	19	n/a	n/a	n/a	n/a
egg white & roasted red pepper	2	170	8	5.0	470	11	0	3	12	n/a	n/a	n/a	n/a
kale & portabella mushroom	2	230	14	9.0	340	11	2	1	15	n/a	n/a	n/a	n/a
Spinach, feta & egg white wrap	1	290	8	3.5	840	34	3	5	20	n/a	n/a	n/a	n/a
Strawberry overnight grains	1 order	300	16	11.0	15	35	4	20	5	n/a	n/a	n/a	n/a
Bagels													
Cheese, onion & garlic	1	300	5	2.0	530	50	3	5	12	n/a	n/a	n/a	n/a
Cinnamon raisin	1	270	1	0.0	370	58	3	11	9	n/a	n/a	n/a	n/a
Everything	1	290	3	1.0	530	57	3	5	10	n/a	n/a	n/a	n/a
Plain	1	280	2	0.0	620	56	2	2	9	n/a	n/a	n/a	n/a
Sprouted grain	1	330	6	0.5	490	57	7	4	12	n/a	n/a	n/a	n/a

RESTAURANT & FAST FOOD CHAINS

Starbucks

	Amount	Calories	Fat (g)	Saturated Fat (g)	Sodium (mg)	Carbohydrate (g)	Fiber (g)	Sugar (g)	Protein (g)	Vitamin D (mcg)	Calcium (mg)	Iron (mg)	Potassium (mg)
Bakery													
Blueberry muffin	1	320	14	2.5	240	49	2	20	5	n/a	n/a	n/a	n/a
Cake pops													
birthday	1	170	9	5.0	110	23	0	18	1	n/a	n/a	n/a	n/a
chocolate	1	160	8	4.5	80	23	1	18	2	n/a	n/a	n/a	n/a
cookie dough	1	180	9	5.0	80	23	0	12	2	n/a	n/a	n/a	n/a
unicorn	1	150	7	4.0	95	20	0	14	1	n/a	n/a	n/a	n/a
Cheese danish	1	290	14	9.0	400	33	1	11	7	n/a	n/a	n/a	n/a
Chocolate chip cookie	1	360	18	11.0	220	47	2	31	6	n/a	n/a	n/a	n/a
Cinnamon coffee cake	1	330	15	8.0	270	43	1	21	4	n/a	n/a	n/a	n/a
Croissants													
almond	1	420	25	11.0	390	40	2	13	8	n/a	n/a	n/a	n/a
butter	1	260	15	10.0	320	27	1	5	5	n/a	n/a	n/a	n/a
chocolate	1	340	20	12.0	280	38	2	13	5	n/a	n/a	n/a	n/a
ham & Swiss	1	320	17	9.0	490	28	1	5	14	n/a	n/a	n/a	n/a
Double chocolate brownie	1	480	28	9.0	220	55	3	37	6	n/a	n/a	n/a	n/a
Glazed doughnut	1	480	27	13.0	410	56	1	30	5	n/a	n/a	n/a	n/a
Loaves													
banana nut	1	420	22	3.0	320	52	2	30	6	n/a	n/a	n/a	n/a
iced lemon	1	470	20	9.0	310	68	1	42	6	n/a	n/a	n/a	n/a
pumpkin	1	410	15	2.5	500	63	2	39	6	n/a	n/a	n/a	n/a
Marshmallow dream bar	1	230	5	3.5	220	44	0	24	1	n/a	n/a	n/a	n/a
Scones													
blueberry	1	380	17	10.0	350	54	2	22	6	n/a	n/a	n/a	n/a
petite vanilla bean	1	120	4.5	2.0	95	18	0	8	2	n/a	n/a	n/a	n/a
Lunch													
Chicken & quinoa protein bowl w/ black beans & greens	1	420	17	3.0	1030	42	9	11	27	n/a	n/a	n/a	n/a
Crispy grilled cheese sandwich	1	520	27	16.0	1040	47	4	1	21	n/a	n/a	n/a	n/a
Paninis													
chicken & bacon	1	600	25	8.0	1460	65	3	12	29	n/a	n/a	n/a	n/a
chicken caprese	1	540	20	7.0	1100	57	3	3	32	n/a	n/a	n/a	n/a
ham & Swiss	1	480	23	10.0	1210	41	2	2	24	n/a	n/a	n/a	n/a
tomato & mozzarella	1	370	14	6.0	760	42	3	2	18	n/a	n/a	n/a	n/a
turkey & pesto	1	550	21	7.0	1200	53	3	3	34	n/a	n/a	n/a	n/a
Protein Boxes													
Cheddar & uncured salami	1	470	31	11.0	810	31	3	14	20	n/a	n/a	n/a	n/a
Cheese & fruit	1	470	28	16.0	770	37	3	17	20	n/a	n/a	n/a	n/a
Cheese trio	1	520	24	14.0	710	59	5	40	20	n/a	n/a	n/a	n/a
Chickpea bites & avocado	1	560	37	4.5	710	43	13	7	15	n/a	n/a	n/a	n/a
Eggs & cheddar	1	470	25	7.0	460	40	5	21	23	n/a	n/a	n/a	n/a
Eggs & Gouda	1	540	28	10.0	800	30	5	23	27	n/a	n/a	n/a	n/a
Grilled chicken & hummus	1	300	9	2.0	780	32	7	6	22	n/a	n/a	n/a	n/a
PB&J	1	520	27	8.0	630	51	6	30	20	n/a	n/a	n/a	n/a

RESTAURANT & FAST FOOD CHAINS

Starbucks	Amount	Calories	Fat (g)	Saturated Fat (g)	Sodium (mg)	Carbohydrate (g)	Fiber (g)	Sugar (g)	Protein (g)	Vitamin D (mcg)	Calcium (mg)	Iron (mg)	Potass.
Snacks & Sweets													
Butter gourmet popcorn	1 pkg	140	5	1.0	180	20	4	1	2	n/a	n/a	n/a	n/a
Chocolate covered espresso beans	1 pkg	260	15	8.0	10	29	3	22	3	n/a	n/a	n/a	n/a
Dark chocolate grahams	2	140	8	4.5	30	18	2	11	2	n/a	n/a	n/a	n/a
Kettle corn	1 pkg	130	5	0.0	130	21	3	7	2	n/a	n/a	n/a	n/a
Madeleines	3	220	11	7.0	120	28	0	17	3	n/a	n/a	n/a	n/a
dipped	3	280	15	9.0	100	35	1	24	3	n/a	n/a	n/a	n/a
Potato chips													
BBQ	1 pkg	270	13	1.5	410	35	2	3	5	n/a	n/a	n/a	n/a
salt & vinegar kettle	1 pkg	270	13	1.5	640	34	2	0	5	n/a	n/a	n/a	n/a
simply salted kettle	1 pkg	280	14	1.5	240	34	2	0	5	n/a	n/a	n/a	n/a
sweet potato	1 pkg	300	18	1.5	140	33	5	9	3	n/a	n/a	n/a	n/a
Salted almond & chocolate bites	1 pkg	300	22	7.0	200	24	4	19	7	n/a	n/a	n/a	n/a
Seasonal fruit blend	1 order	90	0	0.0	0	24	4	19	1	n/a	n/a	n/a	n/a
Shortbread	2	170	9	6.0	0	21	1	8	2	n/a	n/a	n/a	n/a
String cheese	1	80	6	3.5	200	1	0	0	7	n/a	n/a	n/a	n/a
Vanilla biscotti w/ almonds	1	200	9	3.0	135	25	1	10	5	n/a	n/a	n/a	n/a
Subway*													
Breakfast													
Bacon, egg & cheese	6 in	710	42	11.0	1230	48	4	5	35	n/a	60	12	n/a
Black Forest ham, egg & cheese	6 in	670	38	10.0	1230	49	4	5	35	n/a	60	12	n/a
Egg & cheese	6 in	640	37	10.0	980	48	4	4	30	n/a	60	10	n/a
Steak, egg & cheese	6 in	700	40	11.0	1260	49	4	4	40	n/a	60	13	n/a
Protein Bowls													
Black Forest ham	1	170	5	1.5	1050	12	3	6	21	n/a	40	5	n/a
Buffalo chicken	1	370	20	4.0	2160	13	3	7	35	n/a	60	1	n/a
Chicken & bacon ranch	1	600	40	13.0	1450	12	3	8	52	n/a	20	1	n/a
Cold cut combo	1	260	16	3.5	1310	9	3	5	20	n/a	10	1	n/a
Italian B.M.T.	1	410	29	11.0	1670	13	3	5	25	n/a	60	3	n/a
Meatball marinara	1	520	32	13.0	1520	33	8	14	28	n/a	150	3	n/a
Oven roasted chicken	1	200	6	2.0	660	11	3	6	27	n/a	40	1	n/a
Oven roasted turkey	1	160	3	0.0	960	11	3	4	25	n/a	40	5	n/a
Spicy Italian	1	550	45	17.0	1910	12	3	4	24	n/a	80	1	n/a
Steak & cheese	1	380	19	9.0	1150	12	4	5	42	n/a	200	9	n/a
Sweet onion chicken teriyaki	1	300	5	1.5	1020	33	3	22	34	n/a	60	1	n/a
Tuna	1	550	47	8.0	660	8	3	4	26	n/a	40	1	n/a
Sandwiches													
Black Forest ham	6 in	270	4	1.0	810	41	4	6	18	n/a	20	3	n/a
Buffalo chicken	6 in	330	11	2.5	1400	39	2	4	24	n/a	0	8	n/a

* Subs, salads, and sandwiches do not include cheese, mayonnaise, oil, or sauce unless indicated.

RESTAURANT & FAST FOOD CHAINS

	Amount	Calories	Fat (g)	Saturated Fat (g)	Sodium (mg)	Carbohydrate (g)	Fiber (g)	Sugar (g)	Protein (g)	Vitamin D (mcg)	Calcium (mg)	Iron (mg)	Potassium (mg)
Subway													
Chicken & bacon ranch	6 in	500	25	10.0	1130	39	2	5	36	n/a	150	8	n/a
Cold cut combo	6 in	280	10	2.5	980	38	1	4	17	n/a	40	8	n/a
Italian B.M.T.	6 in	360	16	6.0	1160	39	2	4	19	n/a	20	8	n/a
Meatball marinara	6 in	400	17	7.0	1080	46	3	6	20	n/a	60	8	n/a
Oven roasted chicken	6 in	280	5	1.0	620	41	4	6	21	n/a	20	2	n/a
Oven roasted turkey	6 in	270	3	0	760	41	4	5	20	n/a	20	3	n/a
Spicy italian	6 in	420	24	9.0	1280	39	2	4	18	n/a	40	8	n/a
Steak & cheese	6 in	320	10	4.5	1020	37	1	3	25	n/a	40	10	n/a
Sweet onion chicken teriyaki	6 in	330	4	1.0	790	52	4	14	24	n/a	40	2	n/a
Tuna	6 in	430	25	4.5	650	37	1	4	19	n/a	0	8	n/a
Veggie delite	6 in	200	2	0.0	320	39	4	5	8	n/a	20	1	n/a
Individual Components													
Bread													
artisan flatbread	6 in	230	4	0.5	330	43	4	3	8	n/a	0	2	n/a
artisan Italian	6 in	160	2	0.5	350	34	0	2	7	n/a	0	7	n/a
hearty multigrain	6 in	190	2	0	310	36	3	3	7	n/a	0	1	n/a
Italian herbs & cheese	6 in	200	4	2.0	550	36	1	2	9	n/a	0	8	n/a
spinach wrap	6 in	290	8	3.5	780	48	2	1	8	n/a	100	2	n/a
tomato basil wrap	6 in	290	8	0.5	730	49	2	1	8	n/a	80	2	n/a
Cheese													
American	1 order	40	4	2.0	210	1	0	0	2	n/a	40	0	n/a
Monterey cheddar	1 order	50	5	3.0	90	0	0	0	3	n/a	80	0	n/a
pepper Jack	1 order	40	4	2.0	180	1	0	0	2	n/a	0	0	n/a
provolone	1 order	50	4	2.0	125	0	0	0	4	n/a	80	0	n/a
Swiss	1 order	50	5	2.5	30	0	0	0	4	n/a	100	0	n/a
Veggies													
banana peppers	1 order	0	0	0.0	65	0	0	0	0	n/a	0	0	n/a
black olives	1 order	0	0	0.0	25	0	0	0	0	n/a	0	0	n/a
cucumbers	1 order	0	0	0.0	0	1	0	0	0	n/a	0	0	n/a
green peppers	1 order	0	0	0.0	0	0	0	0	0	n/a	0	0	n/a
jalapeños	1 order	0	0	0.0	70	0	0	0	0	n/a	0	0	n/a
lettuce	1 order	0	0	0.0	0	0	0	0	0	n/a	0	0	n/a
pickles	1 order	0	0	0.0	115	0	0	0	0	n/a	0	0	n/a
red onions	1 order	0	0	0.0	0	1	0	0	0	n/a	0	0	n/a
spinach	1 order	0	0	0.0	5	0	0	0	0	n/a	0	0	n/a
tomatoes	1 order	5	0	0.0	0	1	0	1	0	n/a	0	0	n/a
Extras													
bacon	1 order	80	7	2.5	180	1	0	1	5	n/a	0	1	n/a
guacamole	1 order	70	6	1.0	105	3	2	0	1	n/a	0	0	n/a
pepperoni	1 order	80	7	2.5	290	1	0	0	3	n/a	0	0	n/a
Sauces													
Caesar	1 order	80	9	1.5	130	0	0	0	0	n/a	0	0	n/a

RESTAURANT & FAST FOOD CHAINS

Subway

	Amount	Calories	Fat (g)	Saturated Fat (g)	Sodium (mg)	Carbohydrate (g)	Fiber (g)	Sugar (g)	Protein (g)	Vitamin D (mcg)	Calcium (mg)	Iron (mg)	Potassium (mg)
chipotle southwest	1 order	60	7	1.0	110	1	0	1	0	n/a	0	0	n/a
honey mustard	1 order	20	0	0.0	80	4	0	4	0	n/a	0	0	n/a
mayonnaise	1 order	100	11	2.0	65	0	0	0	0	n/a	0	0	n/a
light	1 order	50	5	1.0	100	1	0	0	0	n/a	0	0	n/a
oil	1 order	45	5	1.0	0	0	0	0	0	n/a	0	0	n/a
ranch	1 order	70	8	1.5	140	1	0	1	0	n/a	0	0	n/a
red wine vinegar	1 order	0	0	0.0	0	0	0	0	0	n/a	0	0	n/a
Subway vinaigrette	1 order	35	4	0.5	110	1	0	1	0	n/a	0	0	n/a
sweet onion sauce	1 order	30	0	0.0	75	8	0	7	0	n/a	0	0	n/a
yellow mustard	1 order	10	1	0.0	170	1	0	0	0	n/a	0	0	n/a

Wraps

	Amount	Calories	Fat (g)	Saturated Fat (g)	Sodium (mg)	Carbohydrate (g)	Fiber (g)	Sugar (g)	Protein (g)	Vitamin D (mcg)	Calcium (mg)	Iron (mg)	Potassium (mg)
Black Forest ham	1	440	12	4.5	1720	57	4	5	29	n/a	100	6	n/a
Cold cut combo	1	530	24	7.0	1970	54	3	4	27	n/a	150	3	n/a
Italian B.M.T.	1	680	36	14.0	2330	57	4	4	32	n/a	100	5	n/a
Meatball marinara	1	770	39	16.0	2160	75	8	10	34	n/a	200	5	n/a
Oven roasted chicken	1	470	13	5.0	1390	55	4	5	35	n/a	100	3	n/a
Oven roasted turkey	1	440	10	3.5	1690	56	3	3	33	n/a	100	7	n/a
Spicy Italian	1	810	52	20.0	2580	57	4	3	31	n/a	150	4	n/a
Sweet onion chicken teriyaki	1	540	12	4.5	1670	70	4	14	42	n/a	100	3	n/a
Tuna	1	820	54	11.0	1380	52	3	3	33	n/a	100	4	n/a
Veggie delite	1	330	8	3.5	750	56	5	5	10	n/a	100	3	n/a

Salads

	Amount	Calories	Fat (g)	Saturated Fat (g)	Sodium (mg)	Carbohydrate (g)	Fiber (g)	Sugar (g)	Protein (g)	Vitamin D (mcg)	Calcium (mg)	Iron (mg)	Potassium (mg)
Black Forest ham	1	120	3	1.0	570	12	4	6	13	n/a	40	3	n/a
Buffalo chicken	1	220	11	2.0	1120	12	4	6	20	n/a	60	1	n/a
Chicken & bacon ranch	1	460	33	11.0	1000	13	4	7	32	n/a	200	2	n/a
Cold cut combo	1	160	9	2.0	700	10	4	5	12	n/a	80	2	n/a
Italian B.M.T.	1	240	15	5.0	880	12	4	5	14	n/a	60	3	n/a
Meatball marinara	1	290	17	7.0	800	22	7	9	16	n/a	100	3	n/a
Oven roasted chicken	1	130	4	1.0	370	11	4	6	16	n/a	60	1	n/a
Oven roasted turkey	1	110	2	0.0	520	11	4	5	14	n/a	40	3	n/a
Spicy Italian	1	300	23	8.0	1000	12	4	5	14	n/a	60	2	n/a
Steak & cheese	1	210	9	4.0	740	12	4	6	21	n/a	80	5	n/a
Sweet onion chicken teriyaki	1	210	3	1.0	630	30	4	20	19	n/a	60	2	n/a
Tuna	1	310	24	4.0	370	10	4	5	15	n/a	40	2	n/a
Veggie delite	1	50	1	0.0	75	9	4	5	3	n/a	40	1	n/a

Taco Bell

Breakfast

	Amount	Calories	Fat (g)	Saturated Fat (g)	Sodium (mg)	Carbohydrate (g)	Fiber (g)	Sugar (g)	Protein (g)	Vitamin D (mcg)	Calcium (mg)	Iron (mg)	Potassium (mg)
Breakfast Crunchwrap													
bacon	1	670	41	12.0	1270	50	4	3	21	n/a	300	3	n/a
sausage	1	720	47	15.0	1210	51	4	3	21	n/a	350	3	n/a
steak	1	660	38	12.0	1300	51	4	3	24	n/a	350	3	n/a

RESTAURANT & FAST FOOD CHAINS

	Amount	Calories	Fat (g)	Saturated Fat (g)	Sodium (mg)	Carbohydrate (g)	Fiber (g)	Sugar (g)	Protein (g)	Vitamin D (mcg)	Calcium (mg)	Iron (mg)	Potassium (mg)
Cheesy toasted breakfast burrito													
bacon	1	350	16	4.5	870	36	2	3	13	n/a	100	2	n/a
fiesta potato	1	340	14	3.5	750	43	3	3	10	n/a	150	3	n/a
sausage	1	340	17	5.0	730	36	2	3	11	n/a	100	3	n/a
Grande toasted breakfast burrito													
bacon	1	560	30	10.0	1290	49	4	3	24	n/a	300	3	n/a
sausage	1	560	31	10.0	1150	49	4	3	22	n/a	300	3	n/a
steak	1	560	28	9.0	1310	50	4	3	27	n/a	350	3	n/a
Hash brown	1	160	12	1.0	270	13	2	0	1	n/a	0	0	n/a
Hash brown toasted breakfast burrito													
bacon	1	570	33	10.0	1270	49	4	2	21	n/a	300	3	n/a
sausage	1	570	34	10.0	1130	49	4	2	18	n/a	300	3	n/a
steak	1	570	30	9.0	1290	50	4	2	24	n/a	300	3	n/a
Burritos													
Bean	1	350	9	3.5	1000	54	11	3	13	n/a	200	3	n/a
Beef	1	430	19	5.0	970	51	4	3	12	n/a	100	3	n/a
Beefy 5-Layer	1	490	18	7.0	1250	63	9	5	18	n/a	250	3	n/a
Black Bean Crunchwrap Supreme	1	510	17	4.5	1080	77	8	6	13	n/a	250	4	n/a
Burrito Supreme													
beef	1	390	14	6.0	1110	51	9	4	16	n/a	200	3	n/a
chicken	1	370	11	4.5	1110	49	8	4	19	n/a	200	3	n/a
steak	1	370	12	5.0	1090	49	7	4	18	n/a	200	3	n/a
Cheesy bean & rice	1	420	16	4.0	880	56	7	3	10	n/a	150	3	n/a
Cheesy roll up	1	180	9	5.0	430	15	2	0	9	n/a	200	1	n/a
Chicken chipotle melt	1	190	9	3.0	530	15	1	0	12	n/a	100	1	n/a
Quesaritos													
beef	1	650	33	12.0	1390	67	6	5	22	n/a	350	3	n/a
black bean	1	630	29	10.0	1260	73	7	5	19	n/a	400	3	n/a
chicken	1	620	29	11.0	1390	66	4	4	25	n/a	350	3	n/a
steak	1	630	30	11.0	1370	66	4	4	24	n/a	400	3	n/a
Nachos													
Chips & nacho cheese sauce	1 order	220	13	1.5	250	24	2	2	2	n/a	40	0	n/a
Grande nachos box	1	1120	61	13.0	1620	116	21	6	26	n/a	200	3	n/a
Nachos BellGrande													
beef	1 order	740	38	7.0	1050	82	15	5	16	n/a	100	3	n/a
chicken	1 order	720	35	6.0	1050	81	14	5	20	n/a	100	2	n/a
steak	1 order	720	36	6.0	1030	81	14	5	19	n/a	150	2	n/a
Power Menu Bowls													
Chicken	1	470	19	6.0	1200	50	7	2	26	n/a	150	1	n/a
Steak	1	480	20	7.0	1150	51	7	2	25	n/a	200	2	n/a
Veggie	1	430	17	5.0	810	57	10	2	12	n/a	200	1	n/a

Taco Bell

	Amount	Calories	Fat (g)	Saturated Fat (g)	Sodium (mg)	Carbohydrate (g)	Fiber (g)	Sugar (g)	Protein (g)	Vitamin D (mcg)	Calcium (mg)	Iron (mg)	Potassium
Quesadillas													
Black Bean Quesarito	1	630	29	10.0	1260	73	7	5	19	n/a	400	3	n/a
Cheese	1	470	25	12.0	990	37	4	2	19	n/a	450	2	n/a
Chicken	1	510	26	12.0	1250	38	4	2	27	n/a	450	2	n/a
Steak	1	520	27	12.0	1230	38	4	2	27	n/a	500	3	n/a
Tacos													
Chalupas													
black bean	1	330	15	3.0	430	39	5	3	10	n/a	150	2	n/a
Supreme beef	1	350	18	5.0	560	33	4	3	13	n/a	100	2	n/a
Supreme chicken	1	330	15	3.5	560	31	2	3	16	n/a	100	1	n/a
Supreme steak	1	330	16	4.0	530	32	2	3	15	n/a	150	2	n/a
Cheesy gordita crunch	1	500	28	10.0	850	41	5	4	20	n/a	300	2	n/a
Crunchy taco	1	170	9	3.5	310	13	3	0	8	n/a	50	1	n/a
Supreme	1	190	11	4.5	340	15	3	2	8	n/a	80	1	n/a
Nacho Cheese Doritos Locos	1	170	9	3.5	360	13	3	0	8	n/a	60	1	n/a
Supreme	1	190	11	4.5	380	15	3	2	8	n/a	80	1	n/a
Naked chicken chalupa	1	470	30	6.0	1300	31	6	0	21	n/a	60	1	n/a
Soft tacos													
beef	1	180	9	4.0	500	17	3	1	9	n/a	100	1	n/a
chicken	1	160	5	2.5	500	16	1	1	12	n/a	100	1	n/a
spicy potato	1	230	12	3.0	460	27	2	1	5	n/a	100	1	n/a
Supreme beef	1	210	10	5.0	520	20	3	2	10	n/a	100	1	n/a
Supreme chicken	1	180	7	3.5	520	18	2	2	13	n/a	100	1	n/a
Sides & Desserts													
Black beans	1 order	50	1	0.0	135	8	3	0	2	n/a	40	1	n/a
w/ rice	1 order	170	4	0.0	320	31	4	0	4	n/a	40	1	n/a
Cheesy fiesta potatoes	1 order	230	12	2.0	520	28	2	2	3	n/a	40	1	n/a
Cinnabon delights	2 pcs	160	9	2.0	80	17	0	10	2	n/a	20	1	n/a
Cinnamon twists	1 order	170	6	0.0	210	27	0	13	1	n/a	0	0	n/a
Drinks													
Baja Colada	16 oz	210	1	0.5	50	52	0	50	0	n/a	0	0	n/a
Blue raspberry freeze	16 oz	120	0	0.0	35	30	0	30	0	n/a	0	0	n/a
Mountain Dew Baja Blast freeze	16 oz	150	0	0.0	45	41	0	41	0	n/a	0	0	n/a
Wild strawberry freeze	16 oz	150	0	0.0	40	41	0	41	0	n/a	0	0	n/a

Tim Hortons

	Amount	Calories	Fat (g)	Saturated Fat (g)	Sodium (mg)	Carbohydrate (g)	Fiber (g)	Sugar (g)	Protein (g)	Vitamin D (mcg)	Calcium (mg)	Iron (mg)	Potassium
Breakfast													
Oatmeal, maple	1 order	220	3	0.5	220	49	4	20	5	n/a	40	1	n/a
Oatmeal, mixed berry	1 order	210	3	0.5	220	44	6	14	6	n/a	40	1	n/a
Hash brown	1	130	7	0.5	280	16	1	0	1	n/a	20	0	n/a
Strawberry Greek yogurt	1	250	5	0.0	110	29	3	21	14	n/a	150	5	n/a
Vanilla Greek yogurt	1	250	5	0.0	110	29	3	21	14	n/a	150	5	n/a

RESTAURANT & FAST FOOD CHAINS

	Amount	Calories	Fat (g)	Saturated Fat (g)	Sodium (mg)	Carbohydrate (g)	Fiber (g)	Sugar (g)	Protein (g)	Vitamin D (mcg)	Calcium (mg)	Iron (mg)	Potassium (mg)
Bagels													
4 cheese	1	320	5	2.0	580	57	2	3	12	n/a	100	3	n/a
12 grain	1	350	9	1.0	450	55	6	8	11	n/a	80	3	n/a
Blueberry	1	300	3	0.0	450	59	3	8	11	n/a	40	3	n/a
Caramel apple	1	340	4	1.0	520	67	3	16	9	n/a	60	3	n/a
Cinnamon raisin	1	300	2	0.0	390	61	2	10	9	n/a	60	3	n/a
Everything	1	300	3	0.5	450	58	3	6	11	n/a	60	3	n/a
Jalapeño Asiago mozzarella	1	310	4	1.5	730	58	3	2	12	n/a	150	3	n/a
Maple cinnamon French toast	1	350	4	1.5	540	67	2	15	10	n/a	80	3	n/a
Plain	1	300	3	0.0	490	59	3	6	10	n/a	60	3	n/a
Pretzel-style	1	300	3	0.0	850	60	2	4	11	n/a	60	3	n/a
Sundried tomato Asiago parm	1	320	5	2.0	860	59	3	4	12	n/a	150	3	n/a
Bakery													
Cinnamon rolls													
frosted	1	400	14	6.0	380	60	2	24	7	n/a	40	2	n/a
glazed	1	350	13	5.0	350	51	2	16	7	n/a	40	2	n/a
Croissants	1	280	15	6.0	280	30	1	3	6	n/a	20	1	n/a
cheese	1	310	17	8.0	330	30	1	3	7	n/a	80	1	n/a
Danishes													
cherry cheese	1	370	16	6.0	310	50	1	24	5	n/a	40	1	n/a
maple pecan	1	400	19	6.0	270	53	2	21	7	n/a	20	1	n/a
Nutella pastry pocket	1	150	9	4.0	105	16	1	8	2	n/a	20	0	n/a
Ultimate cinnamon bun	1	570	21	10.0	670	89	3	50	8	n/a	150	3	n/a
Donuts													
Apple fritter	1	290	8	3.5	330	38	2	15	7	n/a	40	2	n/a
caramel	1	300	8	3.5	390	52	2	17	7	n/a	40	2	n/a
Blooms													
blueberry	1	240	9	4.5	180	37	1	15	3	n/a	20	1	n/a
strawberry	1	350	7	3.5	190	66	1	44	4	n/a	20	1	n/a
Boston cream	1	220	6	2.5	250	35	1	13	5	n/a	20	1	n/a
Cake													
blueberry	1	370	19	9.0	180	46	1	31	3	n/a	20	1	n/a
chocolate glazed	1	280	14	6.0	320	37	1	19	4	n/a	20	1	n/a
cinnamon sugar	1	220	10	5.0	270	28	1	10	3	n/a	40	1	n/a
double chocolate	1	270	15	6.0	330	32	2	13	4	n/a	20	1	n/a
old fashion	1	210	10	5.0	260	25	1	8	3	n/a	40	1	n/a
dip	1	250	11	5.0	270	33	1	15	4	n/a	20	1	n/a
glazed	1	270	10	5.0	270	41	1	23	3	n/a	40	1	n/a
peanut crunch	1	300	14	5.0	270	39	1	20	5	n/a	40	1	n/a
sour cream	1	270	16	8.0	210	27	1	11	3	n/a	40	1	n/a
cinnamon	1	270	16	8.0	210	29	1	12	3	n/a	40	1	n/a
glazed	1	340	15	8.0	220	46	1	29	3	n/a	40	1	n/a

Tim Hortons	Amount	Calories	Fat (g)	Saturated Fat (g)	Sodium (mg)	Carbohydrate (g)	Fiber (g)	Sugar (g)	Protein (g)	Vitamin D (mcg)	Calcium (mg)	Iron (mg)	Potassium
strawberry double chocolate	1	280	15	6.0	330	33	2	14	4	n/a	20	2	n/a
Canadian maple	1	210	6	2.5	250	35	1	14	5	n/a	20	1	n/a
Chocolate caramel	1	280	9	4.0	330	47	1	23	5	n/a	20	1	n/a
Filled													
blueberry	1	200	5	2.0	230	34	1	12	4	n/a	20	1	n/a
Nutella	1	290	14	4.5	180	34	2	14	6	n/a	40	1	n/a
strawberry	1	200	5	2.0	230	34	1	14	5	n/a	20	1	n/a
Honey cruller	1	310	18	9.0	200	37	0	22	2	n/a	20	0	n/a
Oreo	1	420	18	7.0	270	60	1	33	5	n/a	20	1	n/a
Strawberry cream	1	290	10	4.0	230	45	1	25	4	n/a	20	1	n/a
Yeast													
dip													
chocolate	1	190	7	2.5	210	29	1	8	5	n/a	20	1	n/a
honey	1	190	6	2.5	210	31	1	11	4	n/a	20	1	n/a
maple	1	190	6	2.5	210	29	1	9	4	n/a	20	1	n/a
strawberry	1	210	6	2.5	210	35	1	14	4	n/a	20	1	n/a
vanilla w/ colored sprinkles	1	270	9	3.5	220	45	1	22	4	n/a	20	1	n/a
sugar loop	1	180	6	2.5	210	28	1	8	4	n/a	20	1	n/a
Timbits													
Apple fritter	1	50	2	1.0	40	9	0	4	1	n/a	0	0	n/a
Cake													
birthday	1	80	3	1.5	60	12	0	8	1	n/a	0	0	n/a
blueberry	1	90	5	2.5	45	11	0	7	1	n/a	0	0	n/a
chocolate glazed	1	70	3	1.5	85	10	0	5	1	n/a	0	0	n/a
cinnamon French toast	1	70	4	1.5	65	8	0	3	1	n/a	20	0	n/a
cinnamon sugar	1	60	3	1.0	75	8	1	3	1	n/a	0	0	n/a
double chocolate	1	70	3	1.5	85	9	0	4	1	n/a	0	0	n/a
old fashion	1	50	3	1.0	75	7	0	2	1	n/a	0	0	n/a
glazed	1	70	3	1.0	75	10	0	5	1	n/a	0	0	n/a
salted caramel	1	70	3	1.5	120	11	0	6	1	n/a	0	0	n/a
sour cream glazed	1	90	5	2.0	55	12	0	7	1	n/a	0	0	n/a
Strawberry filled	1	50	1	0.5	35	8	0	4	1	n/a	0	0	n/a
Honey dip yeast	1	45	1	0.5	30	8	0	4	1	n/a	0	0	n/a
Muffins													
Chocolate caramel	1	410	15	4.0	480	64	2	35	5	n/a	40	2	n/a
Chocolate chip	1	420	16	4.5	330	66	2	35	6	n/a	40	3	n/a
Cran apple walnut bran	1	350	14	2.0	370	54	8	20	5	n/a	40	2	n/a
Cranberry white chocolate	1	370	12	2.5	370	60	2	30	5	n/a	60	1	n/a
Fruit explosion	1	340	10	1.5	470	58	2	25	5	n/a	60	1	n/a
Lemon blueberry Greek yogurt	1	360	12	2.0	400	58	5	24	6	n/a	60	2	n/a
Whole grain carrot orange	1	350	11	1.5	360	59	6	26	5	n/a	60	2	n/a
Whole grain pecan banana	1	350	11	1.5	400	60	5	27	6	n/a	40	2	n/a
Wild blueberry	1	340	11	2.0	430	57	2	25	5	n/a	20	1	n/a

RESTAURANT & FAST FOOD CHAINS

Tim Hortons

	Amount	Calories	Fat (g)	Saturated Fat (g)	Sodium (mg)	Carbohydrate (g)	Fiber (g)	Sugar (g)	Protein (g)	Vitamin D (mcg)	Calcium (mg)	Iron (mg)	Potassium (mg)
Sandwiches													
Aged cheddar biscuit	1	540	37	19.0	1220	30	1	4	20	n/a	200	2	n/a
Angus steak & egg	1	400	20	12.0	1200	34	2	5	21	n/a	150	3	n/a
Bacon	1	420	23	13.0	1110	33	2	4	19	n/a	150	3	n/a
Bagel B.E.L.T.	1	560	24	8.0	1140	62	7	11	24	n/a	200	3	n/a
Croissant	1	600	42	19.0	1040	36	2	6	19	n/a	150	2	n/a
Sausage	1	530	34	17.0	1180	33	2	4	19	n/a	150	3	n/a
Steak & four cheese bagel	1	510	17	7.0	1360	62	2	5	27	n/a	250	4	n/a
Turkey sausage	1	350	16	6.0	960	31	1	3	20	n/a	200	2	n/a
Grilled Wraps													
Chicken fajita	1	430	19	8.0	1060	39	3	4	28	n/a	350	2	n/a
Farmer's breakfast	1	680	42	12.0	1150	54	3	3	21	n/a	250	3	n/a
Steak fajita	1	430	20	8.0	1140	40	3	4	26	n/a	350	3	n/a
Steak & cheddar breakfast	1	440	21	8.0	1130	40	2	4	22	n/a	300	3	n/a
Soups & Sides													
Soups													
broccoli cheddar	1 order	180	9	4.0	680	16	2	6	8	n/a	200	0	n/a
chicken noodle	1 order	120	2	0.0	710	21	1	2	5	n/a	20	0	n/a
clam chowder	1 order	190	7	2.0	680	23	1	6	9	n/a	150	1	n/a
hearty vegetable	1 order	80	0	0.0	590	14	2	3	4	n/a	40	0	n/a
potato bacon cheddar	1 order	260	15	8.0	820	22	1	5	7	n/a	150	0	n/a
roasted red pepper & Gouda	1 order	220	14	6.0	680	17	3	11	6	n/a	100	0	n/a
turkey & wild rice	1 order	130	2	0.0	660	25	1	1	3	n/a	20	0	n/a
Chili	1 order	330	18	7.0	960	18	5	5	23	n/a	100	2	n/a
Homestyle soft bun													
white	1	210	1	0.0	450	42	2	1	7	n/a	0	3	n/a
whole wheat	1	200	1	0.0	430	40	4	1	8	n/a	0	2	n/a
Macaroni & cheese	1 order	490	27	10.0	1120	48	1	7	16	n/a	300	1	n/a
Drinks													
Apple cider	medium	250	0	0.0	10	66	0	66	0	n/a	0	0	n/a
caramel supreme	medium	350	5	5.0	30	75	0	45	0	n/a	20	0	n/a
Brewed iced tea													
sweetened	medium	130	0	0.0	20	34	0	33	0	n/a	0	0	n/a
unsweetened	medium	0	0	0.0	20	0	0	0	0	n/a	0	0	n/a
Café mocha	medium	240	9	8.0	240	38	2	32	2	n/a	20	1	n/a
Cappuccino	medium	100	0	0.0	150	15	0	14	9	n/a	350	0	n/a
Coffee	medium	5	0	0.0	10	0	0	0	0	n/a	0	0	n/a
iced	medium	110	7	4.5	30	11	0	9	1	n/a	40	0	n/a
Frozen hot chocolate	medium	570	27	18.0	360	80	2	71	4	n/a	100	1	n/a
Frozen lemonade	medium	190	0	0.0	20	46	0	43	0	n/a	0	0	n/a
strawberry	medium	190	0	0.0	20	47	0	43	0	n/a	0	0	n/a
Frozen strawberries & cream	medium	530	27	18.0	130	70	0	62	4	n/a	150	0	n/a

	Amount	Calories	Fat (g)	Saturated Fat (g)	Sodium (mg)	Carbohydrate (g)	Fiber (g)	Sugar (g)	Protein (g)	Vitamin D (mcg)	Calcium (mg)	Iron (mg)	Potassium
Tim Hortons													
Frozen sugar cookie & cream	medium	540	28	19.0	135	71	0	63	4	n/a	150	0	n/a
Frozen vanilla & cream	medium	530	27	18.0	135	70	0	64	4	n/a	150	0	n/a
Fruit smoothies													
pineapple orange	medium	260	0	0.0	75	56	0	55	8	n/a	80	0	n/a
strawberry banana	medium	230	0	0.0	65	52	1	47	8	n/a	100	0	n/a
Hot chocolate	medium	300	7	6.0	460	57	3	49	2	n/a	20	2	n/a
caramel	medium	400	13	11.0	430	68	3	57	3	n/a	20	3	n/a
Iced capp	medium	430	22	14.0	55	55	0	50	4	n/a	100	0	n/a
caramel	medium	500	28	19.0	70	60	0	53	4	n/a	100	0	n/a
mocha	medium	550	28	19.0	80	72	1	62	4	n/a	100	1	n/a
Oreo	medium	560	30	19.0	115	69	0	59	4	n/a	150	1	n/a
Latte	medium	100	0	0.0	160	15	0	15	10	n/a	350	0	n/a
iced	medium	240	7	4.0	170	35	0	34	12	n/a	450	0	n/a
Cookies													
Chocolate chunk	1	210	9	5.0	240	32	1	17	2	n/a	20	1	n/a
Double chocolate w/ peanut butter filling	1	360	20	11.0	290	40	2	23	5	n/a	20	2	n/a
Lemon shortbread w/ raspberry filling	1	280	10	7.0	250	44	1	21	3	n/a	0	1	n/a
Nutella filled	1	360	18	7.0	190	44	1	25	4	n/a	40	1	n/a
Oatmeal raisin spice	1	210	8	4.5	190	32	1	19	3	n/a	20	0	n/a
Peanut butter	1	250	15	6.0	240	24	2	14	5	n/a	20	0	n/a
Red velvet w/ cream cheese filling	1	300	13	9.0	250	42	1	23	3	n/a	20	1	n/a
Smile	1	300	12	7.0	370	47	1	27	3	n/a	20	1	n/a
White chocolate macadamia nut	1	220	11	5.0	240	29	1	15	2	n/a	20	0	n/a
Uno Pizzeria & Grill													
Appetizers													
Bites													
Buffalo boneless	1 order	1450	97	21.0	4460	67	2	4	75	n/a	n/a	n/a	n/a
honey BBQ boneless	1 order	850	94	19.0	3390	86	2	21	73	n/a	n/a	n/a	n/a
red chili glazed	1 order	1530	95	19.0	3800	98	2	31	73	n/a	n/a	n/a	n/a
Buffalo chicken quesadillas	1 order	860	30	15.0	2610	81	4	11	46	n/a	n/a	n/a	n/a
Cheesy garlic bread	1 order	1180	33	9.0	2330	126	6	10	52	n/a	n/a	n/a	n/a
Giant fried ravioli	1 order	680	37	16.0	1660	63	2	8	26	n/a	n/a	n/a	n/a
Grilled shrimp w/ orange cilantro dipping sauce	1 order	200	1	0.0	930	27	0	18	32	n/a	n/a	n/a	n/a
Muchos Nachos	1 order	1700	61	14.0	3930	199	1	13	66	n/a	n/a	n/a	n/a
Pizza Skins	1 order	1970	131	43.0	2800	146	7	8	53	n/a	n/a	n/a	n/a
Dips													
shrimp & crab	1 order	1160	84	40.0	2300	66	2	13	32	n/a	n/a	n/a	n/a
spinach artichoke deep	1 order	1710	114	28.0	3250	123	7	7	34	n/a	n/a	n/a	n/a
Wings													
Buffalo	1 order	1130	89	23.0	3890	6	2	4	71	n/a	n/a	n/a	n/a
honey BBQ	1 order	1170	86	21.0	2820	25	2	21	69	n/a	n/a	n/a	n/a

RESTAURANT & FAST FOOD CHAINS

Uno Pizzeria & Grill

	Amount	Calories	Fat (g)	Saturated Fat (g)	Sodium (mg)	Carbohydrate (g)	Fiber (g)	Sugar (g)	Protein (g)	Vitamin D (mcg)	Calcium (mg)	Iron (mg)	Potassium (mg)
Burgers													
Aged cheddar & mushroom	1	1120	81	31.0	1250	37	2	3	53	n/a	n/a	n/a	n/a
½ lb	1	1000	72	25.0	1070	35	2	2	46	n/a	n/a	n/a	n/a
gluten sensitive	1	1030	74	24.0	1160	46	6	7	45	n/a	n/a	n/a	n/a
½ lb cheddar	1	1110	81	30.0	1250	35	2	2	53	n/a	n/a	n/a	n/a
gluten sensitive	1	1140	83	29.0	1340	46	6	7	52	n/a	n/a	n/a	n/a
Bacon cheddar	1	1350	99	36.0	2070	35	2	2	71	n/a	n/a	n/a	n/a
gluten sensitive	1	1380	101	35.0	2160	46	6	7	70	n/a	n/a	n/a	n/a
Classic Beyond Burger	1	560	32	10.0	920	42	4	3	26	n/a	n/a	n/a	n/a
Pasta													
Chicken Spinoccoli	1 order	1260	62	29.0	2850	105	7	13	77	n/a	n/a	n/a	n/a
Chicken & broccoli Alfredo	1 order	1450	73	26.0	2150	132	7	13	68	n/a	n/a	n/a	n/a
Deep dish ravioli lasagna	1 order	1190	65	25.0	3240	3	7	14	60	n/a	n/a	n/a	n/a
Macaroni & cheese	1 order	1740	103	52.0	2640	140	6	14	70	n/a	n/a	n/a	n/a
Buffalo	1 order	2200	133	58.0	4310	160	6	14	96	n/a	n/a	n/a	n/a
Romano-crusted chicken parm	1 order	1260	39	7.0	2390	125	7	15	82	n/a	n/a	n/a	n/a
Rattlesnake Pasta	1 order	1410	70	25.0	2120	126	6	10	67	n/a	n/a	n/a	n/a
Shrimp scampi	1 order	1190	54	18.0	1540	128	6	10	44	n/a	n/a	n/a	n/a
Pizza, Deep Dish*													
Cheese & tomato	1 slice	410	20	3.0	650	27	1	1	13	n/a	n/a	n/a	n/a
Chicago classic	1 slice	540	38	12.0	1070	28	1	2	22	n/a	n/a	n/a	n/a
Chicago meat market	1 slice	570	35	9.0	1240	30	1	3	22	n/a	n/a	n/a	n/a
Farmer's market	1 slice	400	22	4.0	510	31	2	3	10	n/a	n/a	n/a	n/a
Four cheese & pesto	1 slice	476	28	7.0	691	28	0	3	16	n/a	n/a	n/a	n/a
Meatball & ricotta	1 slice	515	33	4.0	818	28	0	3	15	n/a	n/a	n/a	n/a
New York deli	1 slice	454	25	6.0	838	30	0	3	16	n/a	n/a	n/a	n/a
Numero Uno	1 slice	440	28	6.0	820	29	2	3	13	n/a	n/a	n/a	n/a
Prima pepperoni	1 slice	420	23	4.0	690	27	1	1	13	n/a	n/a	n/a	n/a
Pizza, Gluten Sensitive**													
Cheese	1 slice	160	6	3.0	200	23	1	2	6	n/a	n/a	n/a	n/a
Pepperoni	1 slice	200	9	4.0	350	23	1	2	8	n/a	n/a	n/a	n/a
Veggie	1 slice	160	6	3.0	200	24	1	3	7	n/a	n/a	n/a	n/a
Pizza, Thin Crust***													
BBQ chicken	1 slice	130	5	2.0	260	15	0	3	8	n/a	n/a	n/a	n/a
cauliflower crust	1 slice	100	5	2.5	240	8	1	3	7	n/a	n/a	n/a	n/a
Bianco Love	1 slice	149	6	2.0	206	14	0	1	6	n/a	n/a	n/a	n/a
Cheese Please!	1 slice	110	5	2.0	180	13	1	1	6	n/a	n/a	n/a	n/a
cauliflower crust	1 slice	80	5	2.5	170	6	1	1	5	n/a	n/a	n/a	n/a

* 8 slices per pie.
** 6 slices per pie.
*** 9 slices per pie.

RESTAURANT & FAST FOOD CHAINS

	Amount	Calories	Fat (g)	Saturated Fat (g)	Sodium (mg)	Carbohydrate (g)	Fiber (g)	Sugar (g)	Protein (g)	Vitamin D (mcg)	Calcium (mg)	Iron (mg)	Potas...
Margherita	1 slice	103	1	0.0	182	13	0	3	5	n/a	n/a	n/a	n/a
Nashville hot	1 slice	189	9	2.0	492	18	0	2	7	n/a	n/a	n/a	n/a
Spicy Hawaiian	1 slice	150	6	2.0	390	19	1	6	7	n/a	n/a	n/a	n/a
cauliflower crust	1 slice	120	6	2.5	380	12	1	6	6	n/a	n/a	n/a	n/a
Super Roni	1 slice	150	8	3.0	310	13	1	1	7	n/a	n/a	n/a	n/a
cauliflower crust	1 slice	120	8	3.5	300	6	1	1	7	n/a	n/a	n/a	n/a
Veggie extravaganza	1 slice	130	5	2.0	200	15	1	2	6	n/a	n/a	n/a	n/a
cauliflower crust	1 slice	100	6	2.5	190	7	1	1	6	n/a	n/a	n/a	n/a
Windy City Works	1 slice	150	7	3.0	270	14	1	1	8	n/a	n/a	n/a	n/a
cauliflower crust	1 slice	120	8	3.5	260	7	1	1	7	n/a	n/a	n/a	n/a
Sandwiches													
BBQ bacon chicken	1	910	43	15.0	2540	52	0	18	74	n/a	n/a	n/a	n/a
Caprese	1	450	18	8.0	770	52	0	3	21	n/a	n/a	n/a	n/a
Chicken parm	1	940	48	12.0	2740	60	0	5	65	n/a	n/a	n/a	n/a
Fish	1	670	35	5.0	1210	68	1	4	21	n/a	n/a	n/a	n/a
Steak, Seafood & Chicken													
Baked haddock	1 order	530	33	6.0	490	12	1	2	48	n/a	n/a	n/a	n/a
Chicken tender platter	1 order	1600	106	18.5	3510	88	7	0	72	n/a	n/a	n/a	n/a
Fish & chips	1 order	1350	93	14.0	2360	106	6	17	32	n/a	n/a	n/a	n/a
Grilled shrimp & sirloin	1 order	690	45	16.0	1400	1	0	0	66	n/a	n/a	n/a	n/a
Lemon basil salmon	1 order	490	38	6.0	700	0	0	0	40	n/a	n/a	n/a	n/a
Lemon herb chick skewers	1 order	440	28	4.5	1170	2	0	0	40	n/a	n/a	n/a	n/a
Mediterranean chicken	1 order	560	21	10.0	1940	43	1	5	49	n/a	n/a	n/a	n/a
Sirloin tips	1 order	470	20	5.0	500	4	1	2	62	n/a	n/a	n/a	n/a
Top sirloin steak	1 order	560	37	15.0	880	0	0	0	52	n/a	n/a	n/a	n/a
Salads													
Berry & goat cheese	1	340	21	5.0	240	34	3	25	7	n/a	n/a	n/a	n/a
Chicken Caesar	1	560	41	9.0	1280	17	5	5	33	n/a	n/a	n/a	n/a
gluten sensitive	1	440	32	7.0	1140	5	5	5	32	n/a	n/a	n/a	n/a
Chopped honey crisp chicken	1	1320	90	24.0	2000	67	5	18	53	n/a	n/a	n/a	n/a
House	1	270	13	6.0	510	30	4	6	14	n/a	n/a	n/a	n/a
Italian chopped	1	680	48	14.0	3130	29	5	13	32	n/a	n/a	n/a	n/a
Side salads													
berry & goat cheese	1	170	10	2.5	130	18	2	13	4	n/a	n/a	n/a	n/a
Caesar	1	220	19	4.5	330	9	3	2	5	n/a	n/a	n/a	n/a
gluten sensitive	1	160	15	3.5	260	5	2	2	4	n/a	n/a	n/a	n/a
house w/o dressing	1	90	5	1.0	95	10	2	3	2	n/a	n/a	n/a	n/a
gluten sensitive	1	25	0	0.0	20	6	2	3	1	n/a	n/a	n/a	n/a
wedge	1	230	19	5.0	550	10	3	5	7	n/a	n/a	n/a	n/a
Sides													
French fries	1 order	450	33	4.5	1550	35	7	0	5	n/a	n/a	n/a	n/a
Loaded mashed potato	1 order	420	26	12.0	850	37	3	4	13	n/a	n/a	n/a	n/a

RESTAURANT & FAST FOOD CHAINS

	Amount	Calories	Fat (g)	Saturated Fat (g)	Sodium (mg)	Carbohydrate (g)	Fiber (g)	Sugar (g)	Protein (g)	Vitamin D (mcg)	Calcium (mg)	Iron (mg)	Potassium (mg)
Uno Pizzeria & Grill													
Red bliss mashed potatoes	1 order	280	14	4.5	560	36	3	3	5	n/a	n/a	n/a	n/a
Roasted seasonal vegetables	1 order	70	4	0.0	105	8	2	5	2	n/a	n/a	n/a	n/a
Steamed broccoli	1 order	70	6	1.0	420	5	3	0	3	n/a	n/a	n/a	n/a
Sweet potato fries	1 order	430	25	3.5	740	47	7	19	2	n/a	n/a	n/a	n/a
Soups													
Broccoli & cheddar	1 order	310	21	10.0	1580	18	3	4	11	n/a	n/a	n/a	n/a
French onion	1 order	450	30	14.0	2070	25	2	6	19	n/a	n/a	n/a	n/a
Desserts													
Awesome chocolate cake	1 slice	1740	79	32.0	770	241	10	168	20	n/a	n/a	n/a	n/a
Brownies	1 order	520	23	7.0	310	77	3	42	5	n/a	n/a	n/a	n/a
Chocolate brownie sundae	1	1130	53	25.0	480	152	4	113	12	n/a	n/a	n/a	n/a
Chocolate chip cookies	1 order	550	27	13.0	310	78	3	46	7	n/a	n/a	n/a	n/a
Crazy-good caramel cake	1 slice	640	25	6.0	930	96	1	67	8	n/a	n/a	n/a	n/a
Deep dish sundae	1	1520	74	39.0	700	206	5	139	19	n/a	n/a	n/a	n/a
Gluten sensitive ice cream sundae	1	890	38	21.0	230	126	0	107	9	n/a	n/a	n/a	n/a
Ooey Gooey Dough Bites	1 order	1370	39	11.0	1080	230	4	107	23	n/a	n/a	n/a	n/a
Shooters													
brownie chocolate	1	230	16	9.0	150	23	1	19	2	n/a	n/a	n/a	n/a
strawberry	1	220	11	7.0	135	30	0	25	2	n/a	n/a	n/a	n/a
Wendy's													
Breakfast													
Bacon, egg & cheese													
biscuit	1	420	27	11.0	1240	28	1	3	16	n/a	130	3	220
classic sandwich	1	320	17	6.0	850	25	1	2	18	n/a	130	3	240
Bacon, egg & Swiss croissant	1	410	23	11.0	890	34	1	6	18	n/a	104	3	230
Breakfast Baconator	1	730	50	19.0	1750	37	1	7	34	n/a	260	4	520
Honey butter biscuit	1	310	19	7.0	670	32	1	8	3	n/a	52	2	55
Honey butter chicken biscuit	1	500	29	9.0	1260	44	2	9	14	n/a	52	3	290
Maple bacon chicken croissant	1	560	30	11.0	1200	51	1	13	22	n/a	52	3	380
Sausage biscuit	1	470	35	13.0	980	27	1	3	12	n/a	78	2	250
Sausage, egg & cheese													
biscuit	1	610	45	17.0	1370	29	1	3	20	n/a	195	3	350
burrito	1	340	20	7.0	920	25	1	2	15	n/a	195	3	180
classic sandwich	1	500	35	12.0	980	26	1	3	22	n/a	195	3	370
Sausage, egg & Swiss croissant	1	600	41	17.0	1030	34	1	7	22	n/a	130	3	360
Sausage gravy & biscuit	1	450	29	11.0	1390	41	1	3	7	n/a	52	2	290
Burgers													
Bacon Double Stack	1	450	26	11.0	820	26	1	6	26	n/a	130	4	350
Baconator	1	960	66	26.0	1540	36	1	7	57	n/a	260	7	750
Son of the Baconator	1	630	40	16.0	1210	36	1	7	32	n/a	195	4	430
Big Bacon Classic	1	650	41	16.0	1230	37	2	8	33	n/a	260	4	530

RESTAURANT & FAST FOOD CHAINS

Wendy's	Amount	Calories	Fat (g)	Saturated Fat (g)	Sodium (mg)	Carbohydrate (g)	Fiber (g)	Sugar (g)	Protein (g)	Vitamin D (mcg)	Calcium (mg)	Iron (mg)	Potassium
double	1	910	62	25.0	1400	37	2	8	53	n/a	260	7	780
triple	1	1220	86	36.0	1770	38	2	9	75	n/a	325	9	1050
Bourbon bacon cheeseburger	1	710	41	16.0	1400	51	2	15	34	n/a	260	5	470
double	1	970	62	25.0	1570	51	2	15	34	n/a	260	7	720
triple	1	1280	86	36.0	1940	52	2	16	75	n/a	325	9	990
Dave's	1	590	37	14.0	1030	37	2	8	29	n/a	260	5	460
double	1	860	57	23.0	1200	37	2	8	49	n/a	260	6	710
triple	1	1160	81	34.0	1570	38	2	8	70	n/a	325	9	980
Double stack	1	410	24	10.0	690	26	1	6	23	n/a	130	4	310
Jr. cheeseburger	1	290	14	6.0	610	26	1	6	15	n/a	130	3	200
Jr. cheeseburger deluxe	1	340	20	7.0	610	27	1	6	15	n/a	130	3	260
Jr. bacon cheeseburger	1	370	23	8.0	650	26	1	5	18	n/a	130	3	290
Jr. hamburger	1	250	11	4.0	420	25	1	5	13	n/a	52	3	170
Pretzel bacon pub cheeseburger	1	840	52	20.0	1310	53	3	6	40	n/a	325	5	300
double	1	1180	79	32.0	1630	53	3	6	64	n/a	520	8	780
triple	1	1520	106	45.0	1940	54	4	6	89	n/a	650	11	1050
Chicken													
Asiago ranch chicken club													
classic	1	630	31	8.0	1800	50	2	6	36	n/a	195	3	550
grilled	1	490	21	7.0	1190	34	1	6	40	n/a	195	3	580
spicy	1	630	30	8.0	1400	52	3	6	36	n/a	195	3	550
Chicken nuggets													
crispy	6 pcs	270	17	3.5	570	14	1	0	15	n/a	0	0	220
spicy	6 pcs	280	18	4.0	720	13	1	0	15	n/a	0	0	210
Chicken sandwich													
classic	1	490	21	3.5	1450	49	2	5	28	n/a	78	3	470
crispy	1	340	17	3.0	680	33	1	4	14	n/a	52	2	210
grilled	1	350	8	1.5	850	35	2	7	33	n/a	78	3	510
spicy	1	500	19	3.5	990	51	3	5	28	n/a	78	3	450
Crispy chicken BLT	1	420	23	6.0	1010	35	1	5	19	n/a	130	2	330
Jalapeño popper sandwich													
classic	1	600	28	10.0	2060	51	2	6	37	n/a	260	3	510
grilled	1	460	18	8.0	1450	35	1	6	41	n/a	195	3	540
spicy	1	600	26	9.0	1660	54	3	6	37	n/a	195	3	510
Pretzel bacon pub													
classic	1	830	43	13.0	2190	69	4	6	43	n/a	325	4	590
grilled	1	700	33	11.0	1580	53	3	6	47	n/a	325	4	620
spicy	1	840	42	13.0	1790	71	5	6	42	n/a	325	4	590
Salads													
Apple pecan	1	550	26	10.0	1280	42	5	33	39	n/a	390	3	860
Jalapeño popper	1	670	41	11.0	1590	39	5	6	37	n/a	377	3	890

RESTAURANT & FAST FOOD CHAINS

Wendy's

	Amount	Calories	Fat (g)	Saturated Fat (g)	Sodium (mg)	Carbohydrate (g)	Fiber (g)	Sugar (g)	Protein (g)	Vitamin D (mcg)	Calcium (mg)	Iron (mg)	Potassium (mg)
Parmesan Caesar	1	440	28	9.5	1110	7	3	3	42	n/a	572	2	730
Southwest avocado	1	560	39	11.5	1250	16	6	6	40	n/a	377	3	1160
Summer strawberry	1	450	23	8.0	1070	25	5	17	41	n/a	390	3	870
Taco	1	690	34	13.0	1870	68	12	16	30	n/a	520	5	1420
Sides													
Apple bites	1 order	35	0	0.0	0	8	1	6	0	n/a	52	0	65
Baked potato	1	270	0	0.0	40	61	7	3	7	n/a	78	3	1560
bacon cheese	1	440	13	6.0	610	64	7	4	17	n/a	195	4	1660
cheese	1	450	14	8.0	710	65	7	4	15	n/a	195	3	1600
chili & cheese	1	500	14	7.0	850	74	9	7	20	n/a	195	5	1860
sour cream & chive	1	310	3	1.5	55	63	7	4	8	n/a	104	3	1610
Chili	large	340	15	6.0	1270	31	8	8	22	n/a	104	5	790
Fries													
Baconator	1 order	470	27	9.0	810	43	4	1	14	n/a	130	1	790
cheese	1 order	450	27	10.0	880	40	3	1	11	n/a	195	1	670
chili cheese	1 order	530	28	10.0	1050	53	7	4	17	n/a	195	3	1000
French	medium	360	17	3.0	280	47	4	0	5	n/a	26	1	830
pub	1 order	480	28	10.0	860	44	4	1	14	n/a	260	1	810
Oatmeal bar	1	270	10	4.0	230	44	4	23	3	n/a	26	3	110
Seasoned potatoes	medium	330	14	2.5	900	46	4	1	4	n/a	0	1	660
Strawberries	1 order	20	0	0.0	0	5	1	3	0	n/a	0	0	105
Desserts													
Chocolate chunk cookie	1	330	16	8.0	210	43	2	26	3	n/a	0	3	95
Classic chocolate frosty	medium	470	12	8.0	210	79	0	65	13	n/a	585	2	840
Vanilla frosty	medium	450	12	8.0	210	75	0	63	12	n/a	585	0	730
Sugar cookie	1	330	16	8.0	300	44	1	24	3	n/a	0	1	35

SALADS

	Amount	Calories	Fat (g)	Saturated Fat (g)	Sodium (mg)	Carbohydrate (g)	Fiber (g)	Sugar (g)	Protein (g)	Vitamin D (mcg)	Calcium (mg)	Iron (mg)	Potassium (mg)
Caesar w/ dressing	1 cup	160	13	3.0	384	8	2	2	3	0	83	1	204
Carrot-raisin	½ cup	208	15	2.5	176	17	2	11	1	0	30	1	309
Chef													
w/ dressing	1 cup	312	23	7.5	924	9	2	5	17	1	150	2	566
w/o dressing	1 cup	178	11	5.5	496	3	2	4	17	1	28	1	306
Chicken w/ mayonnaise	½ cup	236	18	3.0	351	3	0	2	16	0	14	0	199
Coleslaw													
w/ mayonnaise	½ cup	98	7	1.0	178	9	1	8	1	0	35	0	165
w/ vinaigrette	½ cup	41	2	0.0	14	7	1	6	1	0	36	0	179
Cucumber													
creamy w/ mayonnaise	½ cup	59	4	3.0	13	5	1	2	1	0	35	0	124
w/ vinegar	½ cup	26	0	0.0	188	6	0	4	0	0	11	0	98
Egg w/ mayonnaise	½ cup	286	26	5.0	420	1	0	1	11	2	47	1	117
Fruit, fresh	½ cup	40	0	0.0	3	10	1	7	1	0	7	0	143
Gelatin w/ fruit	½ cup	73	0	0.0	30	18	1	9	1	0	10	2	125

SALADS

	Amount	Calories	Fat (g)	Saturated Fat (g)	Sodium (mg)	Carbohydrate (g)	Fiber (g)	Sugar (g)	Protein (g)	Vitamin D (mcg)	Calcium (mg)	Iron (mg)	Potassium (mg)
Ham	½ cup	273	20	6.0	1360	13	0	0	11	1	10	1	152
Lobster	½ cup	170	14	2.0	459	1	0	1	9	0	56	1	170
Macaroni w/ mayonnaise	½ cup	163	4	1.0	214	27	1	3	4	0	8	1	52
Pasta primavera	½ cup	152	4	1.0	311	26	2	2	4	0	45	1	184
Potato													
German-style	½ cup	95	3	1.0	158	15	2	1	3	0	15	1	390
w/ mayonnaise	½ cup	231	15	2.0	245	22	2	2	2	0	14	0	359
w/ eggs & mayonnaise	½ cup	216	13	2.0	453	22	2	7	3	0	21	1	333
Seafood													
w/ mayonnaise	½ cup	191	16	2.5	579	1	0	1	10	0	67	1	166
w/ pasta, vinaigrette	½ cup	126	7	1.0	524	11	1	1	5	1	5	1	132
Shrimp w/ mayonnaise	½ cup	204	10	1.5	299	21	0	2	7	0	28	1	53
Spinach w/o dressing	1 cup	60	4	1.0	146	2	1	0	5	0	61	2	342
Tabbouleh	1 cup	202	16	2.0	792	15	3	2	3	0	32	1	246
Taco													
w/ salsa	1 (16 oz)	170	9	3.0	363	15	3	1	7	0	95	2	229
w/ salsa & shell	1 (19 oz)	400	22	7.0	720	39	5	3	11	0	166	4	290
Three bean w/ oil	½ cup	81	4	0.5	200	10	3	3	3	0	20	1	158
Tortellini, cheese	½ cup	189	14	3.0	561	14	2	1	5	0	95	1	87
Tossed w/o dressing	1 cup	28	0	0.0	24	7	2	3	1	0	41	1	219
Tuna w/ mayonnaise	½ cup	233	19	3.0	493	3	0	2	12	1	24	1	184
Waldorf w/ dressing	½ cup	118	10	1.0	59	8	1	6	1	0	11	0	99

SALAD DRESSINGS*

	Amount	Calories	Fat (g)	Saturated Fat (g)	Sodium (mg)	Carbohydrate (g)	Fiber (g)	Sugar (g)	Protein (g)	Vitamin D (mcg)	Calcium (mg)	Iron (mg)	Potassium (mg)
Blue cheese	1 T	74	8	1.5	98	1	0	1	0	0	6	0	14
fat-free	1 T	18	0	0.0	135	4	0	1	0	0	8	0	32
light	1 T	15	1	0.5	144	0	0	0	1	0	14	0	1
Buttermilk	1 T	63	7	1.0	132	1	0	1	0	0	4	0	9
Caesar	1 T	80	9	1.5	178	0	0	0	0	0	7	0	4
fat-free	1 T	18	0	0.0	177	4	0	1	0	0	5	0	7
light	1 T	16	0	0.0	172	3	0	2	0	0	4	0	4
Catalina	1 T	65	6	1.0	103	3	0	3	0	0	4	0	17
fat-free	1 T	40	0	0.0	300	10	0	6	0	0	1	0	13
Chipotle ranch	1 T	150	15	2.5	190	3	0	2	0	0	26	0	51
Creamy parmesan	1 T	70	8	1.0	135	1	0	1	1	0	4	0	5
French	1 T	73	7	1.0	134	3	0	3	0	0	4	0	11
fat-free	1 T	132	0	0.0	853	32	0	16	0	0	5	1	84
light	1 T	222	12	0.0	838	31	0	17	1	0	11	1	107
Green Goddess	1 T	65	7	1.0	133	1	0	1	0	0	5	0	9
Honey mustard	1 T	72	6	1.0	80	4	0	2	0	0	2	0	3

* For mayonnaise/Miracle Whip, see Fats, Oils, Cream & Gravy.

SALAD DRESSINGS	Amount	Calories	Fat (g)	Saturated Fat (g)	Sodium (mg)	Carbohydrate (g)	Fiber (g)	Sugar (g)	Protein (g)	Vitamin D (mcg)	Calcium (mg)	Iron (mg)	Potassium (mg)
Italian	1 T	35	3	0.5	146	2	0	2	0	0	2	0	12
creamy	1 T	63	7	1.0	132	1	0	1	0	0	4	0	9
fat-free	1 T	7	0	0.0	158	1	0	1	0	0	4	0	14
light	1 T	14	1	0.0	125	1	0	1	0	0	2	0	13
Oil & vinegar	1 T	43	4	0.5	243	2	0	1	0	0	1	0	7
Peppercorn parmesan	1 T	60	6	1.0	135	1	0	1	1	0	2	0	9
Ranch	1 T	65	7	1.0	135	1	0	1	0	0	4	0	10
fat-free	1 T	17	0	0.0	126	4	0	1	0	0	7	0	16
light	1 T	30	3	1.0	155	2	0	1	0	0	7	0	14
Russian	1 T	54	4	0.5	173	5	0	3	0	0	2	0	27
light	1 T	23	1	0.0	139	4	0	4	0	0	3	0	25
Sesame seed	1 T	66	7	1.0	150	1	0	1	0	0	3	0	24
Thousand Island	1 T	60	5	1.0	150	2	0	2	0	0	3	0	17
fat-free	1 T	21	0	0.0	126	5	1	3	0	0	2	0	20
light	1 T	30	2	0.0	146	4	0	3	0	0	4	0	31
Vinaigrette													
balsamic	1 T	45	4	1.0	155	2	0	2	0	0	0	0	0
raspberry, light	1 T	30	1	0.0	240	5	0	5	0	0	0	0	0
red wine	1 T	60	5	0.5	210	6	0	5	0	0	0	0	0
fat-free	1 T	15	0	0.0	115	4	0	3	0	0	0	0	0
light	1 T	23	2	0.5	160	2	0	1	0	0	0	0	0
Western	1 T	170	12	2.0	250	13	0	12	0	0	4	0	10
fat-free	1 T	25	0	0.0	140	6	0	1	0	0	1	0	13

SOUPS

Canned & Prepared

Bean													
w/ bacon	1 cup	172	6	1.5	896	23	8	4	8	0	84	2	496
w/ franks	1 cup	280	8	2.0	960	38	8	14	12	0	80	2	560
Beef barley w/ veg	1 cup	127	2	1.0	725	19	2	3	7	0	27	1	295
Beef broth	1 cup	17	1	0.5	893	0	0	0	3	0	14	0	130
reduced sodium	1 cup	14	0	0.0	540	0	0	0	3	0	7	0	48
Beef consommé	1 cup	7	0	0.0	372	0	0	0	1	0	6	0	54
Beef noodle	1 cup	171	6	1.5	793	11	1	1	18	0	34	2	320
Black bean	1 cup	114	2	0.5	1200	19	8	8	6	0	47	2	309
Cheddar cheese	1 cup	166	7	4.5	926	20	3	11	5	1	201	0	241
Chicken alphabet	1 cup	140	3	0.5	960	24	2	2	6	0	0	0	1660
Chicken & dumplings	1 cup	99	3	1.5	737	11	2	1	7	0	27	1	282
Chicken & rice	1 cup	82	2	0.5	783	14	1	0	2	0	53	0	41
Chicken & stars	1 cup	140	2	0.5	790	10	0	0	3	0	10	0	60
Chicken broth	1 cup	14	1	0.0	890	1	0	1	2	0	10	0	43
reduced sodium	1 cup	17	0	0.0	554	1	0	1	3	0	19	1	204
Chicken gumbo	1 cup	56	1	0.5	954	8	2	2	3	0	24	1	76

SOUPS

	Amount	Calories	Fat (g)	Saturated Fat (g)	Sodium (mg)	Carbohydrate (g)	Fiber (g)	Sugar (g)	Protein (g)	Vitamin D (mcg)	Calcium (mg)	Iron (mg)	Potassium (mg)
Chicken noodle	1 cup	58	2	0.5	834	7	1	0	3	0	12	1	58
Chili beef w/ beans	1 cup	272	9	3.0	1140	33	8	5	15	0	84	3	671
Chunky, Campbell's													
chicken & dumplings	1 cup	170	9	2.0	890	14	6	1	7	0	30	1	150
chicken corn chowder	1 cup	190	9	2.0	890	20	2	3	6	0	30	1	290
chicken noodle	1 cup	120	3	1.0	790	14	1	2	8	0	20	1	510
grilled chicken & sausage gumbo	1 cup	140	3	1.5	850	21	2	3	6	0	40	1	240
hearty beef barley	1 cup	140	2	1.0	790	23	4	5	7	0	20	1	340
New England clam chowder	1 cup	180	10	1.5	790	16	2	1	6	0	30	1	210
savory chicken w/ rice	1 cup	120	2	0.0	790	20	1	1	6	0	30	1	250
savory vegetable	1 cup	90	1	0.0	770	19	3	5	3	0	50	1	430
sirloin burger w/ veg	1 cup	130	4	1.5	790	18	3	3	6	0	30	1	340
steak & potato	1 cup	120	3	1.0	870	17	1	1	6	0	10	1	300
Clam chowder													
Manhattan	1 cup	134	3	2.0	1000	19	3	4	7	0	67	3	384
New England	1 cup	151	5	2.5	682	19	1	7	8	1	176	3	466
Corn chowder	1 cup	91	5	2.0	312	8	1	4	4	1	92	1	219
Cream of asparagus	1 cup	149	7	2.5	880	17	1	7	6	1	184	1	365
Cream of broccoli	1 cup	68	4	1.5	353	6	1	4	3	1	80	0	174
Cream of celery	1 cup	151	8	3.0	687	15	1	8	6	1	196	1	315
Cream of chicken	1 cup	120	4	2.0	880	13	1	6	7	1	162	1	252
Cream of mushroom	1 cup	161	9	2.5	903	15	1	7	6	2	171	0	275
condensed	1 cup	158	10	2.0	1382	14	2	0	2	0	24	0	128
low-fat	1 cup	120	4	1.0	1500	18	2	0	2	0	20	0	100
low-fat	1 cup	140	5	1.0	820	20	0	4	2	0	20	0	960
reduced sodium	1 cup	126	5	2.0	523	16	1	9	6	1	171	1	657
Cream of potato	1 cup	154	5	2.5	796	22	1	8	6	1	176	0	399
Cream of shrimp	1 cup	151	8	5.0	878	14	0	7	7	1	171	1	236
Double Noodle	1 cup	100	2	0.5	790	17	1	0	3	0	10	1	40
Escarole	1 cup	74	2	1.0	446	7	2	4	7	1	179	3	698
French onion	1 cup	369	16	7.5	1030	39	2	6	17	0	328	3	374
Gazpacho	1 cup	95	6	1.0	625	10	3	6	2	0	34	1	508
Green pea	1 cup	320	6	2.5	1740	52	10	17	17	0	54	4	372
Healthy Request													
chicken w/ whole grain pasta	1 cup	80	2	0.5	410	11	2	2	6	0	20	1	710
cream of mushroom	1 cup	140	6	1.0	820	20	0	4	2	0	20	0	960
homestyle chicken noodle	1 cup	120	4	1.0	820	16	2	0	6	0	20	0	980
homestyle savory chicken & brown rice	1 cup	110	3	0.5	410	16	1	4	5	0	0	0	740
Mexican-style chicken tortilla	1 cup	140	3	0.5	410	22	3	3	7	0	49	1	851
tomato	1 cup	140	0	0.0	820	32	2	16	4	0	20	2	1200
vegetable beef	1 cup	160	2	0.0	820	28	4	4	10	0	40	2	1400

SOUPS

Canned & Prepared

	Amount	Calories	Fat (g)	Saturated Fat (g)	Sodium (mg)	Carbohydrate (g)	Fiber (g)	Sugar (g)	Protein (g)	Vitamin D (mcg)	Calcium (mg)	Iron (mg)	Potassium (mg)
Hot & sour	1 cup	95	3	0.5	917	11	1	1	6	0	46	2	134
Italian-style wedding	1 cup	120	4	1.5	690	15	1	2	6	0	0	0	320
Lentil	1 cup	159	4	0.5	464	22	8	3	10	0	30	3	342
Lobster bisque	1 cup	129	6	3.5	600	4	1	3	13	0	131	1	362
Matzo ball	1 cup	145	5	1.0	831	19	1	2	6	1	34	1	154
Minestrone	1 cup	82	2	0.5	629	11	1	2	4	0	39	1	308
Mushroom	1 cup	95	6	1.0	830	8	1	0	2	0	17	0	76
Oyster stew	1 cup	194	12	7.0	786	10	0	9	10	2	260	4	394
Pasta e fagioli	1 cup	228	6	1.5	531	33	6	2	12	0	134	3	423
Pepper pot	1 cup	47	2	1.5	174	3	0	1	3	0	18	0	180
Scotch broth	1 cup	97	4	1.0	156	7	1	2	7	0	10	1	189
Seafood chowder	1 cup	273	15	9.0	339	15	2	2	20	1	44	1	622
Split pea w/ ham	1 cup	195	4	1.5	762	28	4	5	12	0	35	2	321
Tomato													
bisque	1 cup	220	5	3.0	1740	42	2	30	2	0	40	1	520
creamy, ready to serve	1 cup	83	5	3.5	208	8	2	4	1	0	12	0	154
reduced sodium	1 cup	57	1	0.5	33	9	1	7	2	0	66	1	185
regular w/ milk	1 cup	58	1	0.5	211	10	1	7	2	1	66	0	352
regular w/ water	1 cup	32	0	0.0	186	8	1	4	1	0	8	0	275
w/ water & rice	1 cup	116	3	0.5	788	21	2	7	2	0	27	1	319
Turkey noodle	1 cup	58	2	0.5	834	7	1	0	3	0	12	1	58
Vegetable	1 cup	94	1	0.0	643	19	3	4	3	0	43	1	434
Vegetable beef	1 cup	141	4	2.5	923	16	2	7	10	1	171	1	365
Vegetable broth	1 cup	12	0	0.0	710	2	0	1	1	0	7	0	46
Vegetarian vegetable	1 cup	72	2	0.5	629	12	1	4	2	0	24	1	207
Wild rice w/ chicken	1 cup	143	5	1.0	848	13	1	2	12	0	28	1	219

Dehydrated/Boxed

	Amount	Calories	Fat (g)	Saturated Fat (g)	Sodium (mg)	Carbohydrate (g)	Fiber (g)	Sugar (g)	Protein (g)	Vitamin D (mcg)	Calcium (mg)	Iron (mg)	Potassium (mg)
Beef noodle	½ cup	190	7	3.5	790	26	1	1	4	0	0	2	85
Bouillon, dry													
regular	1 cube	10	1	0.0	966	1	0	1	1	0	15	0	15
beef	1 cube	6	0	0.0	864	1	0	1	1	0	2	0	15
chicken	1 cube	10	0	0.0	1150	1	0	0	1	0	9	0	18
vegetable	1 cup	13	0	0.0	269	2	0	0	0	0	2	0	24
sodium free													
beef	1 tsp	10	0	0.0	0	2	0	1	0	0	0	0	380
chicken	1 tsp	10	0	0.0	0	2	0	1	0	0	0	0	380
Chicken noodle	1 cup	56	1	0.5	561	9	0	1	2	0	4	0	32
Chicken rice	1 cup	58	1	0.5	931	9	1	0	2	0	7	0	11
Cup-a-Soup													
chicken noodle	1 cup	80	2	0.0	640	12	0	0	3	0	0	1	0
cream of chicken	1 cup	70	2	1.5	640	13	0	1	0	0	0	0	0

SOUPS

	Amount	Calories	Fat (g)	Saturated Fat (g)	Sodium (mg)	Carbohydrate (g)	Fiber (g)	Sugar (g)	Protein (g)	Vitamin D (mcg)	Calcium (mg)	Iron (mg)	Potassium
Cup Noodles													
beef	1 (14 oz)	290	11	5.0	1150	41	2	2	7	0	0	3	180
chicken	1 (14 oz)	290	11	5.0	1160	41	2	2	6	0	0	3	260
Leek	1 cup	171	8	3.0	838	20	1	11	7	1	188	1	315
Minestrone	1 cup	90	1	0.0	560	20	3	3	4	0	30	1	300
Miso	1 cup	79	4	0.5	1460	6	1	2	6	0	38	1	127
Onion	1 cup	30	0	0.0	851	7	1	0	1	0	22	0	76
Ramen noodle													
beef	1 cup	190	7	3.5	790	26	1	0	5	0	0	2	85
chicken	1 cup	190	7	3.5	790	26	1	0	5	0	0	2	90
shrimp	1 cup	190	7	3.5	860	26	1	0	5	0	0	2	90
Tomato	1 cup	101	2	1.0	943	19	1	10	2	0	77	0	294
Vegetable	1 cup	101	6	1.5	893	12	1	4	2	0	38	1	94
Vegetable beef	1 cup	110	1	0.0	790	22	3	2	4	0	40	1	182

VEGETABLES*

	Amount	Calories	Fat (g)	Saturated Fat (g)	Sodium (mg)	Carbohydrate (g)	Fiber (g)	Sugar (g)	Protein (g)	Vitamin D (mcg)	Calcium (mg)	Iron (mg)	Potassium
Alfalfa sprouts, raw	½ cup	4	0	0.0	1	0	0	0	1	0	5	0	13
Artichokes													
boiled/steamed	1 medium	64	0	0.0	72	14	7	1	3	0	25	1	343
hearts, marinated	½ cup	58	4	0.0	244	7	2	0	2	0	7	0	120
Asparagus, cooked	½ cup	44	2	0.5	114	4	2	2	2	0	23	2	194
Bamboo shoots, raw	½ cup	21	0	0.0	3	4	2	2	2	0	10	0	405
Bean sprouts, raw	½ cup	14	0	0.0	3	3	1	2	1	0	6	0	67
Beets, pickled	½ cup	55	0	0.0	127	14	1	9	1	0	9	0	98
Bok choy, cooked	½ cup	12	0	0.0	160	2	1	1	1	0	93	1	223
Broccoli													
cooked	½ cup	49	3	0.0	120	5	2	1	2	0	38	1	255
florets, raw	½ cup	10	0	0.0	10	2	1	1	1	0	21	0	142
w/ cheese sauce, cooked	½ cup	90	5	3.0	260	7	2	1	5	0	132	1	241
Brussels sprouts, cooked	½ cup	35	0	0.0	114	7	3	2	3	0	34	1	313
Cabbage													
Chinese, cooked	½ cup	12	0	0.0	160	2	1	1	1	0	93	1	223
green, cooked	½ cup	40	2	0.0	105	5	2	3	1	0	31	0	133
red, raw	½ cup	14	0	0.0	12	3	1	2	1	0	20	0	110
Carrots													
cooked	½ cup	49	0	0.0	221	11	3	6	1	0	39	0	382
raw	1 large	30	0	0.0	50	7	2	3	1	0	24	0	230
Cauliflower													
cooked	½ cup	41.6	3	0.0	118	4	2	2	2	0	18	0	242
raw	½ cup	14	0	0.0	17	3	1	1	1	0	12	0	165
w/ cheese sauce, cooked	½ cup	85	6	1.5	310	7	1	3	3	1	247	0	149

* For dried beans, peas, and lentils, see Vegetarian Foods & Legumes.

VEGETABLES

VEGETABLES	Amount	Calories	Fat (g)	Saturated Fat (g)	Sodium (mg)	Carbohydrate (g)	Fiber (g)	Sugar (g)	Protein (g)	Vitamin D (mcg)	Calcium (mg)	Iron (mg)	Potassium (mg)
Celery													
cooked	½ cup	30	2	0.5	166	2	1	1	1	0	33	0	210
raw	1 medium	6	0	0.0	32	1	1	1	0	0	16	0	104
Chinese-style, frozen	½ cup	40	1	0.0	10	8	2	4	1	0	40	0	320
Chives, raw	1 T	1	0	0.0	0	0	0	0	0	0	3	0	9
Corn, cooked													
cream-style, can	½ cup	92	1	0.0	365	23	2	4	2	0	4	1	168
on the cob	1 (4 oz)	86	1	0.0	15	29	3	3	3	0	2	1	270
w/ butter sauce, frozen	½ cup	91	1	0.0	394	20	1	6	2	0	0	4	0
whole kernel, can	½ cup	55	1	0.0	168	12	2	4	2	0	2	0	108
whole kernel, frozen	½ cup	80	1	0.0	3	18	2	2	3	0	4	0	195
Cucumbers, raw													
w/ skin	½ large	23	0	0.0	3	5	1	3	1	0	24	0	221
w/o skin	½ large	14	0	0.0	3	3	1	2	1	0	20	0	191
Eggplant, cooked	½ cup	13	0	0.0	61	3	2	2	1	0	5	0	117
Endive, raw	1 cup	9	0	0.0	11	2	2	0	1	0	7	0	39
Green beans, cooked													
French	½ cup	20	0	0.0	380	3	1	1	1	0	40	0	100
snap	½ cup	22	0	0.0	150	5	2	2	1	0	28	1	91
Green onions, raw	¼ cup	8	0	0.0	4	2	1	1	0	0	18	0	69
Greens, cooked													
beet	½ cup	35	2	0.5	275	3	3	0	2	0	92	2	595
collard	½ cup	22	0	0.0	93	4	3	0	2	0	162	0	148
dandelion	½ cup	39	2	0.5	116	5	2	0	2	0	107	1	228
mustard	½ cup	20	0	0.0	102	4	2	1	2	0	86	1	289
turnip	½ cup	15	0	0.0	73	2	2	0	1	0	69	1	101
Hominy, cooked	½ cup	75	2	1.0	428	12	2	1	1	0	9	1	8
Jicama													
cooked	½ cup	25	0	0.0	3	6	3	1	1	0	7	0	89
raw	½ cup	25	0	0.0	3	6	3	1	0	0	8	0	98
Kale, cooked	½ cup	25	1	0.0	118	3	3	1	2	0	177	1	243
Kohlrabi, cooked	½ cup	43	2	0.5	125	5	3	2	1	0	21	0	300
Leeks, raw	¼ cup	14	0	0.0	5	3	0	1	0	0	13	0	41
Lettuce, raw	1 cup	5	0	0.0	7	1	0	0	0	0	9	0	59
Mixed vegetables, frozen	½ cup	83	3	0.5	135	12	4	3	3	0	22	1	152
Mushrooms													
can	½ cup	38	2	0.5	338	4	2	2	1	0	9	1	101
fried	5 medium	216	13	2.0	317	21	1	1	5	0	25	2	186
raw	½ cup	8	0	0.0	2	1	0	1	1	0	1	0	112
Okra, cooked	½ cup	28	0	0.0	106	6	3	1	2	0	71	1	257
Onions													
chopped, raw	½ cup	32	0	0.0	3	7	1	3	1	0	18	0	117
rings, breaded & fried	5 medium	175	10	1.5	288	20	1	2	2	0	36	0	76

VEGETABLES

VEGETABLES	Amount	Calories	Fat (g)	Saturated Fat (g)	Sodium (mg)	Carbohydrate (g)	Fiber (g)	Sugar (g)	Protein (g)	Vitamin D (mcg)	Calcium (mg)	Iron (mg)	Potassium (mg)
Parsley, raw	¼ cup	5	0	0.0	8	1	1	0	0	0	21	1	83
Parsnips, cooked	½ cup	73	2	0.5	106	13	3	4	1	0	29	0	285
Pea pods, cooked	½ cup	35	0	0.0	100	6	2	3	2	0	36	2	167
Peas, green, cooked	½ cup	89	3	0.5	101	12	5	5	5	0	21	1	203
Peppers, raw													
bell, green/red/yellow	½ cup	15	0	0.0	2	3	1	2	1	0	8	0	131
chile, green, diced	½ cup	30	0	0.0	5	7	1	4	2	0	14	1	255
jalapeño	1 medium	5	0	0.0	1	1	0	1	0	0	2	0	43
Pimientos, can	¼ cup	11	0	0.0	7	2	1	1	1	0	3	1	76
Potatoes, cooked													
au gratin, box	½ cup	164	9	6.0	530	14	2	0	6	0	146	1	485
baked w/ skin	1 (4 oz)	214	0	0.0	416	49	3	4	4	0	12	1	895
blintz, frozen													
w/ cheese	1 (2.2 oz)	130	5	1.5	301	14	0	7	6	0	81	1	82
w/ fruit	1 (2.2 oz)	122	4	1.0	133	17	0	12	4	1	38	1	81
boiled w/o skin	1 (4 oz)	108	0	0.0	301	25	3	1	2	0	10	0	410
French fries, frozen	14 medium	45	3	0.5	74	5	0	0	1	0	2	0	87
hash browns, frozen	½ cup	174	9	1.0	319	23	3	0	2	0	14	0	393
knish, frozen	1 (2 oz)	213	12	2.5	223	21	1	0	5	1	13	1	95
mashed w/ margarine & milk	½ cup	119	4	1.0	350	18	2	1	2	0	22	0	343
O'Brien, frozen	½ cup	171	12	1.5	382	16	2	2	2	0	11	1	346
pancakes, homemade	1 medium (70 g)	126	8	1.5	283	14	2	1	3	0	16	1	314
scalloped, box	½ cup	210	12	6.5	520	17	1	3	9	1	231	0	303
steak fries	7 medium	138	4	0.5	347	25	2	0	2	0	9	1	427
tater tots, frozen	10	189	12	2.0	337	20	2	0	2	0	10	0	194
twice baked w/ cheese	1 (5 oz)	146	6	3.5	442	18	2	2	5	1	274	1	473
Pumpkin, can	½ cup	69	3	1.0	18	10	3	4	1	0	32	2	245
Radishes, raw	10 medium	8	0	0.0	20	2	1	1	0	0	13	0	116
Rutabagas, cooked	½ cup	55	3	0.5	126	8	2	4	1	0	39	0	278
Salad greens, raw	1 cup	6	0	0.0	13	1	0	0	1	0	16	0	95
Sauerkraut, can	½ cup	14	0	0.0	470	3	4	1	1	0	21	1	121
Scallions, raw	1 T	2	0	0.0	1	0	0	0	0	0	4	0	17
Shallots, raw	1 T	7	0	0.0	1	2	0	1	0	0	4	0	33
Spinach													
cooked	½ cup	52	4	0.5	206	4	2	0	3	0	105	3	590
creamed	½ cup	86	6	3.5	431	7	2	1	2	0	82	2	409
raw	1 cup	6	0	0.0	20	1	1	0	1	0	25	1	140
Squash													
acorn, cooked	½ cup	58	0	0.0	4	15	5		1	0	45	1	448
butternut, cooked	½ cup	41	0	0.0	4	11	3	2	1	0	42	1	291
spaghetti	½ cup	38	2	0.5	108	5	1	2	1	0	16	0	89
summer, cooked	½ cup	47	3	0.5	128	4	1	3	1	0	19	0	255
summer, raw	½ cup	11	0	0.0	1	2	1	2	1	0	12	0	128

VEGETABLES

	Amount	Calories	Fat (g)	Saturated Fat (g)	Sodium (mg)	Carbohydrate (g)	Fiber (g)	Sugar (g)	Protein (g)	Vitamin D (mcg)	Calcium (mg)	Iron (mg)	Potassium (mg)
winter, cooked	½ cup	42	0	0.0	132	10	3	4	1	0	25	0	270
zucchini, cooked	½ cup	19	0	0.0	128	4	1	3	1	0	20	0	255
zucchini, raw	½ cup	11	0	0.0	5	2	1	2	1	0	10	0	162
Succotash, cooked	½ cup	81	0	0.0	132	17	3	2	4	0	15	1	235
Sweet potatoes													
baked w/ skin	1 (4 oz)	135	0	0.0	285	31	5	10	3	0	57	1	710
candied, frozen	½ cup	223	4	1.0	178	47	2	36	1	0	25	1	206
mashed w/o fat	½ cup	129	0	0.0	96	30	2	7	3	0	38	2	268
Swiss chard, cooked	½ cup	18	0	0.0	363	4	2	1	2	0	51	2	481
Tomatoes													
cherry, raw	6 medium	18	0	0.0	5	4	1	3	1	0	10	0	237
paste, can	½ cup	108	1	0.0	47	25	5	16	6	0	47	4	1325
puree, can	½ cup	48	0	0.0	253	11	2	6	2	0	23	2	550
stewed, can	½ cup	33	0	0.0	282	8	1	4	1	0	43	2	264
sun-dried	½ cup	71	1	0.0	29	15	3	10	4	0	30	3	940
whole, can	½ cup	21	2	0.5	67	2	1	1	0	0	18	0	103
whole, raw	1 medium	23	0	0.0	6	5	2	3	1	0	13	0	296
Turnips, cooked	½ cup	42	2	0.5	161	5	2	3	1	0	26	0	159
Water chestnuts, can	½ cup	35	0	0.0	6	9	2	3	1	0	5	1	145
Watercress, raw	½ cup	2	0	0.0	7	0	0	0	0	0	20	0	56
Wax beans, cooked	½ cup	36	2	0.5	95	5	2	1	1	0	35	1	89
Yams, cooked													
baked w/ skin	1 (4 oz)	92	0	0.0	246	21	3	6	2	0	38	1	475
mashed	½ cup	92	0	0.0	246	21	3	6	2	0	38	1	475

VEGETARIAN FOODS & LEGUMES

	Amount	Calories	Fat (g)	Saturated Fat (g)	Sodium (mg)	Carbohydrate (g)	Fiber (g)	Sugar (g)	Protein (g)	Vitamin D (mcg)	Calcium (mg)	Iron (mg)	Potassium (mg)
Aduki/adzuki beans													
dry, cooked	½ cup	147	0	0.0	9	29	8	0	9	0	32	2	612
sweetened, can	½ cup	351	0	0.0	323	82	4	27	6	0	33	2	176
Bacon, vegetarian	2 slices	60	5	0.5	220	2	0	0	2	0	4	0	10
Baked beans, vegetarian, can	½ cup	150	0	0.0	570	30	5	13	7	0	50	2	390
Beyond meatless products													
beef crumbles	½ cup	90	3	0.0	140	2	0	0	14	0	40	5	190
burger/ground beef	1 patty (4 oz)	230	14	5.0	390	7	2	0	20	0	100	4	330
chicken tenders	2 pcs	210	12	2.0	450	15	3	2	11	0	20	1	290
meatballs	5	190	21	7.0	500	9	3	0	19	0	110	5	460
sausage	1 link	190	12	5.0	500	5	3	0	16	0	60	4	200
Black beans													
can	½ cup	121	0	0.0	313	22	9	0	8	0	46	3	408
dry, cooked	½ cup	114	0	0.0	204	20	8	0	8	0	23	2	306
Black-eyed peas/cowpeas													
can	½ cup	93	1	0.0	352	16	4	3	6	0	24	1	207
dry, cooked	½ cup	100	1	0.0	218	17	3	3	7	0	22	3	321

VEGETARIAN FOODS & LEGUMES

	Amount	Calories	Fat (g)	Saturated Fat (g)	Sodium (mg)	Carbohydrate (g)	Fiber (g)	Sugar (g)	Protein (g)	Vitamin D (mcg)	Calcium (mg)	Iron (mg)	Potassium (mg)
Black turtle beans													
can	½ cup	109	0	0.0	461	20	8	0	7	0	42	2	370
dry, cooked	½ cup	120	0	0.0	221	23	8	0	8	0	51	3	401
Boca meatless products													
burger	1 (2.5 oz)	70	1	0.0	450	6	4	0	13	0	60	2	0
Chik'N Nuggets	4 (3 oz)	160	5	0.5	420	16	3	1	14	0	40	2	0
Chik'N Patties	1 (2.5 oz)	130	4	0.5	640	13	3	0	11	0	40	2	0
spicy	1 (2.5 oz)	140	6	1.0	420	11	2	0	12	0	40	2	0
ground crumbles	½ cup	60	0	0.0	210	5	3	1	11	0	60	1	0
Broad/fava beans													
can	½ cup	91	0	0.0	580	16	5	0	7	0	33	1	310
dry, cooked	½ cup	94	0	0.0	205	17	5	2	6	0	31	1	228
Butter beans, can	½ cup	29	2	1.0	213	3	1	1	1	0	26	1	69
Calico beans, dry, cooked	½ cup	142	1	0.0	226	26	9	0	9	0	46	2	434
Cannellini beans, can	½ cup	90	0	0.0	310	16	8	1	6	0	70	2	370
Chickpeas/garbanzo beans													
can	½ cup	132	3	0.5	295	20	7	4	7	0	52	2	216
dry, cooked	½ cup	135	2	0.0	200	22	6	4	7	0	40	2	239
Chili, vegetarian, can	1 cup	126	1	0.0	453	11	3	1	10	0	18	2	161
Chili beans, can	½ cup	120	1	0.0	410	21	8	1	7	0	60	2	380
Cranberry/Roman beans													
can	½ cup	108	0	0.0	432	20	8	0	7	0	44	2	338
dry, cooked	½ cup	121	0	0.0	210	22	8	0	8	0	44	2	343
Crowder peas, can	½ cup	131	1	0.0	378	24	6	4	8	0	23	2	371
Falafel patties	1 (0.6 oz)	333	18	2.5	294	5	0	0	13	0	54	3	585
Gardenburger burgers													
black bean chipotle	1 (2.5 oz)	90	3	0.0	390	16	4	3	5	0	30	2	160
regular	1 (2.5 oz)	110	4	1.5	490	17	3	1	5	0	40	1	110
Great Northern beans													
can	½ cup	150	1	0.0	485	28	6	2	10	0	70	2	460
dry, cooked	½ cup	105	0	0.0	211	19	6	0	7	0	60	2	346
Ground meat alternative	¾ cup	120	2	0.0	360	7	5	1	18	0	80	2	560
Hot dogs													
tofu	1 (1.5 oz)	60	3	0.0	270	0	1	0	7	0	20	1	50
veggie	1 (1.5 oz)	60	1	0.0	370	5	0	2	9	0	10	1	30
Hummus	½ cup	312	21	3.0	578	24	7	3	10	0	136	4	301
Kidney beans													
can	½ cup	122	1	0.0	280	22	7	3	8	0	43	2	390
dry, cooked	½ cup	113	0	0.0	211	20	7	0	8	0	25	3	357
Lentils, cooked	½ cup	113	0	0.0	236	19	8	2	9	0	19	3	366

VEGETARIAN FOODS & LEGUMES

	Amount	Calories	Fat (g)	Saturated Fat (g)	Sodium (mg)	Carbohydrate (g)	Fiber (g)	Sugar (g)	Protein (g)	Vitamin D (mcg)	Calcium (mg)	Iron (mg)	Potassium (mg)
Lima beans													
baby, frozen	½ cup	108	0	0.0	43	21	5		6	0	29	2	371
can	½ cup	113	3	0.5	346	17	5	1	5	0	28	2	271
dry, cooked	½ cup	105	0	0.0	215	20	5	1	6	0	27	2	485
Miso, brown	1 T	34	1	0.0	644	4	1	1	2	0	10	0	36
Morningstar Farms burgers													
garden veggie patties	1 (2.4 oz)	110	5	0.5	390	9	4	1	11	0	60	1	150
spicy black bean	1 (2.4 oz)	110	5	0.5	320	13	4	1	9	0	50	2	250
Veggie Grillers original	1 (2.3 oz)	130	5	0.5	390	8	4	1	16	0	60	1	120
Morningstar Farms meatless products													
Chik'N Nuggets	4 (0.8 oz)	190	8	1.0	300	18	4	2	13	0	30	2	200
Chik'N Strips	12 (1.4 oz)	140	4	0.0	410	4	2	0	23	0	150	2	40
Mung beans, dry, cooked	½ cup	144	6	1.0	202	16	7	2	6	0	23	1	229
Natto	½ cup	186	10	1.5	6	11	5	4	17	0	191	8	640
Navy beans													
can	½ cup	148	1	0.0	440	27	7	0	10	0	62	2	378
dry, cooked	½ cup	128	1	0.0	216	24	10	0	8	0	63	2	354
Pigeon peas													
can	½ cup	100	1	0.0	290	17	4	2	5	0	31	2	391
dry, cooked	½ cup	110	1	0.5	257	20	4	2	6	0	41	2	453
Pink beans, dry, cooked	½ cup	182	6	1.0	202	24	5	0	8	0	45	2	437
Pinto beans													
can	½ cup	124	1	0.0	284	23	7	2	7	0	70	2	413
dry, cooked	½ cup	123	1	0.0	204	22	8	0	8	0	39	2	373
Red beans, dry, cooked	½ cup	113	0	0.0	211	20	7	0	8	0	25	3	357
Refried beans, can	½ cup	185	2	0.5	955	30	10	1	12	0	78	4	765
fat-free	½ cup	91	1	0.0	404	16	5	1	6	0	39	2	398
Sausages, vegetarian													
ground	2 oz	80	3	0.0	320	5	3	1	9	0	42	2	218
links	2 (1.6 oz)	70	3	0.0	300	3	1	0	9	0	10	3	40
patties	1 (1.3 oz)	80	3	0.0	230	5	2	1	9	0	30	1	110
Seitan													
chicken-style	5 oz	110	2	0.0	770	4	2	1	20	0	40	1	66
stir-fry strips	⅓ cup	120	2	0.0	380	5	1	2	21	0	20	0	100
traditional	3 oz	90	1	0.0	380	3	1	0	18	0	40	1	60
Soy meal, defatted	½ cup	206	1	0.0	2	22	11	13	30	0	149	8	1520
Soy protein													
concentrate	1 oz	93	0	0.0	1	7	2	6	18	0	103	3	624
isolate	1 oz	95	1	0.0	284	0	0	0	25	0	51	4	23
Soybeans													
green, cooked	½ cup	127	6	0.5	225	10	4	2	11	0	131	2	485
mature, cooked	½ cup	148	8	1.0	204	7	5	2	16	0	86	4	443
mature, roasted, salted	¼ cup	202	11	1.5	70	13	8	2	17	0	59	2	633

VEGETARIAN FOODS & LEGUMES

	Amount	Calories	Fat (g)	Saturated Fat (g)	Sodium (mg)	Carbohydrate (g)	Fiber (g)	Sugar (g)	Protein (g)	Vitamin D (mcg)	Calcium (mg)	Iron (mg)	Potassium (mg)
Split peas, dry, cooked	½ cup	114	0	0.0	233	20	8	3	8	0	14	1	355
Tempeh													
flax	4 oz	160	7	1.0	10	9	7	1	15	0	80	3	260
soy	4 oz	140	5	1.0	10	10	7	0	16	0	60	2	280
wild rice	3 oz	170	5	1.0	10	18	7	1	14	0	60	2	290
Tofurky													
deli slices	5 (0.4 oz)	100	4	0.0	310	4	1	1	13	0	20	1	430
franks	1 link (2.8 oz)	180	9	1.0	630	7	2	2	18	0	20	2	270
original sausage	1 link (3.5 oz)	250	13	1.0	570	10	2	2	24	0	50	2	680
Tofu													
firm, lite	1 slice (3 oz)	45	2	0.0	65	1	0	0	8	0	150	1	48
firm, regular	1 slice (3 oz)	71	4	0.5	28	1	1	0	9	0	125	1	70
flavored, baked	1 slice (3 oz)	90	5	1.0	250	3	1	1	8	0	10	1	120
silken, lite	1 slice (3 oz)	30	1	0.0	50	0	0	0	6	0	37	1	56
silken, regular	1 slice (3 oz)	50	2	0.0	25	1	1	0	6	0	37	1	167
soft, regular	1 slice (3 oz)	50	2	0.5	29	2	1	0	5	0	66	1	110
TVP (textured vegetable protein)	¼ cup	90	0	0.0	5	9	5	2	12	0	62	2	643
White beans, dry, cooked	½ cup	125	0	0.0	217	22	6	0	9	0	81	3	500
Winged beans, dry, cooked	½ cup	127	5	0.5	214	13	2	0	9	0	122	4	241
Yeast													
brewer's buds/flakes	3 T	117	3	0.0	18	15	10	0	15	0	11	1	345
nutritional flakes	3 T	60	0	0.0	2	12	4	0	7	0	6	1	264

Nutrients

CHOLINE

Choline is necessary for your brain and nervous system to manage functions like mood, memory, and muscle control. Your body can make a small amount of choline in your liver, but most comes from your diet.

Did you know? Most multivitamins, including prenatal supplements, do not contain choline, and most adults do not get enough choline overall. More research is being done to help us better understand how a low choline intake may impact our overall health, especially brain health.

The good news is . . . Choline is found in many foods, and deficiency symptoms are very rare in healthy adults.

Tips

1. Reach for proteins like beef (72 mg in 3 oz lean ground beef), chicken (72 mg in 3 oz chicken breast), turkey (72 mg in 3 oz turkey breast), fish (187 mg in 3 oz salmon), dairy products, and eggs (147 mg in 1 egg).

2. Snack on nuts such as almonds (15 mg in 1 oz).

3. Try veggies like shiitake mushrooms (145 mg in 1 cup), cauliflower (72 mg in 1 cup), brussels sprouts (30 mg in 1 cup), or broccoli (30 mg in 1 cup).

4. Say yes to beans, including soybeans (214 mg in 1 cup), kidney beans (54 mg in 1 cup), and lima beans (75 mg in 1 cup).

5. Choose quinoa (43 mg in 1 cup).

6. Sprinkle wheat germ (153 mg in 3 oz) on yogurt, oatmeal, smoothies, or salads.

Adequate Intake (AI) for Choline

Age	Male	Female	Pregnancy	Lactation
19+	550 mg	425 mg	450 mg	550 mg

Note: Getting too much choline has been linked to higher cardiovascular disease risk. Therefore, there's an upper limit for choline from food and supplements: 3,500 mg for adults over 19.

FIBER

More than 90 percent of Americans do not eat enough fiber. But fiber is important for feeling full after eating, managing weight, lowering cholesterol, keeping blood sugars within a healthy range, and maintaining gut health.

Did you know? Dietary fiber is found in plant foods like fruits, vegetables, beans, lentils, whole grains, nuts, and seeds and includes the parts of plant foods your body can't digest or absorb. Typically, the more a food is refined, the less fiber it has. There are two types of dietary fiber: soluble and insoluble. Both are important for good health.

The good news is . . . You can easily get fiber in your diet by choosing whole unprocessed plant foods. Eating too much fiber too quickly can cause gas, bloating, and discomfort, so increase fiber gradually over a few weeks. Drink plenty of water, too, as fiber works best when it absorbs water.

Tips

1. Reach for foods that are higher in prebiotics (a type of fiber that's beneficial for gut health), like Jerusalem artichokes, asparagus, plantains, onions, garlic, leeks, chicory root, bananas, and chickpeas.
2. Make at least half your grains whole grains.
3. Fill half your plate with fruits and vegetables.
4. Choose fresh veggies and fruits as snacks.
5. Sprinkle nuts and seeds on salads, cereals, and yogurt.
6. Check the food label to find high-fiber foods: 20 percent of the Daily Value in one serving is considered a high source of fiber.

Adequate Intake (AI) The Daily Value for fiber is 14 grams per 1,000 calories a day.

IRON

Your body needs iron to grow, develop, and make hemoglobin—the substance in red blood cells that helps transport oxygen from your lungs throughout your body. Without enough oxygen in your blood, you may experience fatigue, dizziness, lightheadedness, headache, and/or shortness of breath.

Women of childbearing age are at higher risk for iron-deficiency anemia because of blood loss during their menstrual periods and pregnancy. Health-care providers often recommend a multivitamin or prenatal vitamin with iron to supplement the iron in foods during these stages of life.

Did you know? Iron in food exists in two different forms: heme and nonheme. Heme iron is only found in animal foods like meats, poultry, and seafood. It is more easily absorbed by your body than the nonheme type, which is found in plant foods like nuts, seeds, lentils, beans, fruits, leafy green vegetables, and fortified cereals. If you don't eat animal foods, you need to consume twice as much iron as someone who eats meat.

The good news is . . . Vitamin C can increase how much iron your body absorbs while you're eating iron-rich vegetarian foods.

Tips

1. A cup of iron-fortified hot cereal contains almost 11 mg of iron. Toss in some dried fruit such as raisins (½ cup has 1.5 mg iron) or dried apricots (½ cup has 3.5 mg iron) for an additional boost. Add some blackberries or orange slices for a colorful burst of vitamin C.

2. A cup of iron-fortified cold cereal has about 18 mg of iron. Wash it down with a chilled glass of citrus juice—an excellent source of vitamin C.

3. Leafy greens like spinach, kale, Swiss chard, collard, and beet greens contain 2.5 to 6 mg of iron per cooked cup. Sauté your greens with a vitamin C–rich food like bell peppers or tomatoes.

4. Grab a handful of seeds or nuts for a snack or toss them into a salad or smoothie. Pumpkin seeds contain 2.7 mg of iron in ½ cup, and 30 peanuts have 1.5 mg.

5. Add beans and lentils to soups and skillet dishes. White, lima, red kidney, and navy beans as well as soybeans, chickpeas, and black-eyed peas are all good sources of iron.

6. Satisfy your sweet tooth with an ounce of dark chocolate (2 mg iron in 1 oz).

Recommended Dietary Allowances (RDAs) for Iron

Age	Male	Female	Pregnancy	Lactation
19–50	8 mg	18 mg	27 mg	9 mg
51+	8 mg	8 mg		

Note: Iron toxicity can be caused by taking high doses of iron supplements for prolonged periods of time or taking a single overdose. Check with your health-care provider before taking an iron supplement.

MAGNESIUM

Many people, especially older adults, don't get enough magnesium. This mineral has an essential role in more than three hundred metabolic pathways in the body, including protein synthesis, muscle and nerve function, blood glucose control, and blood pressure regulation.

Fortunately, healthy people are unlikely to experience magnesium deficiency symptoms. However, it's important to speak with your medical provider if you don't regularly eat foods containing magnesium, have chronic health conditions (like high blood pressure, gastrointestinal diseases, type 2 diabetes, or chronic alcoholism), or take certain medications like antacids and laxatives, all of which can put you at higher risk for deficiency due to poor absorption or increased excretion.

Did you know? The Food and Drug Administration (FDA) does not require food labels to list magnesium content unless it has been added to the food in processing.

The good news is . . . You can find magnesium in many healthy foods like whole unrefined grains, beans, peas, nuts, seeds, legumes, and vegetables.

Tips

1. Nuts and seeds are good sources of magnesium. Examples include 1 T of pumpkin seeds (156 mg), chia seeds (111 mg), or almonds (80 mg).
2. Foods rich in magnesium are also good sources of other nutrients like fiber. To get more fiber, try 1 cup of black beans (120 mg), ½ cup of cooked brown rice (42 mg), or 1 slice of whole grain bread (23 mg).

3. Upgrade your greens to dark leafy greens—a magnesium power player—with 1 cup of spinach (156 mg), Swiss chard (121 mg), or kale (58 mg).

4. Dark chocolate (64 mg in 1 square/oz) is nutritious, delicious, and rich in magnesium.

Recommended Dietary Allowances (RDAs) for Magnesium

Age	Male	Female	Pregnancy	Lactation
19–30	400 mg	310 mg	350 mg	310 mg
31–50	420 mg	320 mg	360 mg	320 mg
51+	420 mg	320 mg		

OMEGA-3 FATTY ACIDS

Omega-3 fatty acids are "essential fats," meaning your body cannot make them from other fats. You must get them from the foods you eat, such as fatty fish and other seafood (like salmon, tuna, trout, crab, oysters, and mussels), nuts and seeds (like walnuts, flaxseeds, chia seeds, and hemp seeds), plant oils (like flaxseed, soybean, and canola oil), seaweed, and fortified foods or supplements. Omega-3s keep your cell membranes, heart, lungs, blood vessels, and immune system healthy and reduce inflammation.

Did you know? There are three main omega-3 fatty acids:

1. Alpha-linolenic acid (ALA)
2. Eicosapentaenoic acid (EPA)
3. Docosahexaenoic acid (DHA)

ALA is found mainly in plant oils, while DHA and EPA are found in fish and other seafood. Your body needs all three to function.

The good news is . . . If you do not eat seafood or you follow a vegan diet, you can still get DHA and EPA by eating nuts, seeds, and plant oils because your body can partially convert ALA to EPA and DHA.

Tips

1. Add 1 T of chia or hemp seeds to your favorite smoothie.
2. Toss some chopped walnuts into salads, oatmeal, or yogurt.

3. Use flaxseed (linseed oil) as a salad dressing oil or add it to juices, smoothies, and shakes. (Do not use it for stir-frying or baking, as it does not react well when heated.)

4. Eat a variety of fish containing omega-3 at least twice a week.

Adequate Intakes (AIs) for Omega-3s (as ALA)

Age	Male	Female	Pregnancy	Lactation
19+	1.6g	1.1g	1.4g	1.3g

Note: Recommended daily amounts for omega-3 fatty acids have not been established for EPA and DHA. The FDA recommends no more than 5 g per day of combined EPA and DHA from dietary supplements, as high doses can be harmful and can interact with some medications such as anticoagulants. Check with your health-care provider before taking an omega-3 supplement.

OMEGA-6 FATTY ACIDS

Omega-6 fatty acids are good for heart health and circulation, and they're necessary for your cells to function properly. Our bodies cannot make omega-6 fats—we need to get them from food. They come from vegetable oils (like corn, safflower, soybean, and sunflower oil), sunflower seeds, pumpkin seeds, walnuts, meat, poultry, fish, and eggs. It's recommended that you eat these types of polyunsaturated fats (generally liquid at room temperature) in place of saturated fats (generally hard at room temperature).

Did you know? You won't find omega-6 or omega-3 fats on food labels. Instead, you can read the label for unsaturated fats versus saturated fats and use that as a guide. Subtract grams of saturated fats and trans fat from total fat grams to see how much of the healthy unsaturated variety is present. Most American adults consume about ten times more omega-6 fats than omega-3 fats.

The good news is . . . Experts generally agree that consuming too little omega-3 is a more significant problem than consuming too much omega-6. The goal is to eat more omega-3 fats to bring the two into balance.

Tips

1. Toss walnuts, hemp seeds, or sunflower seeds into a salad.
2. Add 1 T of peanut butter to a smoothie or slice of whole grain bread.
3. Cook with unsaturated fats like avocado oil in place of saturated fats like butter. Avocado oil has a high smoke point, which makes it ideal for roasting, sautéing, and grilling.

Adequate Intake (AI) for Omega-6 Fatty Acids

Age	Male	Female	Pregnancy	Lactation
19–50	17 g	12 g	13 g	13 g
51+	14 g	11 g		

POTASSIUM

Potassium is important for kidney function, heart health, muscle contraction, and nerve transmission.

Did you know? National surveys tracking dietary intake consistently show that people get less potassium than recommended. Why is this important? Getting too little potassium can deplete calcium in bones, increase blood pressure, and increase risk of kidney stones.

The good news is . . . Potassium is found in many foods and is also an ingredient in many salt substitutes.

Tips

1. Try ½ cup of dried fruit like apricots (1,101 mg), prunes (699 mg), or raisins (618 mg) as a snack.
2. Make lentil soup. One cup of cooked lentils has 731 mg potassium, and you can toss in 2 cups of spinach for 334 mg.
3. Have a baked potato (610 mg in 1 medium) or acorn squash (644 mg in 1 cup) as a side dish.
4. Grab a banana (422 mg in 1 medium) when you're on the go.
5. Grill 3 oz of chicken breast (332 mg), salmon (326 mg), or top sirloin (315 mg).

Adequate Intake (AI) for Potassium

Age	Male	Female	Pregnancy	Lactation
19–50	3,400 mg	2,600 mg	2,900 mg	2,800 mg
51+	3,400 mg	2,600 mg		

SODIUM

Your body uses sodium, found in salt, to maintain fluid balance as well as muscle and nerve function. Your body needs some sodium to work properly, but most of us eat too much, which is linked to health problems like high blood pressure, heart disease, and stroke.

Did you know? Most of the sodium we eat comes from processed, packaged, and canned foods, along with condiments, snack foods, and restaurant meals—not just from the salt shaker.

The good news is . . . Because sodium is an acquired taste, once you reduce the amount you eat, your taste buds may actually prefer foods' natural flavors.

Tips

1. Prepare more meals at home, where you can control how much salt is used in cooking and at the table.
2. Remove the salt shaker from your table and replace it with your favorite no-salt-added blend of herbs and spices.
3. Buy fresh or frozen vegetables with no added salt instead of canned veggies.
4. Rinse canned beans, tuna, and vegetables to remove some of the sodium.
5. Cut back on portion sizes for condiments and salad dressings or use a low-sodium variety. Oil, flavored vinegars, and citrus juices are low-sodium alternatives to bottled salad dressings.
6. Choose unsalted or low-sodium snacks such as nuts, chips, pretzels, popcorn, and crackers.
7. Read Nutrition Facts labels and select foods with less than 5 percent of the sodium Daily Value per serving, or 140 mg or less per serving.

How much sodium do you need?

The Dietary Guidelines for Americans recommend that adults limit sodium intake to no more than 2,300 mg per day.

VITAMIN A

Carrots are good for your eyesight because they contain beta-carotene, a red-orange pigment that your body converts into vitamin A. Vitamin A is not only critical for healthy vision; it's also involved in maintaining your immune system, cells, and organs. Vitamin A has antioxidant properties, helping fight cell damage when your body breaks down food or is exposed to pollution, tobacco smoke, or ultraviolet rays.

Did you know? There are two forms of vitamin A: preformed vitamin A found in animal foods like eggs, meat, fish, fish oils, and dairy, and provitamin A carotenoids found in plant foods like orange and yellow vegetables, leafy green vegetables, tomatoes, fruits, and vegetable oils.

The good news is . . . Because your body can convert beta-carotene from plant foods into vitamin A, it is possible to get enough in your diet even if you don't eat animal foods.

Tips

1. Colorize half your plate with red, orange, yellow, green, blue, and purple fruits and veggies.
2. Add a baked sweet potato (1,403 mcg Retinol Activity Equivalent [RAE]) or frozen spinach (573 mcg RAE in ½ cup) to a meal.
3. Cut up cantaloupe (135 mcg RAE in ½ cup), red peppers (117 mcg RAE in ½ cup), or mango (112 mcg in 1 cup) for a snack.

Recommended Dietary Allowances (RDAs) for Vitamin A

Age	Male	Female	Pregnancy	Lactation
19+	900 mcg RAE	700 mcg RAE	770 mcg RAE	1,300 mcg RAE

Note: Because vitamin A is fat soluble, excess amounts are stored in the body and can be toxic. Check with your health-care provider before taking a vitamin A supplement.

VITAMIN B12

Vitamin B12 is naturally found in animal foods like fish, meat, chicken, turkey, eggs, dairy products, and some fortified foods. Plant foods have no vitamin B12 unless it's been added by the manufacturer during processing.

Did you know? After the age of 50, many adults may not have enough hydrochloric acid in their stomach to absorb vitamin B12 from animal foods. If you're older than 50, look for foods fortified with B12 or talk to a medical provider about supplementation.

The good news is . . . Most adults get enough vitamin B12 from their food. However, some may have trouble absorbing it. If you've been diagnosed with pernicious anemia, celiac disease, or Crohn's disease; had stomach or intestinal surgery; or don't consume any animal products, talk to a medical provider about whether you should supplement your current diet with vitamin B12.

Tips

1. Organ meats like liver and kidneys are rich in vitamin B12. 3 oz of beef liver contains 70 mcg.

2. One 3 oz serving of clams has 84 mcg of vitamin B12. Clams are also high in protein, low in fat, and an excellent source of iron.

3. Embrace sardines, a great source of vitamin B12 and calcium. A 100 g serving of canned sardines in oil contains 9 mcg of vitamin B12. Other fish like salmon (4.8 mcg) and trout (3.5 mcg) are good sources, too.

4. Dairy products don't have as much vitamin B12 as meat and fish, but they are still a good source. Try milk (1.2 mcg in 1 cup) or yogurt (1.1 mcg in 1 cup).

5. Nutritional yeast is a great cheese substitute that has 8 mcg vitamin B12 in 2 T. Sprinkle it on pasta dishes or salads.

6. Reach for fortified foods like breakfast cereals, nondairy milk substitutes, meat substitutes, or energy bars. If vitamin B12 has been added to a food, it will be shown on the label.

Recommended Dietary Allowances (RDAs) for Vitamin B12

Age	Male	Female	Pregnancy	Lactation
19+	2.4 mcg	2.4 mcg	2.6 mcg	2.8 mcg

VITAMIN C

Vitamin C is an antioxidant that protects cell health, assists in making collagen, aids in iron absorption, and is important for immune function. Studies have suggested that getting enough vitamin C from fruits and vegetables may reduce your risk of cancer, heart disease, and age-related macular degeneration (a leading cause of vision loss in older adults).

Did you know? Our bodies don't make vitamin C, so you are entirely dependent on food and drinks for this vitamin.

The good news is . . . Most adults get enough vitamin C from their diet. It is rare to see vitamin C deficiencies in developed countries.

Tips

1. Eat five or more servings of fruits and vegetables every day. Citrus fruits (70 mg in 1 medium orange), red and green peppers (95 mg in ½ cup), kiwis (64 mg in 1 medium), broccoli (51 mg in ½ cup), strawberries (49 mg in ½ cup), brussels sprouts (48 mg in ½ cup), tomatoes (17 mg in 1 medium), and cantaloupe (29 mg in ½ cup) are all good sources of vitamin C.

2. Choose raw fruits and vegetables most often. Vitamin C can be destroyed by heat from steaming, boiling, or microwaving food.

3. Select local fruits and vegetables when possible and eat them as soon as you can after purchase. Vitamin C content decreases with prolonged storage.

4. Check food labels—foods and beverages are often fortified with vitamin C.

Recommended Dietary Allowances (RDAs) for Vitamin C

Age	Male	Female	Pregnancy	Lactation
19+	90 g	75 g	85 g	120 g

Note: If you smoke, you need 35 mg more vitamin C per day than nonsmokers.

VITAMIN D

Your body needs Vitamin D to absorb calcium for building and maintaining healthy teeth and bones as well as protecting against weakening bones. Its anti-inflammatory, antioxidant, and neuroprotective properties support your immune system, muscles, nerves, blood vessels, and brain cells.

Did you know? Only a few foods naturally contain vitamin D, including fatty fish (like tuna, salmon, sardines, herring, mackerel, and trout), fish liver oils, beef liver, and egg yolks. Your body can also make vitamin D when your bare skin is exposed to the sun. However, sunscreen, clouds, smog, old age, and having dark skin can limit the amount of vitamin D your body can make.

The good news is . . . Milk and plant-based milk alternatives such as almond, rice, oat, soy, hemp, and coconut milk are generally fortified with about 2.5–3 mcg (100–120 IU) vitamin D. Vitamin D is also added to other foods like breakfast cereals, margarine, some calcium-fortified orange juice, and yogurt.

Tips

1. Start your day with a bowl of vitamin D–fortified cereal and milk (or fortified milk alternative) and two eggs to get almost half of the recommended daily amount of vitamin D.

2. If you are worried about not getting enough vitamin D, you can measure this with a blood test. If your levels are low, your health-care provider can recommend a vitamin D supplement.

Recommended Dietary Allowances (RDAs) for Vitamin D

Age	Male	Female	Pregnancy	Lactation
19–70	15 mcg (600 IU)	15 mcg (600 IU)	15 mcg (600 IU)	15 mcg (600 IU)
71+	20 mcg (800 IU)	20 mcg (800 IU)		

Note: Vitamin D is fat soluble, and excess amounts stored in the body can be harmful and can interact with some medications. Check with your health-care provider before taking a vitamin D supplement.

VITAMIN E

Hailed as one of the big three antioxidant nutrients along with vitamin A (beta-carotene) and vitamin C, vitamin E helps clean up free radicals in your body. Some free radicals are used by immune cells to fight infections; however, too many can increase oxidative stress, which can accelerate aging and a host of diseases. Your immune system also needs vitamin E to fight off infection.

Did you know? Vitamin E is found mainly in fruits and vegetables that contain fat, including nuts, seeds, avocado, vegetable oils, and wheat germ. Some fish (like salmon and tuna) and some leafy green vegetables (such as beets, turnips, and mustard greens) also contain vitamin E.

The good news is . . . As long as you eat a variety of antioxidant-rich foods, you should get enough vitamin E in your diet.

Tips

1. Snack on a handful of almonds or sunflower seeds (over 7 mg per oz) and you'll be more than halfway to meeting your daily goal.
2. Dip into some guacamole or add avocado slices to toast, sandwiches, or dark green salads. One avocado has 4 mg of vitamin E.
3. Enjoy a glass of almond milk with a peanut butter and jelly sandwich for 10 mg of vitamin E.
4. Sprinkle wheat germ on top of your favorite cereal or yogurt (4.5 mg in 2 T).

Recommended Dietary Allowances (RDAs) for Vitamin E

Age	Male	Female	Pregnancy	Lactation
14+	15 mg	15 mg	15 g	19 mg

Note: Because vitamin E is fat soluble, excess amounts are stored in the body and can be harmful. Check with your health-care provider before taking a vitamin E supplement.

WATER

Drinking water every day is critical for overall health. Staying hydrated helps you think clearly, manage mood, avoid overheating, digest food, lubricate joints, keep a normal body temperature, and prevent kidney stones. In fact, every cell, tissue, and organ in your body requires water to work properly. Even mild dehydration can make you feel low on energy.

Did you know? Recommendations for how much water you need vary based on your age, health, eating patterns, body size, activity level, and geographic location. If you're pregnant or breastfeeding, you need even more water every day. Total water recommendations include what you drink as well as the water in foods, which generally makes up about 20 percent of water intake.

The good news is . . . Your fluid intake is most likely in balance if you don't feel thirsty and your urine is colorless or light yellow.

Tips

1. Make water your beverage of choice.
2. Carry a water bottle and sip it while you're on the go.
3. Keep a glass of water on your nightstand.
4. Stay ahead of your thirst—drink water throughout the day, even if you don't feel thirsty.
5. Substitute water for sugar-sweetened beverages to feel better and reduce your calorie intake.

Adequate Intake (AI) for water

Age	Male	Female	Pregnancy	Lactation
19+	3.7 L (16 cups)	2.7 L (11 cups)	3.0 L (13 cups)	3.8 L (16 cups)

References

Calculator.net, "BMR Calculator," calculator.net/bmr-calculator.html.

Fast food franchise nutrition information, 2021.

Food Processor Nutrition Analysis software, ESHA Research, 2021.

Institute of Medicine, Dietary Reference Intakes for Energy, Carbohydrate, Fiber, Fat, Fatty Acids, Cholesterol, Protein, and Amino Acids (Washington, DC: The National Academies Press, 2005).

Institute of Medicine, *Dietary Reference Intakes for Water, Potassium, Sodium, Chloride, and Sulfate* (Washington, DC: The National Academies Press, 2005).

Johnson, Rachel K., et al., "Dietary sugars intake and cardiovascular health: a scientific statement from the American Heart Association." *Circulation* 120, no. 11: 1011–20.

Parker, Suiz. *1000 Best Bartender's Recipes* (Illinois: Sourcebooks, Inc., 2005).

Soliman, Ghada A. "Dietary Cholesterol and the Lack of Evidence in Cardiovascular Disease." *Nutrients* 10, no. 6 (June 2018): 780.

US Department of Agriculture and US Department of Health and Human Services, "Dietary Guidelines for Americans, 2020-2025," 9th Edition, 2020.

US Department of Health and Human Services, "Body Weight Planner," niddk.nih.gov/bwp.

USDA MyPlate, myplate.gov.

About the Authors

JANE STEPHENSON is a learning and development senior specialist for a globally diversified medical device and health care company headquartered in Chicago, Illinois. She spent the first half of her career as a registered dietitian nutritionist (RDN) and certified diabetes educator (CDE) prior to entering the health care industry. She is the author of several nutrition and fitness educational books and tools targeted to helping people take action to live healthier, happier lives. She splits her time between Sedona, Arizona, and Naples, Florida.

REBECCA LINDBERG, MPH, RDN, is a registered dietitian nutritionist, consultant, author, and speaker at Rebecca Lindberg, LLC, and Rumblings Media Consulting, LLC. For thirty years, she's been helping individuals live well by designing initiatives to improve and sustain health. Rebecca is also the cofounder of Rumblings Media, an organization dedicated to empowering women over fifty to reignite and flourish. She lives in Minneapolis, Minnesota.

rumblingsmedia.com | @rumblingsmedia
relindberg | rumblingsmedia